Transfusion Medicine
in Practice

Transfusion Medicine in Practice

Edited by

Jennifer Duguid, MB, FRCPath
Consultant Haematologist,
Wrexham Maelor Hospital, Wrexham, UK

Lawrence Tim Goodnough, MD
Professor of Medicine, Pathology and Immunology,
Division of Laboratory Medicine, Washington
University School of Medicine, St Louis, USA

Michael J Desmond, MB, MRCP
Consultant Cardiothoracic Anaesthetist,
The Cardiothoracic Centre, Liverpool, UK

MARTIN DUNITZ

2002

© 2002 Martin Dunitz Ltd, a member of the Taylor & Francis Group

First published in the United Kingdom in 2002 by Martin Dunitz Ltd, The Livery House, 7–9 Pratt Street, London NW1 0AE

Tel: +44 (0) 20 74822202
Fax: +44 (0) 20 72670159
E-mail: info@dunitz.co.uk
Website: http://www.dunitz.co.uk

Although every effort has been made to ensure that drug doses and other information are presented accurately in this publication, the ultimate responsibility rests with the prescribing physician. Neither the publishers nor the authors can be held responsible for errors or for any consequences arising from the use of information contained herein. For detailed prescribing information or instructions on the use of any product or procedure discussed herein, please consult the prescribing information or instructional material issued by the manufacturer.

A CIP record for this book is available from the British Library.

ISBN 1-84184-204-4

Although every effort has been made to ensure that all owners of copyright material have been acknowledged in this publication, we would be glad to acknowledge in subsequent reprints or editions any omissions brought to our attention.

Distributed in the USA by
Fulfilment Center
Taylor & Francis
7625 Empire Drive
Florence, KY 41042, USA
Toll Free Tel: +1 800 634 7064
E-mail:cserve@routledge_ny.com

Distributed in Canada by
Taylor & Francis
74 Rolark Drive
Scarborough, Ontario M1R 4G2, Canada
Toll Free Tel: +1 877 226 2237
E-mail: tal_fran@istar.ca

Distributed in the rest of the world by
Thomson Publishing Services
Cheriton House
North Way
Andover, Hampshire SP10 5BE, UK
Tel: +44 (0)1264 332424
E-mail: salesorder.tandf@thomsonpublishingservices.co.uk

Composition by Wearset Ltd, Boldon, Tyne and Wear
Printed and bound in Great Britain by Biddles Ltd.

Contents

Contributors

James P AuBuchon, MD
Blood Bank and Transfusion Service
Dartmouth-Hitchcock Medical Center
One Medical Center Drive
Lebanon, NH 03782
USA

Paula HB Bolton-Maggs, MD, FRCP, FRCPath,
FRCPCH
Royal Liverpool Children's Hospital
Alder Hey
Eaton Road
Liverpool, L12 2AP
UK

Frank E Boulton, MD
National Blood Transfusion Service
Coxford Road
Southampton, SO16 5AS
UK

Mark E Brecher, MD
Transfusion Medicine Service
CB 7600 University of North Carolina Hospitals
101 Manning Drive
Chapel Hill, NC 27514
USA

Simon Bricker, FRCA
Department of Anaesthetics
Countess of Chester Hospital
Liverpool Road
Chester, CH2 1UL
UK

Michael J Desmond, MB, MRCP
Department of Anaesthesia
The Cardiothoracic Centre
Liverpool, L14 3PE
UK

Jennifer Duguid, MB, FRCPath
Department of Haematology
Wrexham Maelor Hospital
Croesnewydd Road
Wrexham
Clwyd, LL13 7TD
UK

Lawrence Tim Goodnough, MD
Division of Laboratory Medicine, Box 8118
Washington University School of Medicine
660 South Euclid Avenue
St Louis, MO 63110
USA

Robert R Jeffrey, MB, FRCSEd, FETCS
Aberdeen Royal Infirmary
Grampian University Hospital NHS Trust
Foresterhill
Aberdeen, AB9 2ZB
UK

Susan Knowles, MB, FRCP, FRCPath
Epsom and St Helier NHS Trust
St Helier Hospital
Wrythe Lane
Carshalton, SM5 1AA
UK

Roshni Kulkarni, MD
Department of Pediatrics, Human Development
and Hematology/Oncology
Michigan State University College of Human
Medicine
MSU Subspeciality Clinics
B-220 Clinical Center
Lansing, MI 48824-1313
USA

Ileana López-Plaza, MD
Department of Pathology
University of Pittsburgh School of Medicine
Institute for Transfusion Medicine
3636 Boulevard of the Allies
Pittsburgh, PA 15213
USA

Jeanne M Lusher, MD
Division of Hematology/Oncology
Children's Hospital of Michigan
3901 Beaubien Boulevard
Detroit, MI 48201
USA

Gary Masterson, MRCP, FRCA
Intensive Therapy Unit
Royal Liverpool University Hospital
Prescot Street
Liverpool, L7 8XP
UK

Aleksandar Mijovic PhD, MB, MRCPath
Department of Haematological Medicine
King's College Hospital
Denmark Hill
London SE5 9RS
UK

Terri G Monk, MD
Department of Anaesthesiology
University of Florida
PO Box 100254
Gainesville, FL 36211
USA

Dafydd W Thomas, MB, FRCA
Department of Anaesthesia and Intensive Care
Swansea NHS Trust
Morriston Hospital
Heol Cwmrhydyceirw
Swansea SA6 6PD
UK

Darrell J Triulzi, MD
Department of Pathology
University of Pittsburgh School of Medicine
Institute for Transfusion Medicine
3636 Boulevard of the Allies
Pittsburgh, PA 15213
USA

1 Hospital transfusion practice

Frank E Boulton

INTRODUCTION

There is no doubt that blood transfusion has saved lives. Unfortunately, some recipients have died from transfusion – although not always from administrative or technical 'errors'. Some early recipients were victims of trauma (including obstetric) or had required major surgery, while others had profound 'pernicious' anaemia. A few were babies with haemorrhagic disease.

TRANSFUSION BEFORE 1940

Clinically based transfusion practice, conceived in the 1820s by James Blundell in London, gestated for nearly nine decades. Several Americans, including two Union soldiers in the Civil War, received human blood in the 1850s and 1860s (others got animal blood), with singular lack of success and occasional deaths through incompatibility.[1,2] Braxton Hicks – Blundell's successor – used rather strong solutions of 'phosphate of soda' to prevent troublesome clotting of blood collected for transfusion. This worked, but few patients survived – although some rallied temporarily with the rather small volumes of 'phosphated blood' given. Brakenridge of Edinburgh was more successful with 5% phosphate (one volume to two or three volumes of blood) used within hours of collection for five patients diagnosed with pernicious anaemia.[3] Incompatibility probably killed one. The same anticoagulant was used for a haemophiliac in 1910;[4] this was the last recorded use of 'phosphated blood' being used.

Although defibrinated blood was used by some surgeons, adverse events were frequent and most surgeons at this stage favoured a 'direct' and rapid approach to avoid clotting. In 1905, Alexis Carrel successfully transfused blood from a New York surgeon to his newborn daughter who had haemorrhagic disease[5] by surgically anastomosing donor artery to patient vein. Crile simply used a short metal tube over which the cut ends of the dissected-out vessels were cuffed to join donor to recipient. Elsberg's similar device was used for Duke's thrombocytopenic patient, from whom platelet function and the value of the bleeding time was first demonstrated. A major problem was the inability to measure the amount transfused – indeed, Duke's donor probably gave more than a litre.[6] An ingenious method for transfusing known volumes of unmodified blood was devised by Unger, who connected lines to recipient and donor via a four-way stopcock and a saline syringe.[7] These direct methods (not to be confused with the later 'directed' methods of donor selection) had the major disadvantage of direct contact between donor and patient, and the surgery meant that donors could only be used once.

Incompatibility was still problematic.

Although Landsteiner wrote 'it might be mentioned that the reported observations [of his newly discovered blood groups] may assist in the explanation of various consequences of therapeutic blood transfusions',[8] no action was taken until Ottenburg introduced pre-transfusion compatibility testing.[9] Even then, many surgeons would not wait – their patients were often in extremis. In his textbook (the first definitively on transfusion), Crile only faintly recognized the compatibility problem as 'occasional hemolysis' that occurred unpredictably.[10] Landsteiner thought that blood group status was determined by serum agglutinins (antibodies); this was corrected when von Dungern and Hirschfeld demonstrated the Mendelian nature of ABO inheritance.[11]

Phosphate failed to catch on, but sodium citrate – used for anticoagulating transfused cattle blood in 1911[12] – was first used for humans in Belgium in 1914. Appropriate doses were described by Lewisohn.[13] A better citrate/glucose mix was devised for the Front in 1917.[14] More suitable formulations resulted in Loutit and Mollison's 'ACD'.[15] A few years later, Gibson[16] added small amounts of phosphate in order to enhance the provision of nucleoside phosphate during storage.

Some transfusions were conducted in the interwar years – usually for surgical or obstetric problems, pernicious anaemia, or a few haemophiliacs. In the USA, many donors from the start were 'professional' (i.e. paid). The first 'Blood Bank' at Cook County Hospital, Chicago, in 1936 required the families of each patient to 'deposit' units of blood in exchange for each unit transfused.[17] Following the Spanish Civil War, the onset of the Second World War galvanized a 'regional' system for blood collection from unpaid donors in Britain, which developed into the post-war National Blood Transfusion Services. Military influences were largely behind the drive to fractionate pooled plasma to produce albumin solutions as an alternative to freeze-dried plasma. Addition of mercury to preserve albumin solutions in tropical climes introduced a step that incidentally inactivated microorganisms.[18] This improved when caprylate and heat pasteurization were introduced in the early 1950s. The transmission of hepatitis by blood was increasingly recognized during the Second World War.

DEVELOPMENTS AFTER 1945

Military influences continued during the Korean and Vietnamese wars, when frozen preservation was developed. Although not needed for routine transfusion, freezing proved essential for storing rare blood or stem cells. The invention of the plastic blood pack enabled 'blood component therapy' to develop.[19] This was enhanced by 'optimal additives', which also improved red cell storage as well as increasing plasma yield for fractionation and easing cryoprecipitation for treating haemophiliacs.[20,21] This helped to meet the rapidly increasing demand for clotting factors, which, however, could only be fully met by using commercially donated apheresis plasma. Early apheresis systems operated with separate packs – at considerable risk to donors, who might, in a busy donor 'clinic', get someone else's red cells returned. Machine-operated systems of ever-increasing efficiency were developed,[22] which also enhanced ways of harvesting platelets and haematopoietic progenitor cells, and also of emergency treatment of hyperviscosity syndrome in people with acutely presenting leukaemia or Waldenström's macroglobulinaemia.

Although tests for syphilis and (in some places) for malaria in donations were introduced very early, cytomegalovirus (CMV) was not recognized until 1965.[23] With the discovery of the 'Dane' particle,[24,25] and its association with 'serum hepatitis' (hepatitis B), a new era opened. Within 25 years many more viruses were recognized as transmissible by transfusion; human T-cell leukaemia/lymphoma viruses I and II (human T-lymphotropic viruses, HTLV-I and -II), human immunodeficiency virus (HIV), hepatitis A and C viruses (HAV and HCV), parvovirus, and other herpesviruses, as well as several viruses of uncertain pathogenicity such as 'TTV' and 'HGV'. But it was the onset of HIV/AIDS in the early 1980s which had the most profound impact on transfusion services in the developed world.[26] The most recent development concerning disease transmission – prions – remains very uncertain, but has nevertheless had a profound impact in cost terms to the UK transfusion services through leading to 'universal leukodepletion' (see below).

The last three decades have witnessed astonishing advances. In the early days, cardiac surgery not only required a large amount of blood cover but also was instrumental in revealing transfusion-transmitted CMV infection.[23] Organ transplantation and neonatal intensive care has depended to a large degree on advances in transfusion therapy, as have the developing oncological services, whose patients experienced profound marrow suppression. Communities with significant populations from the Mediterranean littoral, Asia, and sub-Saharan Africa, in whom thalassaemia and haemoglobinopathies are common, also created new demands on the supply of red cells, while people with haemophilia or immunodeficiencies increased the demand for plasma derivatives. A recent pilot study,[27] combining data from a small mix of specialist and general English hospitals indicated an approximately equal usage of blood for medical and surgical patients; of the medical patient use nearly half was for malignancy and 13% for GI bleeding; while of the surgical causes nearly 30% was orthopaedic (including emergencies), a quarter were for cardiac and 9% for arterial surgery. Seventy percent of recipients were older than 50 years and 10% were younger than 20 years. Approximately 17% of blood recipients died within 6 months (of their primary disease). Comparable studies have been made in France and Denmark.[28,29] Surgical use offers an important target for reduction, although blood use for patients in all these categories needs to be scrutinized.

In 1999, in response to the discovery in 1996 that humans could be infected by the BSE prion – giving rise to a new form of Creutzfeld–Jakob disease (vCJD) – the UK Transfusion Services implemented a scheme of 'universal leukodepletion'. This was in response to independent advice[30] that indicated (on the basis that vCJD infectivity was associated with white cells) that leukodepletion was in the public interest. It is still too early to ascertain whether this has had any beneficial effect, but some observers in the UK hope that some 'incidental benefits' – in the shape of fewer non-haemolytic febrile transfusion reactions and reduced alloimmunization – will prove significant; but views from outside are less optimistic, particularly with regard to the cost-efficacy of leukocyte reduction for alleviating such adverse effects, and as to whether there is any significant impact on immunomodulation and post-transfusion bacterial infection.[31–34]

In view of the known infectivity of BSE by (unleukocyte-depleted) blood transfused to sheep,[35] concern is justified even in the absence, so far, of transmission of vCJD through human blood. By April 2002, 117 people in the UK were known to have been infected with vCJD (plus 5 in France, and one each in Italy, the USA and Hong Kong – the last two having had close associations with the UK). Several of these victims had given blood while apparently healthy, and there is understandable concern for the recipients of their blood – of whom over 20 have been identified. Furthermore, with the prospect of a diagnostic test for vCJD in blood,[36] there is a real dilemma for the blood collection services and their management of donor recruitment – and not just in the UK.

TRANSFUSION-TRANSMITTED DISEASES

Although transfusion-related diseases are predominantly infectious in nature, some (e.g. graft-versus-host disease and 'immunomodulation') are not. The following sections summarize the strategies for selecting 'low-risk' donors, with data from the UK and Ireland.

Medical assessment of donors at sessions

Donation–collection organizations within transfusion services have a duty of care for the donors. This includes giving advice concerning incidental conditions with which they present, and some medications that they may be taking, which have an impact on their suitability as donors. It also includes taking responsibility for any adverse consequences of the donation, whether it be injury or iron deficiency. For recipients, the main consideration is whether transfusing the donation would harm them. Causes for permanent exclusion of donors in the UK include a history of injecting non-prescription drugs, and men who have ever had sex with another man. Regular surveys assess the efficacy of such criteria, which are reviewed annually. Causes for short-term exclusion include certain medications, travel to certain countries (usually in relation to malaria), recent sexual contact with a person judged to be 'at risk' of infection with a significant microorganism, short-term or self-resolving medical conditions, needlestick injury, or procedures such as tattooing and ear piercing. These recommendations are based on epidemiological considerations and differ in detail from those in other developed countries. Minor conditions such as allergies do not debar. All donors complete a self-administered questionnaire; first-timers (about 15% in the UK) have a personal interview with a nurse or doctor familiar with the procedure.[37] The standard volume of blood collected from UK donors – including all testing samples – is nearly 500 ml. All donors are screened for anaemia, principally on a sample of freely flowing fingerstick blood by the gravimetric method, equating to haemoglobin concentrations of 12.5 g/dl and 13.5 g/dl for women and men respectively. In the UK, donors who fail have haemoglobin concentration assessed on venous blood at the session (later checked for full blood count). If it is over 12.0 g/dl for women or 13.0 g/dl for men, they are allowed to donate.[38] The deferral rate through low haemoglobin concentration is 5–10% for women, but many are not iron-deficient, since the threshold is above the lower end of the normal range for women. In Australia, the thresholds are 1.0 g/dl lower for each gender, and in the USA, the threshold is 12.5 g/dl for both men and women. In Europe, men can donate up to four times a year, but three times is the maximum allowed for women. Regular donation decreases iron stores; even some men show true iron deficiency after six donations in two years.[39] Diet and body size are important; women who eat red meat are relatively protected.

The acceptability of blood from people who have been venesected for iron excess due to genetic haemochromatosis (GH) is under discussion. Up to 1% of Northern Europeans are homozygous for the mutation in the HFE protein that is most commonly associated with GH (tyrosine instead of cysteine 282). Most are asymptomatic, but could benefit from frequent venesection. However, many factors impacting on the relative safety of such blood need to be considered, although there is no intrinsic reason why donations from people with GH cannot be accepted if the donor passes the medical assessment. Heterozygotes are not specifically capable of giving blood more frequently.[39]

Bacterial infections

Without doubt, the most frequent and morbid infections in blood products are those caused by bacteria; contamination might be as high as 0.3–0.4%,[40,41] especially in platelets. For this reason, the shelf-life of platelets (which are stored at 22°C) has remained at 5 days, although sterile platelet concentrates in modern plasticized containers are viable for much longer. The most common microorganisms in platelets are Gram-positive skin commensals, presumably deriving from donor skin, while those surviving phagocytosis in fresh blood to contaminate red cells stored at 4°C (which inhibits the growth of most bacteria) are usually psychrophilic Gram-negative bacteria such as *Pseudomonas* spp. These generate potentially lethal toxins. Because moderate febrile reactions were commonly observed after platelet infusion – and attributed to a 'non-specific' cause – several true infections may have been undiagnosed. Many patients receiving platelets are being treated for marrow suppression and are also receiving antibiotics that may also disguise a bacterial reaction induced by endotoxins or exotoxins. But the exacerbation of fever in association with platelet therapy should alert attention.

A few organisms (e.g. *Yersinia enterocolitica*) can be minimized by excluding donations from people with recent gastrointestinal upsets and removing the white cells from the donation. However, many other organisms have been reported. Studies are being conducted to see if diverting the first 10 or 20 ml of blood at the beginning of donation may divert any small skin plugs, or free bacteria, away from the final collection. Initial results are promising.[42] When a red cell unit is infected, Gram-negative organisms are the most common, and can cause a fulminating toxaemia and rapid death with disseminated intravascular coagulation (DIC) in a manner very like an acute immune-induced (ABO) haemolysis.[43,44] However, although red cell preparations are not routinely tested prospectively for bacteria, systems for detecting bacteria in platelets have been examined but not yet widely introduced.[45]

Tests for infectious microorganisms: HBV, HCV, HIV, syphilis

In the UK and Ireland between October 1995 and June 2000, when approximately 13 million donations had been collected, the figures of infected donations were as shown in Table 1.1.[46] Analysis of the age distribution among first-time donors (in cohorts <25, 25–34, 35–44, >44 years) shows that the incidence of infection increases with age, except for HCV in which the 35- to 44-year-old cohort are highest, with 229 men and 109 women per 100 000. Men outnumber women in all groups by 2 to 1 – probably because men generally partake in higher-risk activities. Positive markers among repeat donors are spread more evenly through the ages (except for HCV, where the youngest men are most commonly positive, at 3 per 100 000), and men outnumber women by a little less than 2 to 1.

In a study from London[47] in which 9220 patients were recruited, 5579 recipients of 21 913 units of blood were followed up for markers of infection. None were identified.

The incidence of transfusion-transmitted HBV was 0 in 21 043 units (95% confidence interval (CI) for risk 0–1 in 5706 recipients); for HCV, it was 0 in 21 800 units (95% CI 0–1 in 5911 recipients); for HIV, it was 0 in 21 923 units (95% CI 0–1 in 5944 recipients), and for HTLV 0 in 21 902 units (95% CI 0–1 in 5939 recipients). At that time the UK services were not testing for HTLV. It is planned to introduce NAT testing for HTLV I and II during 2002, which would bring UK transfusion service practices in line with the current UK requirement for testing allogeneic stem cells, as well as other national transfusion services, even though it is also recognized that leukodepletion may well reduce the risk of transmitting HTLV. A considerable proportion of patients had pre-existing infections, and hospital-acquired infections may arise from other sources.

HBV

Of the nearly three million donations collected annually in the UK and Ireland, some 50–100 are confirmed to carry HBV. Over

Table 1.1 Donations infected with HBV, HCV, HIV, or *Treponema pallidum*: UK and Ireland, October 1995–June 2000

	HBC	HCV	HIV	*T. pallidum* antibodies
First timers: 1 in	3 263	1 825	23 719	6 918
Repeat donors: 1 in	137 336	39 109	251 296	50 046
Combined: 1 in	24 458	11 869	120 956	29 371

4000 other donors react positively in the enzyme-linked immunosorbent assay (ELISA) test system but are later not confirmed (i.e. are not infectious). Many of these 'falsely reactive' donations do not react with alternative ELISA systems. A few 'truly' positive donations come from people who have been vaccinated with recombinant hepatitis B surface antigen (HBsAg) very recently. Under certain circumstances, and after exhaustive extra tests, some donors are returned to the panel after a time interval. Although all reacting units are discarded, it is estimated that between 10 and 20 non-reactive but infectious units are transfused each year. Such contamination is undetectable even by the best screening tests available, or are missed through testing system failure – although such events are minimized through meticulous attention.

The standard systems test for HBsAg by automated ELISA. Antibody to the HBV core antigen HBcAg (anti-HBc) is also tested for in donors with a past history of adult hepatitis; if positive, the donation is tested for antibody to HBsAg (anti-HBs): if the serum contains more than 100 international units of this per litre, the donor is regarded as having mounted an immune response, which indicates sufficient acquired immunity to render them at no risk.

HCV

In spite of improvements over the years in methods detecting HBsAg, up to 1990 there remained cases of icteric and fatal hepatitis following transfusion with HBsAg-negative blood. In the mid-1970s, post-transfusion incidences of this non-A non-B hepatitis (NANBH) were 5–10% in the USA and 1% in the UK.[48] Although surrogate liver function tests were tried, such as the alanine aminotransferase

(ALT) activity and anti-HBc reactivity, it was not until 1991 that serological screening for HCV (following its identification[49]) could be introduced and a further reduction achieved. Up until then, HCV had been responsible for over 90% of all cases of NANBH. Donor follow-up reveals HCV infection to be commonly associated with past injection of illicit drugs.[50]

A few donors react falsely with the reagents from certain manufacturers; such donors may, with care, be reinstated if they test negative with alternative kits. Various tests for microbiological polymerase chain reaction (PCR) or nucleic acid amplification tests (NAT) have recently been applied, with little increase in the detection,[51] so questions of cost-efficacy are asked. Nevertheless, the UK services are testing each donation for HCV RNA by NAT in 'minipools', and developments are in hand to make this applicable to blood products within 24 hours of collection.

Current ELISA tests on UK donors are reactive in just over 2000 each year, but positivity is confirmed by recombinant immunoblotting assay (RIBA) in only one tenth. Testing by alternative ELISA systems may allow falsely 'reactive' donors to donate. Between April 1999 and September 2000, of over four million donations tested, 314 were confirmed to be HCV-antibody positive, of which approximately two-thirds reacted by NAT; three donors were anti-HCV-negative but NAT-positive. Trials of tests for HCV antigen indicate a slightly lower detection rate than by NAT. In spite of this sensitive screening system, it is estimated now that between 5 and 10 donations each year are infectious for HCV in spite of it not being detected by this screening and confirmation system. This would be mostly due to 'window period' failures.

Other countries in Northern Europe have similar rates. The prevalence of confirmed anti-HCV-positive donors in Germany[52] reached 121 per 100 000 in 1999, and seemed more from women. The estimated risk of transmitting HCV there was estimated to be 1 in 200 000 (1 in 97 000 to 1 in 1 400 000) for repeat donors. In 1995, the calculated risk for first-time donors was 1 in 20 000 (1 in 15 000 to 1 in 28 000).

HIV

ELISA screening and Western blot confirmatory tests for HIV-1 have been available since 1985, and tests for HIV-2 became available in the following year. Since then, only two donations collected in the UK have been found to have transmitted HIV – to five recipients (because two or three components of the donated blood were given to different patients). Several more may have done so, but no infected recipients have yet been found. The calculated transmission rate now is 1 in between 2.5 and 5 million.[53] Currently about 1500 donations are reactive each year, of which about 20 are confirmed true-positive. First-time donors are 5–10 times more likely to be positive than 'accredited' ones.

Follow-up of donors confirmed positive

Donors have a right to medical advice after any unexpected significant medical condition is revealed during or after donation (including sickle cell trait, thalassaemia or GH). For HIV infection, systems for counselling and follow-up may be needed. Any donor with HBV or HCV needs access to specialist care. All such donors should be interviewed – not least to see whether any factors were missed during the medical assessment. About one-third of all UK donors positive for HCV admit to previous drug use, and one-third of HIV-positive donors are gay men (in spite of the exclusion clauses). Such donors either do not regard such factors as significant, or may genuinely fail to recollect them (this may be particularly true for first timers). But the distinct rate of positivity among repeat donors indicates that some are being economical with the truth.

Other infectious hazards

Although no cases of transfusion-transmitted Chagas' disease have been reported in the UK in the last two decades, this parasitic disease, caused by *Trypanosoma cruzi* and endemic to rural parts of South America, has been known to be transmitted by transfusion since 1952;[54] donated blood may be treated with trypanosomicides such as gentian violet, sometimes with added ascorbic acid.[55] Studies from California and New Orleans show that *T. cruzi*-affected donations are strongly associated with a Hispanic origin of the donor – sometimes indicating vertical (female) transmission through three generations.[56] Within non-endemic countries, the best donation-selection strategy is to ask the donors if they have lived in South America, or if they or their mothers were born there, or if they have lived in South America, or if they or their mothers were born there, or if they have received a transfusion there. If their blood contains no detectable antibody to *T. cruzi*, it may be used for transfusion. For European countries, it is not necessary to test most people who have merely paid short visits –

even to 'jungle areas' – but tests can be conducted in cases of doubt.

Serological tests for syphilis are mandatory in most transfusion services, but their value is somewhat limited. The treponeme only survives for a few days at 4°C storage in red cells, and episodes of transmission by transfusion are now very infrequent. The method of testing can pose some problems – the more sensitive (such as TPHA) can reveal past infection decades before, but even donors cured of the infection may not be acceptable according to some national criteria (whereas people with a past history of gonorrhoea may be acceptable). However, relatively less sensitive tests (such as reagin tests) can sometimes detect non-related conditions such as the presence of lupus antibody. Such claims are, however, anecdotal.

There has recently been one UK fatality due to malaria. This seems to have been the fourth in the UK in more than 25 years. Nevertheless, the global significance of this organism means that it has to be considered. For developed countries, the major problem comes through donors holidaying or working for short times in tropical areas. A quarantine period (6 months in Europe, 12 months in North America)[57] is applied to reduce risk, but at considerable cost to the blood supply. A few people who have been treated apparently successfully for malaria harbour organisms for weeks, months, or even years. These can be detected by serological tests for malaria antibodies, but these are less well accredited than, for example, those for *T. cruzi*, although progress is being made.

Viruses known or suspected to cause occasional transmission include hepatitis A (although the major way of transmitting this is by the oral–faecal route), parvovirus B19 (since it is ubiquitous in the community, it cannot be avoided – but the known propensity towards marrow aplasia means that it should be borne in mind under certain circumstances), and – largely by analogy with CMV – herpesviruses. The β or γ subtypes: Epstein–Barr virus, human herpesvirus-8, and CMV itself – seem to be more important in this context than herpes simplex and varicella zoster viruses. The clinical significance of some other viruses occasionally found in the blood of donors ('TTV', 'HGV', etc.) is far from clear;[58] there may be concerns that, although they are not associated with any disease in the persons carrying them, if transmitted by blood to a sick recipient significant morbidity may follow.

Inactivation of viruses and bacteria in blood products

A reduction in infectious risk might be achieved by the addition (followed perhaps by removal) of viricidal chemicals to blood products. Single-donor fresh frozen plasma can be treated with methylene blue and light, or by psoralens and ultraviolet light.[59–61] The 'solvent detergent' approach has also been successfully introduced for the inactivation of lipid-coated organisms in plasma. Psoralens have also been applied to platelet concentrates, and similar treatments of red cells are under development.[62]

NON-INFECTIOUS HAZARDS

Medications taken by donors

With notable exceptions, in principle it is not the drug but the condition for which treatment is required that guides donor acceptance policies. For example, people on short-term antibiotic therapy for an acute infection are not usually acceptable, but those receiving tetracyclines for acne may be. Similarly, hypertension, even when well controlled by diuretics or by beta blockers, may be a reason to defer donation although the medications themselves would not affect the quality of the donation for the recipient. On the other hand, drugs that are teratogenic in trace quantities, such as tamoxifen and some derivatives of vitamin A,[63] render donations unacceptable even if the donor is otherwise healthy and only taking them for prophylaxis. There has to be concern that some recipients – pregnant women, or their fetuses – may be unduly prone to adverse influences. Aspirin-based medications need not prevent donation, but donated blood should not be used for preparing platelet concentrates. Oral contraceptives, or hormone replacement therapy (or some bisphosphonates) to combat osteoporosis, are not reasons for donor deferral.

Immunological complications of transfusion

Serological compatibility is essential for blood safety. For all but those chronically dependent through marrow failure (either through primary disease or therapy), only red cell compatibility is required. Platelet compatibility is confined to those who become refractory to platelet therapy through immune differences, which are usually mediated through HLA antibodies; and (very rarely) some people may need transfused platelets to be typed according to their HPA requirements.

Red cell compatibility

Red cell compatibility testing has come to rely principally on determination of the ABO and Rh D group of the patient, and on screening patient's serum by an antiglobulin test for clinically significant antibodies. This uses a small panel (two or three) of screening cells specially selected to express the most relevant antigens. If an antibody is detected, cells negative for the antigen are chosen, matched with donor red cells by antiglobulin techniques. Emergency procedures can accelerate the delivery of blood. The 'Maximum Surgical Blood Ordering Schedules – MSBOS' determines the number of units initially available for planned surgical procedures.[65] Patients with no antibodies can receive blood selected through computer records, since recent advances in information technology have now made the labelling of blood packs very reliable.[65]

Classic ABO incompatibility still occurs – nearly always through operational rather than technical errors. The symptoms and signs may vary from mild haemolytic jaundice to rapid anaphylactic death. This variation is mostly due to the strengths of antigen–antibody reactions, which is strongest in group O people with relatively high IgM titres of anti-A receiving group A_1 blood. Recipients with low antibody titre (such as elderly men and newborns), or who (by luck) receive units displaying weak group A antigenicity, may escape lightly. Haemoglobinuria may be followed by oliguria or anuria requiring a period of dialysis (occasionally the onset is so severe that there is no period of haemoglobinuria). This is due to renal tubular necrosis resulting from red cell membrane fragments coated with immune complexes, and to the haemoglobin dimers, which go through the glomerular filter and become deposited in the tubular epithelium. Causative errors are usually due to incorrect identification of the patient, either when blood is sampled for pre-transfusion testing or when being transfused. Laboratory errors are usually due to working on incorrectly selected samples.

Delayed haemolytic reactions may occur either through not detecting a reactive antibody (which would represent a laboratory failure) or because the concentration of significant antibodies from previous sensitizing episodes has fallen too low to be detected. These can cause significant morbidity – including jaundice and renal impairment – which can aggravate any morbidity from the primary disorder, as well as producing a suboptimal rise in the patient's haemoglobin concentration. Concerns have recently been expressed that if the antiglobulin phase of the match between donor red cells and patient serum is removed – either with the adoption of an 'immediate spin only' or an 'electronic' match through computerized records – the antibody screen procedure may require greater stringency, possibly by increasing the number of panel test cell samples to four. There is no evidence in the current literature to support the validity of such concerns, nor of concerns that such measures would miss the occasional donation from a donor whose red cells react positively to a direct antiglobulin test.[66]

Histocompatibility
Although the human leukocyte antigen (HLA) systems do not involve red cells, their presence on white cells and platelets can complicate the management of people who receive several transfusions, and also multiparous women through fetal exposure to paternal HLA. Elucidation of HLA was integral to the development of organ and haematopoietic stem cell transplantation, so that histocompatible organs and donors could be selected; but the presence of even non-vital white cells and platelets in red cell products can induce sensitization to HLA. If HLA-reactive blood is given, the symptoms may be relatively nonspecific (fever, headache, etc.) but alarming; they may be accompanied by and compound the effects of the non-immune biological mediators of inflammatory responses such as cytokines and other 'pyrogens'. HLA antibodies in patients receiving therapy with platelets bearing the relevant antigens will be refractory to those platelets; in such cases HLA and HPA (human platelet antigen – see below) antibodies should be sought and histocompatible platelets given if such antibodies are present. Petz et al[67] have devised a system whereby platelets for immune-refractory patients are selected for HLA type according to the specificity of any detected anti-HLA, which enables more compatible donors to be identified than would be available by selecting only those who are of the same HLA type as the patient.

IgA-deficient recipients
People who are congenitally deficient in immunoglobulin A (IgA) are rare (about 1 in 800), but can (even with no history of previous transfusion of pregnancy) possess powerful antibodies to IgA, or one of its subclasses, and react very adversely to IgA infusions in plasma or even fractionated immunoglobulin for intravenous use. Known individuals should be checked before transfusion, but most often the first intimation comes with

transfusion. Tests for anti-IgA should be included for all such cases with the first transfusion, even of red cells in optimal additive, since enough IgA is present in the residual plasma to cause reactions.[68]

Platelet transfusion immunology

Platelet antigens, deriving from genetic polymorphisms among surface glycoproteins, can give rise to antibodies, complicating transfusion. There are eight well-defined systems of human platelet antigens (HPA-1 to HLA-8), each with a pair of alleles (designated 'a' or 'b') to which antibodies can arise in antigen-negative people, and several other rare antigens, not all associated with true membrane proteins.[69] There are two types of clinical response. In post-transfusion purpura (PTP), typical cases occur in people who have been sensitized by past transfusion or more usually by pregnancy, often decades previously. Some days after receiving another transfusion containing platelets (even effete ones, as in red cell preparations), the patient's own platelets seem to become involved as bystanders in a delayed immune response, resulting in thrombocytopenia. The treatment of choice is intravenous immunoglobulin.

In neonatal alloimmune thrombocytopenia (NAITP), the mother becomes exposed to paternal HPA from feto-maternal bleeds during pregnancy. Resulting anti-HPA antibodies may cross the placenta and destroy the baby's platelets, resulting in intrauterine bleeding, including in the baby's brain. This may need managing through intrauterine transfusions of specially prepared platelet concentrates.

Transfusion-related acute lung injury (TRALI)[70]

This is usually caused by the passive transfusion of plasma containing antibodies to HLA and granulocyte antigens (human neutrophil, antigens – HNA), which react with the patient's neutrophils. Agglutinated neutrophils in the pulmonary circulation release their inflammatory mediators, which cause the symptoms of acute respiratory distress. Red cell preparations with reduced plasma content are rarely implicated, and whilst using fresh-frozen plasma and platelet concentrates prepared exclusively from men (especially if they have not been transfused) – since blood from women who have been pregnant may well contain HLA and HNA antibodies – would largely alleviate this risk, such a strategy is not always possible. TRALI has occurred as a result of antileukocyte antibodies in the patient reacting with passively donated white cells, even in red cell preparations that may be partially depleted of leukocytes.

Transfusion-associated immunomodulation (TRIM)

This term has been given to observed and hypothetical immunological events surrounding blood transfusion. The first such to be observed was the apparently paradoxical finding that people awaiting renal transplantation could be relatively 'tolerized' by allogeneic blood, thus enhancing, non-specifically, the chances of successful engraftment. Other examples are less favourable, including possible enhancement of the growth of metastases after surgical removal of primary malignancies when transfusion accompanied the surgery, and also an increase in susceptibility to microbial infections following peri-operative transfusion, both at the surgical site and at remote locations (especially lungs). The component of blood most likely to cause immunomodulation is the white cells. These matters are discussed by Vamvakas, Dzik, and Blajchman.[71] They indicate that the evidence does not support an enhancement by transfusion of the growth of malignant metastases, although they indicate that the three main studies conducted – in which there was reasonable homogeneity of design – may not be sensitive enough to exclude the possibility of an effect of possibly up to 20%. They also addressed the issue of transfusion-related infections, and concluded, from the evidence of somewhat heterogeneous trials, that it seemed doubtful – although the best designed trial (by van der Watering et al) was suggestive. This study also indicated a favourable effect on hospital length of stay. One problem is that many of the comparisons for both themes were between partially leukodepleted preparations derived from buffy-coat depleted blood and fully leukodepleted blood, so the differences may not have been as large as those that could have resulted from comparing fully leukodepleted with non-depleted blood. There is therefore much interest in the results of further observational studies and randomized trials.

Transfusion-associated graft-versus-host disease (TAGvHD)

The ingress of viable incompatible immune-competent cells during transfusion will usually be dealt with by the patient's immune system. If the patient has impaired immunity – either from their primary disease or as a result of drugs such as some nucleoside ana-logues – then transfused alien leukocytes may survive and engraft. The bone marrow is particularly vulnerable; the ensuing reaction – (TAGvHD) – inducing untreatable marrow failure, with uniformly fatal results. Such complications can be avoided by prior gamma-irradiation of the product to be transfused (25 Gy per pack), which prevents any lymphocytes from multiplying.[72] It is possible that leukodepletion may also reduce the chances of engraftment, but this cannot be recommended on its own. Patients in populations with relatively few HLA polymorphisms are more liable to receive HLA-compatible transfusions, even from randomly selected donors. Donor leukocytes in the transfusion may engraft more easily and subsequently recognize host antigens, probably of the 'minor' or 'non-major' histocompatibility types, as 'foreign' thereby inducing TAGvHD. The blood product from any parent-to-child donations should also be irradiated prior to transfusion.

It is of some interest that whereas the first three years of the UK *Serious Hazards of Transfusion* (SHOT) scheme – which were prior to the introduction of universal leukodepletion – reported twelve cases of TAGvHD, there was only one case in the next two years during which universal leukodepletion was applied. This was in a patient for whom the current guidelines did not recommend irradiated cells and who was transfused with blood processed for leukodepletion. (The patient was a young woman with relapsed Acute Lymphoblastic Leukaemia receiving remission–induction chemotherapy which did not include purine antagonists; irradiation is recommended of blood components transfused to patients receiving these agents.) Although the guidelines are being reconsidered, it is still noteworthy that the leukodepletion procedure (which is likely to have been effective) was still insufficient to remove donor lymphocytes.[73]

Effects of biological mediators of inflammation in transfused blood

Non-haemolytic febrile transfusion reactions are common with standard platelet concentrates. These may have a considerable quantity of contaminating leukocytes, particularly when the top of the buffy coat layer of the centrifuged whole blood is taken into the platelet-rich plasma. Viable lymphocytes remaining in the final concentrate, which is kept at 20°C, are still producing cytokines, while those cells that die release their contents into the plasma.[74] When the platelets are transfused after three or four days of storage, the concentrations of these biological mediators in the plasma can be very high. These high concentrations cause fever and headaches upon transfusion, for which corticosteroids and antihistamines, and even reduction of leukocyte content by bedside filtration on platelets four or five days old, have little effect. The symptoms are best managed with non-aspirin antipyretic drugs such as paracetamol (acetaminophen). Effective reduction of leukocytes to less than five million per pack reduces this cause of adverse response; when marked fevers accompany the transfusion of leukocyte-reduced platelets, it is important to eliminate bacterial contamination as a cause, since this can occur in more than one platelet concentrate per thousand.

HAEMOVIGILANCE

Procedures monitoring the frequency and types of adverse events following transfusion have been introduced in several countries, particularly France, and the USA.[75,76] The UK SHOT scheme, which started in 1997, is a voluntary 'no-blame' system in which hospital staff are encouraged to report any adverse event following a transfusion. Participation is increasing – 'nil returns' are encouraged. For 2001, there were incidents from 199 hospitals out of the 379 reporting (180 submitted 'nil returns'). In over half (213 out of the 315), an incorrectly selected component had been transfused, a failure to follow phlebotomy protocols being a common cause, but there were also a significant number of laboratory errors, some of which were committed by experienced staff during the day. In the overall 5-year period, there were 1148 incidents, 699 being of 'wrong blood component'. There were 287 transfusion reactions (of which 223 produced minor morbidity only, but 21 caused major morbidity and there were 6 deaths definitely attributed to the transfusion), 70 diagnoses of TRALI, 40 of post-transfusion purpura, 13 of TAGvHD, and 35 infections (HIV, HTLV-I, and HAV – one case each; HBV – 8 cases; HCV – 2 cases; bacteria – 21 cases (6 deaths); and one fatal case of malaria.[73]

Some of these adverse events were unavoidable or genuinely unpredictable. Others, such as the TRALI (with which blood from female donors is highly associated – presumably because of a distinct rate of pregnancy-associated leukocyte alloimmunization), might have been avoided by more thorough selection of blood product, but there may be operational reasons complicating the intentional selection of male donors only, particularly for platelets. However, human errors were the predominant cause, and although greater training and awareness is essential in order to reduce such episodes, other technological solutions may be needed. Certainly, the record in the UK appears not to have improved even after 5 years of data presentation, which emphasizes the need for a 'new look' at root causes. Although barcoding for individual patient identification, utilizing wristbands and IT software to ensure that the right patient gets the blood, appears to be a promising approach, there are several hurdles to overcome – not least the habit of anaesthetists and others of removing the wristbands in order to gain access to a vein for administering the blood.

COSTS

Over 30 million blood donations are collected annually over the world, proportionally most in the developed nations of the West. North America and north-west Europe alone account for at least 22 million. Although the bulk of donations require little more than basic medical management at the sessions, the small minority of donors with conditions requiring further interpretation or intervention add a disproportionate cost. Hence, even where donors are unremunerated – as in the UK for over 70 years – 'handling costs' are considerable. Although organizations differ widely between nations, many have reorganized their transfusion services in the AIDS era as it has been realized that what had traditionally been regarded as semicharitable concerns for the voluntary provision of blood actually require highly sophisticated management structures. The radical restructuring of transfusion services in the UK in the mid-1990s, which produced the National Blood Authority for

England (and analogous bodies for Scotland, Wales, and Northern Ireland) is mirrored elsewhere. Ever-increasing requirements of accountability are directing a more 'pharmaceutical' style of service provision, with documented 'Good Manufacturing Practices' and 'Good Laboratory Practices' that provide a basis for inspection by Standards Bodies. This is also part of a more general tightening of scrutiny of professional performances internationally, and not only in health service provision, with similar responses developing in Europe, Canada, Australia, and New Zealand. In the USA, where the concept of public accountability of management is no stranger, there are, however, still many separate small 'blood banks' serving communities and/or hospitals, in which collection and clinical services are closely linked.

In the UK, with a population of 56 million and where about 2.5 million blood donations are collected, tested, and transfused each year (on about 1.5 million occasions to about 700 000 patients), the 1990s also saw radical changes in blood processing. More sophisticated systems, such as computerized documentation of records, new processes of platelet production, and, particularly, 'universal leukodepletion', were introduced. In 1994 – the year before the reorganization of the English transfusion services was effected – all standard donations were processed into red cell preparations, over one million platelet concentrates (for about 200 000 infusions), about 250 000 units of fresh-frozen plasma, and about 25 000 units of cryoprecipitated plasma. A few platelet-pheresis donations were collected separately, and some plasma-pheresis conducted – mainly for hyperimmune plasma. The raw cost for this provision was about £120 million, almost half being required for the payroll for the collection teams, other transport, clerical, and managerial staff, doctors, scientists, and nurses. Twelve million pounds alone was required for the purchase of the blood collection packs, and up to £4 million was spent on the mandatory microbiology tests. Up to 1996, some costs were offset by remuneration to the transfusion services for the plasma supplied for fractionation – about 500 metric tonnes a year. The average charge to the hospitals for each unit of red cell concentrate supplied was about £35. At the hospitals, costs include those for storage of blood packs, data logging, patient testing, and staff, and add between £20 and £40 per unit.

In 1999, the introduction of leukodepletion – which, like the withdrawal of UK plasma from the world fractionation market, was a response to finding the first cases of vCJD among young adults in the UK – vastly increased the cost of producing blood components, quite apart from the loss of the value of 500 tonnes of donor plasma (which including the hyper-immune plasma collections, were worth about £17 million).[77] The collection packs alone (now with integral filters) tripled in price. English hospitals are now charged nearly £100 for each red cell unit, and £160 for each 'Adult Therapeutic Dose' ('ATD') of platelets (equivalent in platelet content to five single-donor packs). Increasing demand for platelet concentrates, the overall quality of which is undoubtedly improved by leukodepletion (on the basis of a reduced rate of febrile reactions alone), has required more platelet 'ATDs' to be collected by apheresis from single donors, who are still unremunerated in spite of increased demands on their time.[33]

The blood collection and processing services in England are usually separate from the services in the hospitals where blood is matched for transfusion to specific patients. However, anticipation that decreasing demand from hospitals (because of greater efficiencies induced, in part, by greater recognition of costs) might result in downsizing of transfusion centres have yet to be realized. Improvements in clinical efficiency of blood use have not generally become rapidly apparent, but it would also be reasonable to expect increasing demands from an aging population who, nevertheless, expect high-quality medical services. There is, however, plenty of room for improvements in clinical blood use, so that only those patients really requiring a transfusion get one. Studies within several UK hospitals are beginning to show this.

REFERENCES

1. Kuhns WJ. Blood transfusion in the Civil War. *Transfusion* 1965; **5**: 92–4.
2. Schmidt PJ. Transfusion in America in the eighteenth and nineteenth centuries. *N Engl J Med* 1968; **279**: 1319–20.
3. Brakenridge DJ. Transfusion of human blood in the treatment of pernicious anaemia. *Edin Med J* 1892; **38b**: 409–29.
4. Addis T. The effect of intravenous injections of fresh human serum and of phosphated blood on the coagulation time of the blood in hereditary haemophilia. *Proc Soc Exp Biol Med* 1916; **14**: 19–23.
5. Lambert SW, quoted in Peterson EW. Results from blood transfusion. *JAMA* 1916; **LXVI**: 1291–5.
6. Duke WW. The relation of blood platelets to hemorrhagic disease. *JAMA* 1910; **LV**: 1185–91.
7. Unger LJ. Transfusion of unmodified blood. *JAMA* 1917; **LXIX**: 2159–65.

8. Landsteiner K. Ueber Agglutinationserscheinungen normalen menschlichen Blutes. *Wien klin Woch* 1901 [translation: *Transfusion* 1961; **1**: 5–8].

9. Ottenberg R. Studies in isoagglutination; I Transfusion and the question of intravascular agglutination. *J Exp Med* 1911; **13**: 425–38.

10. Crile GW. *Hemorrhage and Blood Transfusion, An Experimental and Clinical Approach.* New York: Appleton, 1909.

11. von Dungern EF and Hirschfeld L. Uber Vererbung gruppenspezifischer Strukturen des Blutes II. *Z Immunitatsforsch* 1910; **vi**: 284–92.

12. Todd C, White RG. On the fate of red blood corpuscles when injected into the circulation of an animal of the same species. *Proc R Soc Lond, Ser B* 1911; **84**: 255–9.

13. Lewisohn R. Blood transfusion by the citrate method. *Surg Gynecol Obstet* 1915; **21**: 37–47.

14. Robertson OH. Transfusion with preserved red cells. *BMJ* 1918; **i**: 691–5.

15. Loutit JF, Mollison PL. Advantages of a disodium-citrate–glucose mixture as a blood preservative. *BMJ* 1943; **ii**: 744.

16. Gibson JG, Rees SB, McManus TJ, Scheitlin WA. A citrate–phosphate–dextrose solution for the preservation of human blood. *Am J Clin Pathol* 1957; **28**: 569.

17. Fantus B (ed). The therapy of the Cook County Hospital – Blood preservation. *JAMA* 1937; **109**: 128–31.

18. Foster PR. Letter to Editor, *Newsletter of the British Blood Transfusion Society* (Manchester, UK), February 2001: 21.

19. Walter CW, Murphy WP. A closed gravity technique for the preservation of whole blood in ACD solution utilizing plastic equipment. *Surg Gynecol Obstet* 1952; **94**: 687.

20. Hogman CF, Hedlund K, Zetterstrom H. Clinical usefulness of red cells preserved in protein-poor mediums. *N Engl J Med* 1978; **299**: 1377.

21. Hogman CF, Eriksson L, Ericson A, Reppucci AJ. Storage of saline–adenine–glucose–mannitol-suspended red cells in a new plastic container: polyvinyl-chloride plasticised with butyryl-*n*-trihexyl-citrate. *Transfusion* 1991; **31**: 26–9.

22. Rock G, McCombie N, Tittley P. A new technique for the collection of plasma: machine plasmapheresis. *Transfusion* 1981; **21**: 241–6.

23. Kääriäinen L, Klemola E, Paloheimo J. Rise of cytomegalovirus antibodies in an infectious-mononucleus-like syndrome after transfusion. *BMJ* 1966; **i**: 1270–2.

24. Blumberg BS, Sutnick AI, London WT. Hepatitis and leukaemia: their relation to Australia antigen. *Bull NY Acad Med* 1968; **44**: 1566.

25. Dane DS, Cameron CH, Briggs M. Virus-like particles in serum of patients with Australia-antigen associated hepatitis. *Lancet* 1970; **i**: 695–8.

26. Starr D. *Blood, An Epic History of Medicine and Commerce.* London: Little, Brown, 1999: 217.

27. Llewelyn C, Amin M, Ballard S et al. Transfusion medicine epidemiology pilot study. *Br J Haem* 2002; **117**(Suppl 1): 77.

28. Mathoulin-Pelissier S, Salmi LR, Verret C et al. Blood transfusion in a random sample of hospitals in France. *Transfusion* 2000; **40**: 1140–6.

29. Titlestad K, Georgsen J, Jorgensen J, Kristensen T. Monitoring transfusion practices at two university hospitals. *Vox Sang* 2001; **80**: 40–7.

30. Det Norske Veritas. Assessment of the Risk of Exposure to vCJD Infectivity in Blood and Blood Products – Final Report for the Spongiform Encephalopathy Advisory Committee and the Department of Health. February 1999.

31. Dzik S. Universal leukoreduction: view from across the pond. *Transfus Med* 2000; **10**(Suppl 1): S11 (abst).

32. Goodnough LT. The case against universal

WBC reduction (and for the practice of evidence-based medicine). *Transfusion* 2000; **40**: 1522–7.

33. Blajchman MA. Transfusion-associated immunomodulation and universal white cell reduction: Are we putting the cart before the horse? *Transfusion* 1999; **39**: 665–70.

34. Fergusson D, Hébert PC, Barrington KJ, Shapiro SH. Effectiveness of WBC reduction in neonates: what is the evidence of benefit? *Transfusion* 2002; **42**: 159–65.

35. Houston F, Foster JD, Chang A et al. Transmission of BSE by blood transfusion in sheep [See comments]. *Lancet* 2000; **356**: 999–1000. Comment in ibid: 955–6.

36. Anonymous. Scientists race to develop a blood test for vCJD. *Nature Med* 2001; **7**(3): 261.

37. James V (ed). *Guidelines for the Blood Transfusion Services in the United Kingdom*, 4th edn. London: HMSO, 2000.

38. Boulton FE, Threshold concentration of haemoglobin in donor blood. *Vox Sang* 1999; **77**: 108.

39. Boulton FE, Collis D, Inskip H et al. A study of the iron and *HFE* status of blood donors, including a group who failed the initial screen for anaemia. *Brit J Haematol* 2000; **108**: 434–9.

40. Blajchman MA, Ali AM, Richardson HL. Bacterial contamination of cellular blood components. *Vox Sang* 1994; **67**(Suppl 3): 25–33.

41. Hogman CF, Engstrand L. Serious bacterial complications from blood components – How do they occur? *Transfus Med* 1998; **8**: 1–3.

42. Bruneau C, Perez P, Chassaigne M et al. Efficacy of a new collection procedure for preventing bacterial contamination of whole-blood donations. *Transfusion* 2000; **41**: 74–81.

43. Boulton FE, Chapman ST, Walsh TH. Fatal reaction to transfusion of red-cell concentrate contaminated with *Serratia liquefasciens*. *Transfus Med* 1998; **8**: 15–18.

44. McDonald CP, Hartley S, Orchard K et al. Fatal *Clostridium perfringens* sepsis from a pooled platelet transfusion. *Transfus Med* 1998; **8**: 19–22.

45. Aubert G, Vautrin AC, Michel VP et al. Evaluation of three automated blood culture systems. Bio Argod, Bact T/Alert, bactec. *Pathol Biol* 1993; **41**: 434–40 [in French].

46. Soldan K. NBA/PHLS CDSC Unpublished Quarterly Infection Surveillance Report No. 122, June 2000.

47. Regan FA, Hewitt P, Barbara JA, Contreras M. Prospective investigation of transfusion transmitted infection in recipients of over 20 000 units of blood. *BMJ* 2000; **320**: 403–6.

48. Mollison PL. *Blood Transfusion in Clinical Medicine*, 6th edn. Oxford: Blackwell Science, 1979; 658–9.

49. Choo Q-L, Kuo G, Weiner AJ et al. Isolation of a cDNA clone derived from a blood-borne non-A non-B viral hepatitis genome. *Science* 1989; **244**: 359–61.

50. Van der Poel C, Cuypers H, Reesink H et al. Risk factors in hepatitis C virus-infected blood donors. *Transfusion* 1991; **31**: 777–9.

51. AuBuchon JP. Allocating resources to improve the safety of transfusion. *Transfus Med* 2000; **10**(Suppl 1): 19.

52. Koerner K, Cardoso M, Dengler T et al. Estimated risk of transmission of hepatitis C virus by blood transfusion. *Vox Sang* 1998; **74**: 213–16.

53. Voak D, Caffrey EA, Barbara JAJ et al. Affordable safety for the blood supply in developed and developing countries. *Transfus Med* 1998; **8**: 73–6.

54. Wendel S, Gonzaga AL, Chagas' disease and blood transfusion: a new world problem? *Vox Sang* 1993; **64**: 1–12.

55. Moraes-Sousa H, Bordin JO. Strategies for prevention of transfusion-associated Chagas' disease. *Transfus Med Rev* 1996; **10**: 161–70.

56. Shulman IA. Intervention strategies to reduce the risk of transfusion-transmitted *Try-*

panosoma cruzi infection in the United States. *Transfus Med Rev* 1999; **13**: 227–34.

57. Mungai M, Tegtmeier G, Chamberland M, Parise M. Transfusion-transmitted malaria in the US from 1963 through 1999. *N Engl J Med* 2001; **344**: 1973–8.

58. Poovorawan Y, Tangkijvanich P, Theamboonlers A, Hirsch P. Transfusion transmissible virus TTV and its putative role in the etiology of liver disease. *Hepato-Gastroenterology* 2001; **48**: 256–60.

59. Williamson LM, Allain JP. Virally inactivated fresh frozen pasta. *Vox Sang* 1995; **69**: 159–66.

60. Aznar JA, Bonanad S, Montoro JM et al. Influence of methylene blue photoinactivation on coagulation factors from fresh frozen plasma, cryoprecipitate and cryosupernatants. *Vox Sang* 2000; **79**: 156–60.

61. Lerner RG, Nelson J, Sorcia E et al. Evaluation of solvent/detergent-treated plasma in patients with a prolonged prothrombin time. *Vox Sang* 2000; **79**: 161–7.

62. Corash L. Inactivation of viruses, bacteria, protozoa and leukocytes in platelet and red cell concentrates. *Vox Sang* 2000; **78**(Suppl 2): 205–10.

63. Association of British Pharmaceutical Industries Compendium of Data Sheets 1999–2000: 1346 (Neotigason) and 1356 (Roaccutane).

64. Boral LI, Henry JB. The type and screen: a safe alternative and supplement in selected surgical procedures. *Transfusion*, 1977; **17**: 163.

65. Säfwenberg J, Högman CF, Cassemar B. Computerised delivery control – a useful and safe complement to the type and screen compatibility testing. *Vox Sang* 1997; **72**: 162–8.

66. Issitt PD, Anstee DJ. *Applied Blood Group Serology* 4th edn. Durham, N Carolina: Montgomery Scientific Publications, 1998: 1019.

67. Petz LD, Garratty G, Calhoun L et al. Selecting donors of platelets for refractory patients on the basis of HLA antibody specificity. *Transfusion* 2000; **40**: 1446–56.

68. Mollison PL, Engelfriet CP, Contraras M. *Blood Transfusion in Clinical Medicine*, 10th edn. Oxford: Blackwell Science, 1998: 457 and 499.

69. Ibid: 442.

70. Popovsky MA, Chaplin HC, Moore SB. Transfusion related acute lung injury: a neglected serious complication of hemotherapy. *Transfusion* 1992; **32**: 589–92.

71. Vamvakas EC, Dzik WH, Blajchman MA. Deleterious effects of transfusion-associated immunomodulation: appraisal of the evidence and recommendations for prevention. In: *Immunomodulatory Effects of Blood Transfusion* (Vamvakas EC, Blajchman MA, eds). Bethesda, MD: AABB Press, 1999: 253–85.

72. British Committee for Standards in Haematology, Blood Transfusion Task Force. Guidelines on gamma irradiation of blood components for the prevention of transfusion-associated graft-versus-host disease. *Transfus Med* 1996; **6**: 261–71.

73. Love EM, Soldan K. *Serious Hazards of Transfusion Annual Reports 1998–1999, 1999–2000, and 2000–2001*. Manchester UK: SHOT Office, 2000, 2001, 2002.

74. Heddle NM, Klama LN, Singer J et al. The role of the plasma from platelet concentrates in transfusion reactions. *N Engl J Med* 1994; **331**: 625–8.

75. Debeir J, Noel L, Aullen JP et al. The French haemovigilance system. *Vox Sang* 1999; **77**: 77–81.

76. International Forum. Haemovigilance systems. *Vox Sang* 1999; **77**: 110–20.

77. Dzik S. Universal leukoreduction: view from across the pond. *Transfus Med* 2000; **10**(Suppl 1): S11 (abst).

2 Transfusion products

Susan Knowles

INTRODUCTION

Over the last 60 years, the ability of the transfusion services to provide blood components and blood products for transfusion support has been the cornerstone for many advances in medical practice. For example, during this time, the treatment of haemophilia evolved from giving freshly prepared plasma to cryoprecipitate and eventually to high-purity factor VIII concentrates.

Blood components are those therapeutic constituents that can be prepared by centrifugation, filtration and freezing using conventional blood bank technology. Their development has been dependent upon the availability of preservative solutions for whole blood and, secondly, integral plastic collection containers that enable components to be separated in a closed sterile system.

The transfusion of blood components, rather than whole blood, has several advantages, including the following:

- Optimal preservation of in vitro function of blood constituents; red cells maintain functional capacity best when refrigerated, the quality of plasma constituents is best preserved in the frozen state, and platelet storage is optimal when kept at room temperature with continuous agitation
- More effective treatment by specific replacement of deficiency, and the avoidance and possibly harmful infusion of surplus constituents
- Efficient utilization of blood donations and the provision of surplus plasma for the production of plasma derivatives or blood products

WHOLE BLOOD

Guidelines from the Council of Europe,[1] the UK,[2] and the American Association of Blood Banks (AABB)[3] define a blood donation as 450 ml ±10% of blood collected into citrate anticoagulant also containing phosphate and dextrose (CPD). The red cell and haemoglobin content is variable and dependent upon the donor's haematocrit and precise volume bled. However, the Council of Europe specifies that a unit should contain a minimum of 45 g haemoglobin.

Storage lesions

Whole blood should be stored at $4 \pm 2°C$ to diminish red cell utilization of ATP and preserve red cell viability. If the anticoagulant preservative solution also contains adenine (CPD-A1) to increase red cell ATP, viability is improved, and red cell recovery should be at least 70% at the end of a shelf life of 35 days. The addition of adenine causes a more rapid fall in red cell 2,3-bisphosphoglycerate (2,3-BPG), which in turn causes an increased affinity of haemoglobin for oxygen and decreases oxygen-carrying capacity during storage. After 10 days of storage, all 2,3-BPG is lost, but up to 50% is regenerated within 8 hours of transfusion. The red cell membrane sodium/potassium ion (Na^+/K^+) pump is also paralysed at 4°C. The membrane becomes leaky, with K^+ leaving the cells into the surrounding medium and Na^+ entering the cells. After 35 days' storage in CPD-A1, the plasma K^+ reaches a value of 78.5 mmol/l.

However, whole blood is rarely used, since, within a few hours or days, some coagulation factors (especially V and VIII) and platelets decrease in quantity or lose viability. After a 7-day hold at 4°C, factor VIII levels will have fallen to 0.32 ± 0.09 IU/ml and there is a lesser fall in factor V levels to 0.78 ± 0.15 IU/ml. Other coagulation factors are stable. At 4°C, platelets undergo a shape change from discoid to spherical, which is irreversible after 8 hours, and their in vivo survival is reduced to 2 days. Granulocytes and monocytes also rapidly lose function at 4°C, but, irrespective of the temperature of storage, their function is reduced after 8 hours and disintegration occurs after 24 hours. Microaggregates of platelets and white cells increase in number with storage, and reach levels of greater than 2000/ml by 35 days.

Indications for whole blood

There are no absolute indications for the transfusion of whole blood and little good clinical trial evidence to compare the effectiveness of whole blood with red cell concentrates. However, some physicians continue to use whole blood for selected indications, such as large-volume transfusion in children or exchange transfusion in neonates, where there is a need for red cells and expansion of plasma volume, and the supply of coagulation factors may offset the development of a dilutional coagulopathy.

RED CELL COMPONENTS

Red cells are provided in various formats, which differ with respect to the presence of additive solutions and the extent of white cell removal. Specifications for red cell components are provided in Table 2.1.

Several additive solutions are available (Optisol, SAG-M) that contain combinations of saline, adenine, phosphate, bicarbonate, glucose and mannitol (Table 2.2). These solutions provide better red cell viability during storage, and allow up to a 42-day shelf life (Table 2.3). In preparing red cells in additive solution, blood is collected into a primary pack containing CPD, and all but 10–20 ml plasma is removed and replaced with 80–100 ml additive solution. Red cells and red cells in additive solution can be used interchangeably, with the exception that red cells in additive solution are not recommended for exchange or massive transfusion in neonates.

The white cell content of red cells is reduced either by separating off the buffy coat or by employing filters to which the leukocytes adhere. The residual white cell contents are shown in Table 2.1.

Red cell components may also be divided in a closed 'paedipack' system into four or more aliquots for use in neonates, who may require several transfusions within a period of a few weeks. Using dedicated 'paedipacks' from the same donation, the number of donors whose blood is transfused to the neonate is minimized. Despite concerns of the

Table 2.1 Specifications for red cell components				
Component	Volume (ml)	Minimum Hb (g)	Hct (%)	WBC (per unit)
Red cells (in approximately 80 ml plasma)	230–340	45	0.65–0.75	$>10^9$
Red cells in additive solution	280–420	45	0.5–0.7	$>10^9$
Red cells in additive solution, buffy coat removed	230–340	43	0.5–0.7	$<1.2 \times 10^9$
Red cells in additive solution, leukocyte-depleted	220–340	40	0.5–0.7	$<1 \times 10^6$

Hb, haemoglobin; Hct, haematocrit; WBC, white blood cells.

Table 2.2 Composition of red cell additive solutions		
Substance content	CPD SAG-M	CPD Optisol (AS-5)
NaCl (mmol)	15	15.4
Adenine (mmol)	0.125	0.03
Glucose (mmol)	4.5	6.9
Mannitol (mmol)	2.9	2.7
Volume (ml)	100	100

potential adverse effects of high levels of supernatant K^+ at the end of red cell shelf life, the absolute amount of K^+ administered is far less than the daily requirement of a neonate. Several studies in low-birthweight infants comparing red cells stored for less than 5 days with those up to 35 days old have shown no difference in serum K^+ levels before and after transfusions.[4]

Administering red cells

Bedside identity check

Reports from haemovigilance schemes across the world confirm that the greatest risk of morbidity and mortality from blood transfusion is the administration of the wrong unit to the patient.[5,6] This arises when a patient is transfused with blood intended for another patient who is ABO-incompatible, and can result in an acute haemolytic transfusion reaction. Alternatively, the blood component can be incorrect in that it fails to meet the criteria required (e.g. CMV-seronegative or gamma irradiated). Errors in giving the wrong blood to a patient are preventable.

Failure of some aspect of the pretransfusion bedside identity check is the commonest error leading to the mistransfusion of a unit of

Table 2.3 Biochemical changes in red cells stored for 35 days in CPD-A1 and Optisol (AS-5)		
Variable	CPD-A1	Optisol (AS-5)
Percentage of viable cells (24 hours post transfusion)	71	85
ATP (% initial value)	45	74
23-BPG (% initial value)	<10	<10
K$^+$ (mmol/l)	78.5	46.0

blood. This identity check should involve the following stages:

- Whenever possible, asking the patient to positively identify himself/herself
- Checking the verbal identity given with that on the wristband, the compatibility label on the blood pack, and the compatibility report
- Confirming that the ABO and RhD group are identical on the blood pack, compatibility label, and the compatibility form
- Confirming that any requirements for specialist components have been met.

Systems are available to reinforce the requirement to complete these simple but mandatory steps. One involves a coded locking system such that the blood unit cannot be accessed without matching a three-digit code that can be found only on the patient's wristband.[7] Comprehensive automated systems are also available, involving handheld barcode scanners and label printers that allow the phlebotomist to scan the patient's wristband and generate the specimen collection label, and at administration to automatically match the patient's wristband with the allocated blood units.[8]

Units of red cells should also be inspected to ensure that they are in date and show no signs of leakage, unusual colour or signs of haemolysis.

Time limits for infusing red cells

Red cells should not be taken out of refrigeration until the time of the transfusion, since there is a risk of bacterial proliferation within the pack at room temperature. Red cells that have been out of refrigeration for 30 minutes or more cannot be returned to stock, and if still required, should be transfused immediately. A unit of red cells should be infused over a maximum of 4 hours.

Transfusion equipment

Red cells should be transfused through a sterile blood administration set incorporating a 170–260 µm screen filter and drip chamber that has been primed with saline. Administration sets should be changed at least 12-hourly during red cell infusion, and a new administration set should be used if another fluid is to be infused following the red cells. If red cells are administered to neonates using a syringe, they should also be given through a suitable screen filter.

Blood warmers

Massive rapid infusions of cold blood can

contribute to hypothermia, which in turn is associated with cold-induced coagulopathies and cardiac dysrrhythmias, including cardiac arrest. The use of a blood warmer is often advised for the following:

- adults receiving blood at infusion rates >50 ml/kg/hour
- children infused at rates >15 ml/kg/hour
- infants undergoing exchange transfusions
- patients with cold agglutinins active in vitro at 37°C

No other infusion solutions or drugs should be added to red cells (or any other blood component), since they may contain additives such as calcium, which can cause citrated blood to clot. Dextrose solutions (5%) can lyse red cells. Drugs should never be added to any blood product, since if there is an adverse reaction, it may be impossible to determine if this is due to the blood, to the medication that has been added, or to an interaction of the two.

Indications for red cell transfusion

Given the measurable but small risks of allogeneic blood, the indication for transfusion of red cells (and all other blood components) should be documented in the patient's case notes.

Red cells are primarily used to increase the circulating red cell mass as a means of improving oxygen supply to the tissues, when there has been significant blood loss or there is an intractable symptomatic anaemia. However, since it is difficult to directly measure intracellular oxygen in the clinical setting, surrogate markers such as haemoglobin are often used to judge the need for red cell support, taking into account the patient's clinical condition.

A haemoglobin concentration of 50 g/l is generally considered critical for maintaining bodily functions, and most patients with a haemoglobin less than 60 g/l require red cell support. On the other hand, there is no evidence that cardiovascular function is improved at haemoglobin values above 100 g/l, and hence there is no place for the automatic application of the traditional '100 g/l transfusion trigger'. When making the decision to transfuse, account should be taken of coexistent factors such as age or cardiopulmonary insufficiency that compromise the patient's ability to compensate for an oxygen deficit.

This approach is demonstrated in the Practice Guidelines for Blood Component Therapy sponsored by the American Society of Anaesthesiologists in 1996:[9]

- Red blood cell transfusion is rarely indicated when the haemoglobin is above 100 g/l, and almost always indicated when the haemoglobin is less than 60 g/l.
- When the haemoglobin is between 60 and 100 g/l, consideration should be taken of the patient's individual general risk factors for complications of inadequate oxygenation.
- If possible, red cell transfusion should be avoided by use of other therapeutic measures to minimize blood loss (e.g. preoperative autologous donation and intraoperative blood recovery).

In the perioperative setting, simple algorithms and equations can be used to help guide the need for red cell support.[10] For example:

Number of red cell units required for a specific operation

= predicted fall in haemoglobin (g/l)
  – [preoperative haemoglobin (g/l)
    – threshold haemoglobin for
      transfusion (g/l)]

In patients with haematological diseases receiving intensive chemotherapy, the transfusion 'trigger' is usually in the range of 80–100 g/l. This is not evidence-based, but studies in animal models of thrombocytopenia and evidence from uraemic patients suggest that correction of anaemia also improves the prolonged bleeding time. In chronic anaemias, refractory to haematinic supplements, the decision to transfuse red cells should be based upon the patient's clinical symptoms.[11]

Red cell transfusions are also given in β-thalassaemia major to suppress the patient's own ineffective erythropoiesis and in sickle cell disease to reduce the risk of stroke in children at high risk, in patients with a previous stroke, and to reduce vaso-occlusive events in pregnancy.

Indications for red cells in neonates

There are several guidelines available, from Canada, the USA, and the UK that are based on consensus.[12] An example of current UK recommendations, taken from the *UK Handbook of Transfusion Medicine*,[13] is provided in Table 2.4.

Buffy coat removed red cells

A one-log reduction in the number of contaminating white cells, as can be achieved by removing the buffy coat by centrifugation, is effective in preventing the majority of febrile transfusion reactions accompanying red cell transfusions. However, the white cell content of red cells must be lowered further to have other beneficial effects. (See section below on leukocyte-depleted blood components.)

Washed red cells

Red cells can be depleted of plasma protein and, to a lesser extent, of leukocytes by washing them in up to 2 litres of normal saline using an automated cell washer. Since the process is 'open', the preparation must be given a 24-hour shelf life. Washed red cells

Table 2.4 Red cell transfusions for infants under 4 months of age	
Indication for transfusion	**Suggested transfusion threshold**
Anaemia in the first 24 hours	Haemoglobin <120 g/l
Cumulative blood loss in 1 week	10% blood volume lost
Neonate receiving intensive care	Haemoglobin <120 g/l
Acute blood loss	10% blood volume lost
Chronic oxygen dependency	Haemoglobin <110 g/l
Late anaemia, stable patient	Haemoglobin <70 g/l

are only indicated for patients with uncontrollable febrile or anaphylactic reactions to leukocyte-depleted red cells, who are presumed to have antibodies to plasma proteins. Although they can be used for patients with IgA deficiency and anti-IgA antibodies, it is preferable to use red cells from IgA-deficient donors. Washed red cells are no longer considered necessary for patients with paroxysmal nocturnal haemoglobinuria, for whom leukocyte-depleted components in additive solution are acceptable.

Cryopreserved red cells

Red cells can be stored for years in the vapour phase of liquid nitrogen at −180°C or in mechanical freezers at −80°C, provided they are mixed with a cryoprotectant (usually glycerol) prior to freezing. Since the red cells are washed several times after thawing, they are given a 24-hour shelf life following reconstitution.

Cryopreservation is used to store red cells from donors with a rare antigen composition – either lacking a high-frequency antigen or with the combined absence of several antigens that commonly sensitize patients. Patients who have multiple red cell alloantibodies or rare red cell phenotypes may also have autologous units cryopreserved prior to a planned surgical procedure.

Risks of red cells (other than disease transmission)

- Circulatory overload
- Alloimmunization against red cell antigens
- Haemolytic transfusion reaction
- Febrile non-haemolytic transfusion reaction

- Biochemical imbalance in massive transfusion
- Post-transfusion purpura
- Transfusion-related acute lung injury
- Transfusion-associated graft-versus-host disease

PLATELET CONCENTRATES

Platelets can either be prepared from whole-blood donations or be obtained by apheresis. Apheresis platelets can be human leukocyte antigen (HLA) or human platelet antigen (HPA) matched with the recipient and have the potential advantage of exposing the patient to fewer donors. There are no other qualitative differences between the sources. Platelets can be produced from whole blood either by pooling and centrifuging 4–6 buffy coats or by recentrifuging individual units of platelet-rich plasma (PRP). The former is favoured in Europe, including the UK, whereas the latter PRP method is standard in North America. The PRP method has the disadvantage of higher leukocyte contamination and less plasma is available from the original unit for fractionation. The Council of Europe specifications for platelet concentrates are given in Table 2.5.

Platelets are commonly suspended in donor plasma, but may also be reconstituted in mixtures of plasma and an additive solution, containing acetate, citrate, phosphate and chloride.[14] Platelet additive solutions can maintain platelet viability up to 7 days, enable more plasma to be sent for fractionation, and theoretically reduce the frequency and severity of transfusion complications related to components of the suspending plasma. In practice, in the UK, platelets in additive solution are used for patients experiencing

Table 2.5 The Council of Europe specifications for platelet concentrates

Parameter	PRP	Buffy coat	Apheresis
Volume (ml)	>50	>50/single-unit equivalent	>40 per 60×10^9 platelets
Platelet count	>60×10^9	>60×10^9/single-unit equivalent	>200×10^9/unit
Residual leukocytes, before leukocyte depletion	<0.2×10^9	<0.05×10^9/single-unit equivalent	<1.0×10^9/unit
Residual leukocytes, after leukocyte depletion	<0.2×10^6	<0.2×10^6/single-unit equivalent	<1.0×10^6/unit

reactions to platelet concentrates despite leukocyte depletion. Although it would be useful to have a 7-day shelf life for platelet concentrates, concern has been expressed about the possibility of increased bacterial risk, unless combined with a strategy for screening for bacterial contamination.

Platelets are stored in incubators set at 20–24°C and must be agitated during storage. They have a shelf life of up to 5 days.

Administering platelet concentrates

Although it is not essential to transfuse ABO-identical units, the donor plasma should preferably be compatible, since a dose of platelets will contain 200–300 ml plasma. Particular care should be taken in transfusing group O platelets to non-O recipients, and instances of haemolytic transfusion reactions are particularly likely in paediatric recipients.

Platelets should be administered through a fresh sterile standard blood administration set or platelet infusion set. Platelets are normally infused over not more than 30 minutes.

Indications for platelet transfusion

Platelet transfusions are indicated for the prevention and treatment of haemorrhage in patients with thrombocytopenia or platelet function defects. The recommended therapeutic or prophylactic transfusion 'trigger' is primarily a distinct platelet count. Clinical risk factors and the extent of bleeding also influence the decision as to when and how much to transfuse. There is little evidence from clinical trials on which to base the indications for therapeutic platelet transfusions, and most recommendations are based on observation or consensus. In contrast, there are several randomized trials examining different transfusion thresholds for prophylactic platelet support in haematological and oncological patients that provide evidence that a lower transfusion trigger of 10×10^9/l is not associated with a worse outcome than the traditional trigger of 20×10^9/l.[15]

Several recent guidelines are available, two of which are summarized in Tables 2.6 and 2.7.

Table 2.6 Guidelines on platelet transfusion from the Consensus Conference on Platelet Transfusion, sponsored by the Royal College of Physicians of Edinburgh in 1998[16]

Indications: prophylactic
- Main use: prevention of bleeding in patients with haematological malignancies and bone marrow disease caused by disease/treatment:
  - without risk factors (sepsis, concurrent use of drugs, other abnormalities of haemostasis): threshold of $10 \times 10^9/l$
  - with risk factors: use of a higher threshold of $20 \times 10^9/l$
  - prior to invasive procedure, dependent on the type of procedure (e.g. $>50 \times 10^9/l$ for insertion of intravascular lines or $>100 \times 10^9/l$ for surgery in critical sites)
  - neonates with considerable danger of haemorrhage: 'higher threshold than in adults'

Indications: therapeutic
- Massive haemorrhage: threshold of $50 \times 10^9/l$ 'clinical criteria need to be considered'
- Most major surgery (cardiac and vascular included) can be successfully carried out without platelet support. Patients who have taken aspirin 10 days preoperatively should be evaluated
- Thrombocytopenic purpura: intracranial or eye haemorrhage, severe bleeding from the gut

Contraindications
- Heparin-induced thrombocytopenia
- Thrombotic thrombocytopenic purpura
- Haemolytic uraemic syndrome

Dose
- Recommendation of a 'single therapeutic dose' i.e. $2.5–3 \times 10^9/l$

Indications for platelet concentrates in neonates

The following statements and thresholds are derived from the *UK Handbook of Transfusion Medicine*:[13]

- A threshold of $20 \times 10^9/l$ in otherwise-healthy infants
- A threshold of $30 \times 10^9/l$ in infants with

sepsis, other coagulopathies, and at risk of bleeding due to local tumour infiltration
- A threshold of $30 \times 10^9/l$ may also be appropriate in infants with neonatal alloimmune thrombocytopenia, even in the absence of significant bleeding, since the bound antibody can interfere with platelet function
- A threshold of $50 \times 10^9/l$ in the presence

> **Table 2.7 Practice Guidelines for Blood Component Therapy, sponsored by the American Society of Anaesthesiologists in 1996[9]**
>
> **Prophylactic platelet transfusion is ineffective and rarely indicated:**
> - When thrombocytopenia is due to increased platelet destruction (autoimmune thrombocytopenia)
> - In surgical patients with thrombocytopenia due to decreased platelet production when the platelet count is >100 × 10^9/l
>
> **Prophylactic platelet transfusion is usually indicated:**
> - In surgical patients with thrombocytopenia due to decreased platelet production when the platelet count <50 × 10^9/l
> - Transfusion decision at intermediate counts (50–100 × 10^9/l) should be based on the risk of bleeding
>
> **Therapeutic transfusion:**
> - Surgical and obstetric patients with microvascular bleeding usually require platelet transfusion if the platelet count is <50 × 10^9/l, and rarely require therapy if it is >100 × 10^9/l.
> - 'Platelet transfusion may be indicated despite an apparently adequate platelet count if there is known platelet dysfunction and microvascular bleeding'
>
> **Dose**
> - No recommendation, but a statement that 'one platelet concentrate (i.e. that derived from a single unit of blood) will increase the platelet count by approximately 5–10 × 10^9/l in the average adult' and that the 'usual therapeutic dose is one concentrate per 10 kg'.

of bleeding or prior to lumbar puncture or central venous line insertion
- In infants with intracranial or other life-threatening bleeding to maintain the platelet count above 100 × 10^9/l

Risks of platelet concentrates (other than disease transmission)

- Bacterial contamination
- Febrile non-haemolytic transfusion reactions

- Alloimmunization against HLA and HPA antigens
- Post-transfusion purpura
- Transfusion-related acute lung injury (when platelets are suspended in plasma)

IRRADIATED CELLULAR BLOOD COMPONENTS

Gamma-irradiated cellular blood components are used to prevent the occurrence of transfusion-associated graft-versus-host disease (TA-

GvHD). TA-GvHD is a potential complication of transfusing any blood component containing viable T lymphocytes where there is a degree of disparity in histocompatibility antigens between donor and patient. Interaction between donor T lymphocytes and recipient cells carrying either class I or class II HLA antigens results in cellular damage, in part by direct lymphocytotoxicity and also through the production of cytokines. The major target tissues include the skin, thymus, gastrointestinal tract, liver, spleen, and bone marrow, and within 1–2 weeks following transfusion, this damage results in fever, rash, diarrhoea, hepatitis and profound pancytopenia. TA-GvHD has a mortality rate of over 90%, largely because of overwhelming infection.

Gamma-irradiation at a dose of 25 Gy to all parts of the pack is required to prevent donor lymphocyte proliferation. No part of the pack should be exposed to more than 50 Gy, since this dosage is associated with cellular damage. Dosimetry studies are required to define the best dose field, and the process is ideally carried out in a dedicated blood irradiator.

Shelf life of irradiated blood components

Irradiated red cells have reduced but acceptable in vivo survival rates, depending on their age at the time of irradiation and the duration of post-irradiation storage. The current UK guidelines recommend that red cells should be irradiated at any time up to 14 days after collection, and thereafter can be stored for up to a further 14 days. The American guidelines stipulate that red cells can be stored for only 28 days after irradiation.

Gamma irradiation also causes an acceler-ated loss of intracellular potassium from red cells, with the result that supernatant potassium levels are approximately twice as high as in non-irradiated cells throughout the period of storage. The significance of this depends upon the volume and speed of transfusion, as well as the age of the blood. Infusion of a large potassium load, particularly if given rapidly and/or into a central vein, may cause serious cardiac dysrhythmias. However, it is not recommended that the supernatant potassium be removed by washing, since any manipulation increases the risk of error and the potential for bacterial contamination. However, where the patient is at particular risk from hyperkalaemia (e.g. in intrauterine or exchange transfusion), it is recommended that the red cells be transfused within 24 hours of irradiation.

Gamma irradiation has no untoward effect on the quality of platelet concentrates which can be irradiated at any stage after preparation and retain a normal shelf life of up to 5 days.

Indications for gamma-irradiated blood components[17,18]

There are three categories of blood components:
1. Those that are intrinsically high-risk and should always be irradiated, irrespective of the recipient:
   - Granulocytes are contaminated with large numbers of lymphocytes, and are always transfused within hours of collection. They are also given to recipients with some degree of immuno- suppression.
   - All transfusions of cellular components between family members and

all HLA-selected platelets should be irradiated, because of the importance of HLA haplotype sharing as a risk factor for TA-GvHD.

2. Those with such a low risk that irradiation is never required:
   • Fresh-frozen plasma, cryoprecipitate, and fractionated plasma products.
3. Those cellular components that should be irradiated for susceptible patients, as shown in Table 2.8.

Paediatric transfusion

TA-GvHD following intrauterine transfusion (IUT) from an unrelated donor is very rare. However, TA-GvHD is more likely to be seen in this situation, since the fetus is probably less able to reject allogeneic lymphocytes, which in turn are going to be viable, since blood less than 5 days old is used. Infants who have had an IUT may be more prone to TA-GvHD from any subsequent transfusions, and should continue to receive irradiated components. Cases of TA-GvHD have also been described following exchange transfusion (ET), and, where practical, cases should also receive irradiated blood.

The postirradiation shelf life for IUT and ET blood in the UK is 24 hours, and the blood should be used within 5 days of collection.

There is no need to irradiate units for small-volume transfusions, and, indeed, this practice, by shortening the shelf-life to 14 days, severely limits the potential to reduce donor exposure to these infants by allocating 'paedipacks' from a single donation.

Haematopoietic stem cell allografting and autografting

There is no consensus as to how long irradi-

Table 2.8 Patients who should receive gamma-irradiated cellular blood components		
Universally recommended	Additional recommendation in the UK	Additional recommendations in some countries
Congenital immunodeficiencies affecting T cells	Patients receiving fludarabine and related drugs	HIV positivity and AIDS
Intrauterine and exchange transfusions in neonates		Aplastic anaemia
Allogeneic bone marrow (or PBSC) transplantation		Acute leukaemia
Autologous bone marrow (or PBSC) transplantation		Chronic leukaemias
Hodgkin's disease		Non-Hodgkin's lymphoma All neonatal transfusions

ated components should be given in these situations, and there is considerable variation in practice. In the UK, it is recommended that irradiated blood be provided while the patient requires prophylaxis against transplant-induced GvHD (usually 6 months) or until the lymphocyte count is above 1×10^9/l. Irradiation of blood components may need to be continued for longer if the transplant was performed for a congenital immunodeficiency or if there is chronic GvHD from the allograft.

For autograft recipients, irradiated blood components should be commenced 1 week prior to stem cell harvesting. This is to prevent the harvesting of allogeneic T lymphocytes, which might cause TA-GvHD after infusion. Irradiated blood should be used until there is unequivocal evidence of haematopoietic engraftment and lymphoid reconstitution.

Human immunodeficiency virus infection and acquired immunodeficiency syndrome

Although irradiated components are provided by some blood banks in the USA, individuals with HIV or AIDS appear not to be at increased risk of TA-GvHD. This may be due to virus uptake by donor lymphocytes following transfusion, limiting their capacity to proliferate.

LEUKOCYTE-DEPLETED BLOOD COMPONENTS

Blood components are depleted of leukocytes by means of filtration, which can be effective through several mechanisms, including the following:

- direct adhesion of granulocytes and monocytes to filter fibres
- physical trapping of more rigid lymphoid cells in the fibre mesh
- platelet activation and secondary adhesion of granulocytes and monocytes

The specifications for leukocyte-depleted components vary between countries, but the Council of Europe's standards state that the residual white cell count should be below 1×10^6/l and that this level should be achieved in 90% of the components tested. In contrast, the AABB standards define a leukocyte-depleted component as one with less than 5×10^6 residual white cells/l, and the US Food and Drug Administration (FDA) guidelines state that 100% tested units should meet the standard. The UK's position is that taken by the AABB. Leukocyte removal should be performed while the cells are still intact and blood is filtered as soon as possible after collection, and certainly within 48 hours.

Several countries, including Canada, France, Ireland, Portugal, and the UK, have implemented universal leukocyte depletion of blood components, and it is likely that others will follow. The impetus in the UK and Ireland was the theoretical risk that variant Creutzfeldt–Jakob disease (vCJD) might be transmissible by blood, and in particular by the leukocytes.[19] However, the benefit of leukocyte depletion in reducing the infectivity of blood from individuals with vCJD is unknown, since the distribution of PrP^{sc} (the insoluble form of cellular prion protein) remains uncertain. PrP^c (the normal cellular prion protein) is also known to be expressed in higher quantities on platelets than on white cells or red cells.[20]

The theoretical advantages of leukocyte-depleted blood components[21,22]

Reduction of transmission of leukocyte-associated viruses

These include cytomegalovirus (CMV) and other DNA herpesviruses such as Epstein–Barr virus (EBV), human herpesvirus-8/Kaposi sarcoma-associated herpesvirus (HHV-8/KSHV), and T-cell viruses, such as human T-cell leukaemia virus (HTLV) I and II. A small number of studies of prestorage leukocyte depletion have demonstrated its efficacy in preventing transfusion-transmitted CMV. It is known that CMV-seronegative components are associated with a 4% risk of transmitting infection. Quality control data show that prestorage leukocyte depletion has a failure rate far less than 1%, suggesting that this technology may prove to be superior to serological testing for CMV antibodies for the prevention of CMV transmission. The AABB, the Council of Europe, and the British Standards Committee in Haematology in the UK all consider that components that are leukocyte-depleted at source are equivalent in safety to those tested as CMV-seronegative. However, this view has not yet been endorsed by the FDA or the UK Guidelines for Transfusion Services, and, until more data become available, CMV testing of leukocyte-depleted components continues to be performed by most transfusion services.

Reduction in incidence of HLA alloimmunization

Leukocyte depletion does reduce the incidence of HLA alloimmunization in multitransfused recipients, but residual immunization rates of 10–25% patients are accounted for by women who have already been exposed to HLA alloantigens in pregnancy. However, leukocyte depletion has less impact on refractoriness to random platelet donations in view of the importance of non-immune factors as independent clinical predictors of poor responses to transfused platelets (see below).

Reduction in incidence of non-haemolytic febrile transfusion reactions

Leukocyte reduction is an effective means of preventing these reactions following the transfusion of red cells or platelets. In the former, they are due to a reaction between contaminating leukocytes in the red cells and recipient antibodies, while in the latter they are due to the accumulation of cytokines during storage of the platelet concentrates, which can also be prevented by prestorage leukocyte depletion.

Reduced immunomodulation following transfusion

The beneficial effect of prior transfusion on renal allograft survival has been known for over 20 years, and is still clinically important despite the introduction of potent immunosuppressive drugs. However, the exact mechanism of this benefit remains unknown. There have been many clinical studies examining the possible effect of transfusion on recurrence of cancers, particularly colorectal cancer. Although the majority of retrospective studies have demonstrated an adverse effect of transfusion, there is no evidence of any benefit in using either autologous or leukocyte-depleted blood.[23,24] Several (but not all) studies have suggested a beneficial impact of leukocyte depletion on the rate of postoperative infections.

TA-GvHD

The impact of leukocyte depletion upon the incidence of TA-GvHD is unknown, and this manipulation cannot be relied upon to prevent the condition.

CMV-SERONEGATIVE BLOOD COMPONENTS

CMV-seronegative blood components remain the accepted means of preventing transfusion-transmitted CMV. However, there are several studies that confirm that some healthy individuals who test seronegative for CMV still harbour the virus.[25,26]

The indications for CMV-seronegative components, as outlined in the *UK Handbook of Transfusion Medicine*,[13] include the following:

- transfusion in pregnancy
- intrauterine transfusions
- transfusions to neonates and to infants in the first year of life
- transfusions to the following groups of CMV-seronegative recipients:
  - after allogeneic bone marrow/peripheral blood progenitor transplants where the donor is also CMV-seronegative
  - after autologous bone marrow/peripheral blood progenitor cell transplants
  - potential recipients of allogeneic bone marrow/peripheral blood progenitor cell transplants
  - patients with HIV infection

HLA- (AND HPA-) SELECTED PLATELET CONCENTRATES

HLA-selected platelets are indicated for patients who have HLA alloimmunization and are refractory to the transfusion of random platelet concentrates, i.e. with repeated failure to gain a satisfactory increment after a platelet transfusion.

Definitions of refractoriness are usually based upon the values of corrected count increment (CCI):

- CCI $\leqslant$ 7.5 at less than 1 hour
- CCI $\leqslant$ 4.5 at 20–24 hours

where

$$CCI = \frac{\text{platelet increment } (10^9/l) \times \text{body surface area } (m^2)}{10^{11} \text{ transfused platelets}}$$

Up to 60% patients who have received multiple platelet transfusions will become refractory to the transfusion of a random platelet concentrate. Refractoriness to platelet transfusions can be caused by immune or non-immune factors; the commonest cause of immunological refractoriness is the presence of antibodies directed against HLA class I alloantigens. Additional accepted causes of platelet refractoriness are given in Table 2.9.

In one study of patients refractory to random platelet transfusions, non-immune factors were present alone in 67%, immune factors alone in 25%, and a combination of factors in 21%.[27] Failure to achieve a satisfactory CCI at 1 hour is more in favour of the existence of immune factors, whereas a poor CCI at 24 hours can be the result of non-immune or immune factors.

Prevention of HLA alloimmunization

Prestorage leukocyte depletion below 5×10^6 per transfusion is very effective in the preven-

Table 2.9 Causes of refractoriness to random platelet concentrates	
Immune	Non-immune
HLA class I antibodies	Quality platelet concentrate
HPA antibodies	Disseminated intravascular coagulation
ABO antibodies	Splenomegaly
Platelet autoantibodies	GvHD
Drug-related antibodies: to penicillin, vancomycin, quinine	Drugs: amphotericin
	Veno-occlusive liver disease
	Fever/infections

tion of primary HLA alloimmunization, and results in less than 5% HLA antibody fomation.[28] However, presensitization of mothers to HLA antigens in pregnancy increases the risk of alloimmunization after platelet transfusion, and HLA antibodies develop in up to 44% of women with previous pregnancies who receive leukocyte depleted components during treatment for haematological malignancies.[29] Not all patients who develop HLA alloantibodies become refractory, and results from the TRAP (Trial to Reduce Alloimmunization to Platelet) study indicate that HLA antibodies can be expected to occur in up to 20% of patients receiving leukocyte-depleted blood components, but will contribute to refractoriness in only 5% of patients.[30]

Ultraviolet (UV)-B irradiation can also prevent HLA alloimmunization, since it inactivates donor antigen-presenting cells (APC) at dosages not severely affecting platelet function. In the TRAP study, refractoriness was found in 16% of the patients in the control group receiving standard platelet transfusions, in 10% of the patients in the UV-B-treated group, and in 8% of the patients receiving leukocyte-depleted platelets. Hence UV-B irra-

diation and leukocyte depletion by filtration appear to be equally effective in the prevention of HLA alloimmunization.

Immune factors and refractoriness

Although HLA alloantibodies are the commonest and most important cause of immunological refractoriness, up to 25% patients with HLA antibodies will also possess HPA antibodies. However, their contribution to platelet refractoriness is unclear. Anti-A and/or anti-B antibodies can diminish the survival of antigen-positive platelets, but rarely give rise to refractoriness.

Increased destruction of platelets is often observed following autologous or allogeneic bone marrow transplantation as a result of temporary immune imbalance during the period of reconstitution of the transplanted haematopoietic cells, which can enhance the development of autoantibodies.

Non-immune factors

Several studies have shown a storage-time-related decrease in CCI, particularly in patients with other non-immune factors known to impair platelet survival. The impact of fever or infection on the consumption of platelets is debated, but some studies have shown that post-transfusion increments can be decreased by 20–40%. Circulating immune-complex (CIC) levels are often elevated in patients with infections, and the presence of CICs is inversely correlated with post-transfusion increments. Infection may also be accompanied by disseminated intravascular coagulation (DIC), which leads to increased consumption of platelets.

Acute and chronic GvHD and CMV infection are associated with increased levels of platelet-associated IgG (PAIgG) and consequently increased removal of platelets from the circulation. Irradiation, chemotherapeutic drugs, growth factors, and immune-modulating drugs used to treat GvHD contribute to the vasculopathy that also gives rise to increased platelet consumption.

The spleen normally pools approximately one-third of platelets produced in the marrow as well as those transfused, and platelet recovery may be reduced to 15–20% in patients with splenomegaly.

Drug-induced thrombocytopenia can result from a variety of mechanisms, and it is important to correlate the clinical history of drug administration with the onset of thrombocytopenia or platelet transfusion refractoriness.

Approaches to platelet refractoriness

In the presence of factors associated with increased platelet consumption and a poor 24-hour increment, frequent transfusions of platelets rather than increased dosages are recommended.

If HLA alloantibodies are present, compatible platelet donors have to be selected. Selection of HLA-compatible donors is based either on HLA type selection or on the results of platelet crossmatch techniques. Both require registered apheresis donors, and although the predictability of transfusion efficacy by crossmatching ranges between 60% and 90%, this strategy is limited in that matches can rarely be found from limited available platelet inventories for patients with multispecific HLA antibodies. HLA class I typed donations are matched to the recipient, although in many instances a complete match is not possible and donations are given from donors who possess one or more HLA antigens that, although are not identical, are from the same cross-reactive or public epitopes.[31]

GRANULOCYTE CONCENTRATES

Granulocyte concentrates can be prepared either from apheresis or from pooled buffy coats. The minimum dose of granulocytes required for clinical efficacy has not been established, but encouraging results have been obtained from the use of 5×10^9 granulocytes/m^2 daily.[32] To obtain this dose of granulocytes from apheresis, the donor has to be stimulated with granulocyte colony-stimulating factor (G-CSF) with or without steroids, which gives rise to logistical and ethical issues. Alternatively, this dose can be obtained by pooling the buffy coats from 15–18 donations.[33] Since the component should be irradiated and transfused as soon as possible after collection, and certainly within 24 hours, there are additional problems in completing the mandatory microbiology testing within a short time-frame.

The use of granulocyte concentrates has

declined since the 1970s, with the availability of more effective antimicrobial therapy for neutropenic sepsis. Their use is essentially confined to treating severely neutropenic patients with proven sepsis who are not responding to appropriate and adequate antibiotic therapy. Once initiated, their use should be continued daily for up to 7 days or until there is clinical improvement.

In countries employing routine leukocyte depletion of blood components as a risk-reduction strategy for vCJD, granulocyte concentrates are only provided on a concessionary named-patient basis. With the advent of nucleic acid testing (NAT) for HCV-RNA, which cannot currently be completed in less than a working day, further concessions would become necessary to allow the release of granulocyte concentrates. In such circumstances, the prescribing physician would be entirely liable in the event that the component caused transfusion-transmitted infection.

FRESH-FROZEN PLASMA

Fresh-frozen plasma (FFP) is produced from a single blood donation or from plasma collected by apheresis. Plasma from whole blood should be separated not more than 18 hours after collection and the freezing process should be completed within 1 hour to a temperature below −30°C. Optimal storage is at −30°C or lower, and at this temperature, FFP can be kept for 12 months. At −18°C to −25°C, the storage time should be reduced to 3 months.

The content of coagulation factors varies, reflecting the individual variations between donors. However, the activity of coagulation factors and inhibitors in thawed FFP should be at least 70% of the original individual activity in donor plasma. When stored correctly, FFP contains, in addition to the coagulation and fibrinolytic enzymes, their inhibitors such as antithrombin III, protein S, protein C, α_2-macroglobulin and α_2-antiplasmin. Once thawed, the FFP should be transfused as soon as possible and should not be refrozen.

Indications for FFP

The generally accepted indications, which are covered in both the Practice Guidelines for Blood Component Therapy[9] and the British Committee for Standards in Haematology guidelines[34] are as follows:

- Replacement of single coagulation factor deficiencies, where a specific or combined factor concentrate is unavailable
- Immediate reversal of warfarin effect, when prothrombin complex concentrate and factor VII concentrates are unavailable
- Thrombotic thrombocytopenic purpura (TTP)
- Correction of microvascular bleeding in the presence of elevated (>1.5 times normal) prothrombin time (PT) or partial thromboplastin time (PTT)

The practice guidelines from the American Society of Anesthesiologists also accept that it is reasonable to give FFP to correct microvascular bleeding secondary to coagulation factor deficiencies in patients with more than one blood volume transfused pending the availability of coagulation test results. Although the British guidelines would regard DIC as a definite indication, there is no indication for blood components to normalize laboratory results in chronic DIC or in the absence of haemorrhage in acute DIC.

The initial therapeutic dose of FFP is 10–15 ml/kg. Further infusions should be guided by the results of laboratory monitoring. In the case of TTP, the patient should be exchanged with 3–4 litres of FFP daily.

ABO-compatible FFP should be used, and since there is a small amount of red cell stroma in the preparation, RhD-compatible FFP should, whenever possible, be given to females of childbearing age.

Risks of FFP

- Plasma components do not transmit CMV or HTLV, but other infection risks are in keeping with other blood components
- FFP is also most likely to be responsible for the occurrence of transfusion-related acute lung injury (TRALI)
- Risk of volume overload due to protein content
- Urticaria in 1–3% recipients
- Occasional anaphylactic transfusion reactions with a rapid infusion rate

Virus-inactivated FFP preparations

Viruses in plasma can be inactivated by using either methylene blue (MB) or solvent–detergent (SD) treatment. MB treatment can be applied to single unpooled units of plasma, and requires the prior removal of white cells by filtration or freeze–thawing. The MB may be removed prior to transfusion to the patient, but, at the concentrations used, no toxicity has been demonstrated or is predicted. SD treatment is applied to pools of between 600 and 1500 ABO-identical donations, and carries the additional theoretical risk of transmitting unknown agents to a larger population. Both treatments can still allow the transmission of hepatitis A virus (HAV) and parvovirus B19, and there have been batch withdrawals in the USA because of possible parvovirus B19 transmission. However, there are potential advantages of SD-FFP in that the pooling dilutes antibodies responsible for immune-mediated reactions and probably reduces the risks of mild allergic reactions as well as reducing the incidence of TRALI. SD-FFP may also be advantageous in the treatment of TTP, because of the loss of high-molecular-weight von Willebrand factor (vWF) multimers, which contribute to the excessive platelet activation and consumption.[35]

Both methods are associated with 15–20% loss of labile clotting factors, but are still effective in substituting for standard FFP,[36] although there has been a report of an increased demand for FFP following the introduction of MB-FFP.[37]

CRYOSUPERNATANT PLASMA

This is the supernatant plasma removed during the preparation of cryoprecipitate, which as a consequence contains reduced levels of fibrinogen and factors V and VIII. The only indication for its use is in the treatment of TTP, since it lacks the largest vWF multimers that are present in FFP and cryoprecipitate. However, the evidence for its superiority over standard FFP is controversial, since although one study found an improvement in survival using cryosupernant when compared with historical controls treated with standard FFP,[38] this advantage has not been confirmed in a prospective randomized trial performed by the North American TTP Group.[39]

CRYOPRECIPITATE

Cryoprecipitate contains a major portion of the factor VIII, vWF, fibrinogen, factor XIII, and fibronectin present in freshly drawn and separated plasma. Each unit contains at least 70 IU factor VIIIC and between 200 and 250 mg fibrinogen. It is prepared by allowing frozen plasma to thaw at +2°C to +6°C, recentrifuging at the same temperature, and suspending the cryoglobulin fraction in 10–20 ml plasma. Its storage and stability are as for FFP.

Cryoprecipitate is now primarily used in the treatment of patients with hypofibrinogenaemia which can occur in patients with DIC and advanced liver disease and for reversal of fibrinolytic agents. Plasma levels of fibrinogen greater than 1.0 g/l are generally considered as adequate for haemostasis, and empirically one bag of cryoprecipate is given for every 5 kg body weight. The fibrinogen content is also made use of as a component of fibrin sealant or glue.

PLASMA PRODUCTS

Traditionally, plasma has been fractionated to provide albumin, factor VIII and IX concentrates, and immunoglobulins. However, the range of products has been extended in recent years to include, for example, antithrombin III, prothrombin complex concentrate, and activated protein C. Isolation of individual proteins is primarily based upon the solubility differences using the principles developed by Edwin Cohn in 1925 and chromatography.

ALBUMIN

A unit of albumin usually contains 20 g, either as 400 ml of a 5% solution or 100 ml of a 20% solution. Other constituents include sodium at a concentration of 130–150 mmol/l, other plasma proteins, and stabilizers. The physiological property of albumin to generate and preserve colloid osmotic pressure is the reason for most of its clinical applications. However, the therapeutic indications for albumin solutions are limited – particularly by their cost and the availability of cheaper alternatives.

Furthermore, the Cochrane Injuries Group 1998 systematic review of human albumin concluded that there was no evidence that albumin reduces mortality in patients with hypovolaemia, burns, and hypoalbuminaemia, and also concluded that albumin might increase mortality.[40]

Acute plasma volume replacement

Several trials have compared the use of crystalloids, synthetic colloids, and albumin for vascular loading in peri-operative care. Little difference has been found in clinical outcome, provided that adequate volumes of crystalloids are given and blood volume is maintained. Although there are few guidelines for this situation, most units would recommend a first-line treatment with crystalloids or artificial colloids. Albumin may be administered when the upper limits for synthetic colloids (1.5 g/kg body weight) are reached or when there is concern that coagulation may be impaired by their continued use.

Therapeutic plasma exchange

When repeated and often daily plasma exchanges are used, the plasma oncotic pressure of the patient would soon become critically low if albumin were not the main constituent of the replacement fluid. In these circumstances, a combination of albumin and crystalloids is indicated.

Thermal injuries

There have been no recent randomized trials evaluating the benefit of albumin in adult patients. However, albumin is contraindicated in the first phase of treatment of thermal injuries, when there is increased microvascular permeability both in injured and in healthy tissue. Its use is usually reserved for severely burned patients whose albumin falls to approximately 20 g/l.

Diuretic-resistant oedema in hypoproteinaemic patients

A 20% albumin solution is used in this situation. In the nephrotic syndrome, albumin may be used on a short-term basis for patients with acute, severe peripheral, or lung oedema. In patients with cirrhosis and liver failure, most would recommend that albumin should be reserved for the treatment of impending hepatorenal syndrome.[41]

COAGULATION FACTOR CONCENTRATES (FACTORS VIII AND IX)

These are used in the treatment of patients with congenital factor concentrate deficiencies – haemophilia and von Willebrand disease – and a discussion is beyond the scope of this chapter.

ANTITHROMBIN III

Hereditary deficiencies of this plasma constituent lead to recurrent venous thromboem-

bolism. Antithrombin III is stable in stored blood, but concentrates are needed if clinically significant deficiencies are to be treated effectively. Heat-treated antithrombin III concentrates are available, and are indicated for the prevention and treatment of patients with hereditary antithrombin III deficiency.

Acquired deficiencies of antithrombin III can also occur in DIC coagulation, and concentrates may be used in patients who do not respond to simple replacement therapy with FFP and cryoprecipitate.

PROTHROMBIN COMPLEX CONCENTRATES

Prothrombin complex concentrates (PCC) usually contain variable amounts of factors II, IX, and X, and are administered with specific factor VII concentrates. However, some (e.g. Prothromplex T; Immuno, Vienna) contains factors II, VII, IX, and X.

These concentrates are the treatment of choice for managing excessive oral anticoagulation, when the patient is suffering a potentially life-threatening haemorrhage. Although FFP will provide the necessary clotting factors, large volumes have to be given and factor IX levels are only minimally increased by FFP. The dose of concentrate used is calculated at approximately 50 IU factor IX/kg body weight.

PCCs may also be considered in the management or prevention of bleeding episodes in patients with liver disease undergoing invasive procedures. However, since they carry the risk of inducing thromboembolism (because they often contain activated coagulation components), they should be used with caution in this situation. Patients with liver disease are particularly at risk, since they have impaired clearance of activated clotting factors and reduced levels of antithrombin III.

PROTEIN C CONCENTRATES

Protein C concentrates are available for patients with an inherited deficiency of this inhibitor who are at risk of venous thromboembolism and who may be receiving heparin therapy for spontaneous thrombosis or who are undergoing surgery.

Activated protein C

Recombinant human activated protein C has emerged as a new drug for treating severe sepsis in intensive care patients. Activated protein C is a potent antithrombotic serine protease with substantial anti-inflammatory properties. Pro-inflammatory cytokines released in response to infection can also activate coagulation and inhibit fibrinolysis. A combination of procoagulant and inflammatory stimuli provides a potent mechanism for initiating and perpetuating microvascular injury, intravascular coagulation, inadequate tissue perfusion, and organ failure. Activated protein C inhibits activated factors V and VIII, stimulates fibrinolysis, reduces production of tumour necrosis factor α by monocytes, and reduces interactions between neutrophils and endothelial cells.

In a randomized, double-blind, placebo-controlled, multicentre phase three trial, activated protein C reduced the circulating levels of d-dimer and interleukin-6, confirming its antithrombotic and anti-inflammatory properties. Activated protein C was also associated with a reduction in the relative risk of death of 19.4% and an absolute reduction in the risk of death of 6.1% ($p = 0.005$).[42]

IMMUNOGLOBULINS

Preparations consist of intact IgG molecules (>95%), with a distribution of IgG subclasses corresponding to that in normal human serum. Most preparations contain traces of IgA and soluble CD4, CD8, soluble HLA molecules, and cytokines. Since the product is prepared from pooled plasma, it contains a broad array of immune antibodies against foreign antigens. The final phases of the fractionation process for intravenous immunoglobulin differ in that they are designed to control the anticomplement activity of the purified IgG and to stabilize it with added sucrose.

Intramuscular immunoglobulin

Intramuscular immunoglobulin can passively transfer antibody, and there are two types of preparation – normal human immunoglobulin and specific immunoglobulins. Normal immunoglobulin is used for the protection of susceptible contacts against hepatitis A and measles. Specific immunoglobulins are used when a specific antibody is required to provide short-term protection against infection or as immunotherapy, as in the prevention of RhD alloimmunization.

The available specific preparations are as follows:

- Hepatitis B immunoglobulin, given alongside vaccination in individuals accidentally inoculated with the virus and to infants born to mothers who have been infected during pregnancy or who are high-risk carriers
- Rabies immunoglobulin, given alongside vaccination to individuals who are unim-

munized and have been exposed to an animal from a high-risk country
- Tetanus immunoglobulin, if an individual is non-immune and wound soiling is severe
- Varicella zoster immunoglobulin, for primary infection in immunosuppressed individuals, including those treated with steroids
- Anti-D immunoglobulin for the treatment of RhD haemolytic disease of the newborn

Intravenous immunoglobulin

Intravenous immunoglobulin (IVIG) provides optimal replacement therapy for patients with antibody deficiencies (both primary and secondary), and in high doses is immunomodulatory and is used in the treatment of a variety of autoimmune conditions.

Primary and secondary antibody deficiencies (hypogammaglobuminaemia)

Patients with these disorders present with recurrent bacterial infections, usually of the respiratory tract, which are only partially responsive to treatment with antibiotics. In primary immunodeficiencies in particular, infection can also be a problem at other sites, and can be overwhelming as with bacterial meningitis. Replacement therapy with IVIG ameliorates these problems, with most impact on pulmonary function.

In primary immunodeficiency states, IVIG in doses of 600 mg/kg every 4 weeks is effective. However, in practice, the dose has to be tailored to the patient, and most require infusions of 200–300 mg/kg every 2–3 weeks.

Chronic lymphocytic leukaemia (CLL) is the commonest cause of secondary antibody deficiency, and many of these patients suffer from recurrent bacterial infections. IVIG replacement in doses of 200–400 mg/kg every 3 weeks has been shown to reduce both the incidence and recurrence of serious bacterial infections. Similar findings are available for patients with multiple myeloma, and it is known that the risk of septicaemia or pneumonia can be prevented by regular immunoglobulin infusions. The decision to treat such patients should take into account their immunoglobulin levels and the misery and morbidity caused by recurrent infections that might well be ameliorated or prevented by regular immunoglobulin infusions.

IVIG is also used in bone marrow transplantation to prevent complications stemming from the period of immunodeficiency produced by the procedure, and has been shown to reduce the risk both of Gram-negative septicaemia and of bacterial and fungal infections in allogeneic transplantation. Some HIV-positive children who suffer from recurrent bacterial infections also benefit from IVIG. Although premature infants are often hypogammaglobulinaemic and studies have shown lower infection rates with the use of IVIG, there is no evidence that this therapy reduces mortality, and its routine use cannot be recommended.

Intravenous immunoglobulin in autoimmune and inflammatory diseases[43]

There are several mechanisms by which IVIG exerts an immunomodulatory effect, and the importance of each mechanism will vary according to the clinical condition. Established modes of action are provided in Table 2.10.

Higher doses of IVIG are required for an immunomodulatory effect, and the commonly

Table 2.10 Immunoregulatory effects of immunoglobulin	
Category of effect	Examples of effect
Fc receptor	• Blockade of Fc receptors on macrophages and effector cells • Induction of inhibitory Fcγ receptor IIB
Inflammation	• Attenuation of complement-mediated damage • Induction of anti-inflammatory cytokines
B cells and antibodies	• Control of emergent bone marrow B-cell repertoires • Neutralization of circulating autoantibodies by antiidiotypes
T cells	• Regulation of the production of helper T-cell cytokines • Neutralization of T-cell superantigens
Cell growth	• Inhibition of lymphocyte proliferation

used dose schedule is 0.4 g/kg for 5 successive days.

IVIG is now accepted therapy for a number of autoimmune diseases, including the following:

- autoimmune thrombocytopenia; particularly in childhood and pre-splenectomy
- post-transfusion purpura
- Kawasaki vasculitis
- Guillain–Barré syndrome
- dermatomyositis
- myasthenia gravis
- multiple sclerosis

Side-effects

Mild reactions occur during or after the infusion in up to 5% of patients; symptoms include headache, chills, nausea, fatigue, myalgia, arthralgia, and hypertension. These reactions can be minimized by slowing the infusion rate. Where an anaphylactoid reaction occurs in association with IVIG administration, the infusion should be stopped and, after appropriate resuscitation, investigations undertaken to check for IgA deficiency and anti-IgA antibodies.

Immune complex formation and complement activation can occur and give rise to severe malaise, rigors, and chills. This can be the result of complement-activating IgG aggregates in the preparation or the presence of a high bacterial load in the recipient.

Renal dysfunction

High-dose treatments may cause oliguric renal failure, particularly in the elderly or in patients with pre-existing renal impairment, as a result of tubular damage induced by the high solute load of sugars used to stabilize the IgG.

Aseptic meningitis

Patients receiving high-dose treatments may also develop meningitic symptoms, typically 48–72 hours post infusion. Symptoms can be prevented with non-steroidal anti-inflammatory drugs or can be relieved by employing a very slow infusion rate.

C1 ESTERASE INHIBITOR

A partially purified concentrate of C1 esterase inhibitor is available, and should, whenever possible, be used to treat severe attacks of angioedema in patients with either the hereditary or the acquired deficiency. The concentrate has the advantage over FFP of not providing more complement to fuel further inflammation and tissue oedema if adequate inhibitor levels are not reached.

α_1-ANTITRYPSIN

This substance plays an important role in inhibiting neutrophil elastase, an enzyme involved in the proteolysis of connective tissue, especially in the lung. Hereditary deficiency of α_1-antitrypsin leads to progressive emphysema, and there is some evidence that replacement therapy using a concentrate may halt the progression of the disease. However, since the concentrate has only a 4–5-day half-life and adequate supplies would be dependent upon a recombinant source, its usefulness has still to be defined.

REFERENCES

1. Council of Europe. *Guide to the Preparation, Use and Quality Assurance of Blood Components*, 5th edn. Strasbourg: Council of Europe Publishing, 1999.
2. United Kingdom Blood Transfusion Services/National Institute for Biological Standards and Control, *Guidelines for the Blood Transfusion Services in the United Kingdom*, 4th edn. Norwich: The Stationery Office, 2000.
3. American Association of Blood Banks. *Standards for Blood Banks and Transfusion Services*, 20th edn. Bethesda, MD: AABB, 2000.
4. Liu E, Mannino E, Lane TA. A prospective randomised trial of the safety and efficacy of a limited donor exposure transfusion program for premature infants. *J Pediatr* 1994; **125**: 92–6.
5. Sazama K. Reports of 355 transfusion-associated deaths: 1976 through 1985. Transfusion 1990; **30**: 583–90.
6. Williamson LM, Lowe S, Love E et al. *Serious Hazards of Transfusion Annual Report 2000–2001*. Manchester: SHOT Office, 2002.
7. Wenz B, Burns ER. Improvement in transfusion safety using a new blood unit and patient identification system as part of safe transfusion practice. *Transfusion* 1991; **31**: 401–3.
8. Jensen NJ, Crosson JT. An automated system for bedside verification of the match between patient identification and blood unit identification. *Transfusion* 1996; **36**: 216–21.
9. Practice Guidelines for Blood Component Therapy. A Report by the American Society of Anesthesiologists Task Force on Blood Component Therapy. *Anesthesiology* 1996; **84**: 732–47.
10. Mercurali F, Inghilleri G. Proposal of an algorithm to help the choice of best transfusion strategy. *Curr Med Res Opin* 1996; **13**: 465–78.
11. Murphy MF, Wallington TB, Kelsey P et al. Guidelines for the use of red cells. British Committee for Standards in Haematology, Blood Transfusion Task Force. *Br J Haematol* 2001; **113**: 24–31.
12. Hume H, Bard H. Small volume red blood cell transfusions for neonatal patients. *Transfusion Med Rev* 1995; **9**: 187–99.
13. McClelland DBL (ed). *Blood Transfusion Services of the United Kingdom. Handbook of Transfusion Medicine*, 3rd edn. London: The Stationery Office, 2001.
14. Murphy S. The efficacy of synthetic media in the storage of human platelets for transfusion. *Transfusion Med Rev* 1999; **13**: 153–63.
15. Rebulla P, Finazzi G, Marangoni F et al. Threshold for prophylactic platelet transfusions in adults with acute myeloid leukaemia. *N Engl J Med* 1997; **337**: 1870–5.

16. Norfolk DR, Ancliffe PJ, Contreras M et al. Consensus Conference on Platelet Transfusion, Royal College of Physicians of Edinburgh, 27–28 November 1997. Synopsis of background papers. *Br J Haematol* 1998; **101:** 609–17.

17. Vogelsang GB, Hess AD. Graft-versus-host disease: new directions for a persistent problem. *Blood* 1994; **84:** 2061–7.

18. British Committee for Standards in Haematology. Guidelines for gamma irradiation of blood components for the prevention of transfusion-associated graft-versus-host disease. *Transfusion Med* 1996; **6:** 261–71.

19. Turner ML, Ironside JW. New-variant Creutzfeldt–Jakob disease: the risk of transmission by blood transfusion. *Blood Rev* 1998; **12:** 255–68.

20. Barclay GR, Hope J, Birkett CR et al. Distribution of cell-associated prion in normal adult blood determined by flow cytometry. *Br J Haematol* 1999; **107:** 804–14.

21. Williamson LM. Leucocyte depletion of the blood supply – How will patients benefit? *Br J Haematol* 2000; **110:** 256–72.

22. Dzik S, Aubuchon J, Jeffries L et al. Leucocyte reduction of blood components: Public policy and New Technology. *Transfusion Med Rev* 2000; **14:** 34–52.

23. Blajchman MA. Allogeneic blood transfusions, immunomodulation and postoperative bacterial infection: Do we have the answers yet? *Transfusion* 1997; **37:** 121–5.

24. Vamvakas EC. Transfusion-associated cancer recurrence and postoperative infection: Meta-analysis of randomised controlled clinical trials. *Transfusion* 1996; **36:** 175–86.

25. Stanier P, Taylor DL, Kitchen AD et al. Persistence of cytomegalovirus in mononuclear cells in peripheral blood from blood donors. *BMJ* 1989; **299:** 897–8.

26. Larsson S, Soderberg-Naucler C, Wang FZ et al. Cytomegalovirus DNA can be detected in peripheral blood mononuclear cells from all seropositive and most seronegative healthy blood donors over time. *Transfusion* 1998; **38:** 271–8.

27. Doughty HA, Murphy MF, Metcalfe et al. Relative importance of immune and non-immune causes of platelet refractoriness. *Vox Sang* 1994; **66:** 200–5.

28. Novotny VMJ, van Doorn R, Witvliet MD et al. Occurrence of allogeneic HLA and non-HLA antibodies after transfusion of prestorage filtered platelets and red blood cells: a prospective study. *Blood* 1995; **85:** 1736–41.

29. Sintnicolaas K, van Marwijk Kooij M, van Prooijen HC et al. Leucocyte depletion of random single-donor platelet transfusions does not prevent secondary human leucocyte antigen alloimmunisation and refractoriness: a randomised prospective study. *Blood* 1995: **85:** 824–8.

30. Slichter SJ. The Trial to Reduce Alloimmunisation to Platelets Study Group. Leucocyte reduction and ultraviolet B irradiation of platelets to prevent alloimmunisation and refractoriness to platelet transfusions. *N Engl J Med* 1997; **337:** 1861–9.

31. Novotny VMJ. Prevention and management of platelet transfusion refractoriness. *Vox Sang* 1999; **76:** 1–13.

32. Graw RH Jr, Herzig G, Perry S, Henderson ES. Normal granulocyte transfusion therapy. Treatment of septicaemia due to Gram-negative bacteria. *N Engl J Med* 1972; **287:** 367.

33. Belardinelli A, Beletti D, Nucci S et al. Granulocyte transfusion: Is there a role for buffy coats in the current management of infected neutropenic adult patients? *Vox Sang* 1996; **70:** 45–6.

34. British Committee for Standards in Haematology. Guidelines for the use of fresh frozen plasma. *Transfusion Med* 1992; **2:** 57–63.

35. Harrison CN, Lawrie AS, Iqbal A et al. Plasma exchange with solvent detergent plasma of resistant thrombotic thrombocytopenic purpura. *Br J Haematol* 1996; **94:** 745–56.

36. Williamson LM, Llewelyn CA, Fisher NF et

al. A randomised trial of solvent detergent and standard fresh frozen plasma in the coagulopathy of liver disease and liver transplantation. *Transfusion* 1999; **39**: 1227–34.

37. Atance R, Pereira A, Ramirez B. Transfusing methylene blue-photoinactivated plasma instead of FFP is associated with an increased demand for plasma and cryoprecipitate. *Transfusion* 2001; **41**: 1548–52.

38. Rock G, Shumak KH, Sutton DMC et al. Cryosupernatant as replacement fluid for plasma exchange in thrombotic thrombocytopenic purpura. *Br J Haematol* 1996; **94**: 383–6.

39. Zeigler ZR, Shadduck RK, Gryn JF et al. Cryoprecipitate poor plasma does not improve early response in primary adult thrombotic thrombocytopenic purpura. *J Clin Apheresis* 2001; **16**: 19–22.

40. Cochrane Injuries Group Albumin Reviewers. Human albumin administration in critically ill patients: a systematic review of randomised controlled trials. *BMJ* 1998; **317**: 235–40.

41. Vermeulen LC, Ratko TA, Erstad BL et al. A paradigm for consensus. The University Hospital Consortium guidelines for the use of albumin, nonprotein colloid, and crystalloid solutions. *Arch Intern Med* 1995; **155**: 373–9.

42. Bernard GR, Vincent J-L, Laterre R-F et al. Efficacy and safety of recombinant human activated protein C for severe sepsis. *N Engl J Med* 2001; **344**: 699–709.

43. Mackay IR, Rosen FS. Immunomodulation of autoimmune and inflammatory disease with intravenous immune globulin. *N Engl J Med* 2001; **345**: 747–55.

3 Blood transfusion in patients requiring long-term support

Aleksandar Mijovic

INTRODUCTION

Transfusion of blood products is usually an interim measure until the loss of red cells or platelets is compensated by a normal bone marrow, or until an effective treatment restores normal haematopoiesis. However, a number of congenital or acquired conditions are characterized by chronic anaemia or thrombocytopenia generally unresponsive to treatment (Table 3.1). Patients suffering from those conditions require regular red cell and/or platelet support for extended periods of time, often for a lifetime. This translates into several months or years for patients with myelodysplastic syndromes, or several decades for patients with haemoglobinopathies, as the life expectancy in sickle cell disease has extended into the fifth decade of life[1] and the median survival in thalassaemia major reaches 23–31 years in developed countries.[2]

Implementation of regular long-term transfusion programmes poses numerous medical and psychological problems, and is associated with significant costs. This chapter addresses the aspects of long-term transfusion support in common clinical conditions in which blood transfusion is the cornerstone of treatment, The goals and modalities of transfusion, and the use of appropriate components, are discussed, as are adjuvant and alternative therapies, and the complications of long-term transfusion support. Finally, the problems faced by transfusion-dependent patients in the developing world are briefly discussed.

ACQUIRED DISEASES REQUIRING LONG-TERM TRANSFUSION SUPPORT

The principles of blood transfusion and the use of blood components are similar for this heterogeneous group of diseases. With the exception of myelodysplastic syndromes and bone marrow failure, all are either relatively

Table 3.1 Conditions characterized by long-term transfusion dependence

Acquired
- Myelodysplastic syndromes
- Bone marrow failures: aplastic anaemia, pure red cell aplasia, chemotherapy-induced aplasia
- Primary myelofibrosis
- Chronic haemolytic anaemias: cold haemagglutinin disease, paroxysmal nocturnal haemoglobinuria
- Anaemia of renal failure (unresponsive to erythropoietin)
- Anaemia of chronic inflammatory disease (rarely)

Congenital
- Thalassaemia major
- Sickle cell anaemia
- Congenital aplastic anaemia (Fanconi anaemia)
- Congenital dyserythropoietic anaemia
- Erythropoietic porphyria
- Platelet function disorders

rare, or seldom require transfusion support for extended periods of time.

Indications for transfusion. Blood components

Red cells

The aim of red cell transfusion in patients with chronic anaemia is to maintain the haemoglobin at a level that allows the patient to carry out activities regarded as essential in life. Although there are individual variations in the ability to tolerate anaemia, the trigger for red cell transfusion is usually a haemoglobin level of around 9 g/dl for patients over the age of 60 years; in younger patients with life expectancy of several years, a more restrictive policy may be instituted (a haemoglobin 'trigger' of 7–8 g/dl) in order to limit iron overload. Organ damage due to iron deposition seldom causes clinical problems, at least until ferritin exceeds 2500 ng/ml. Iron chelation is warranted only in selected patients whose red cell transfusion requirements extend over several years.

Packed red cells in additive solution or plasma-reduced red cells are the components used for transfusion. Washing of red cells in saline, once preferred for transfusion in paroxysmal nocturnal haemoglobinuria, is no longer considered necessary. It is important to ensure that blood transfused to patients with cold agglutinin disease is prewarmed to 37°C, using approved blood warmers.

Platelets

In patients with severe thrombocytopenia, without bleeding and/or sepsis, prophylactic platelet transfusions are usually given to maintain the platelet count above $10 \times 10^9/l$. In the presence of fever, splenomegaly, and mucosal damage such as that induced by graft-versus-host disease or cytotoxic drugs, a higher threshold of $15–25 \times 10^9/l$ is desirable. In clinically stable thrombocytopenic patients, the threshold for prophylactic transfusions may be lowered further: Sagmeister et al[3] transfused a group of 25 patients with aplastic anaemia only when the platelet count reached $5 \times 10^9/l$ ($6–10 \times 10^9/l$ if febrile); moreover, they extended the interval between platelet transfusions, irrespective of platelet counts, provided that the patients did not bleed. The authors concluded that this approach was safe, with the only deaths due to bleeding in the group occurring in alloimmunized patients. Although this suggests that an effective regime of chronic platelet transfusions does prevent bleeding, the overall benefit of these programmes is unclear, since there are no controlled studies. However, the findings of Slichter and Harker[4] provide a scientific basis for the use of a platelet count of $5–10 \times 10^9/l$ as the trigger for platelet transfusions in patients with aplastic anaemia, since a significant faecal loss of chromium-labelled red cells was only observed below that count.

Invasive diagnostic procedures (liver biopsy or central venous line insertion) and most surgical interventions require raising the platelet count above $50 \times 10^9/l$; in surgical procedures where even a minimal bleed may be disastrous, such as eye or brain surgery, the platelet count should be raised above $100 \times 10^9/l$.

Prevention of HLA alloimmunization

Leukodepletion of blood products causes a significant reduction of HLA-alloimmunization in previously non-exposed patients.[5] A large randomized study[6] demonstrated a significant reduction in immunization to HLA antigens and platelet refractoriness in acute leukaemia patients transfused with either filtered or ultraviolet light-irradiated platelets. Use of single-donor (apheresis) platelets, as opposed to pooled platelets, would be anticipated to reduce the incidence of HLA alloimmunization by reducing donor exposure; however, the TRAP study[6] found no difference in the cumulative risk of HLA alloimmunization and platelet refractoriness between patients transfused with pooled or single random-donor platelets. Of note, both pooled and single-donor products were *filtered*. Therefore, the routine use of more expensive apheresis platelets to prevent HLA alloimmunization is of dubious value – at least when an effective method of leukodepletion is used.

Once HLA alloimmunization has led to platelet refractoriness, HLA-matched apheresis platelets are generally the only product that can consistently increase platelet counts. Unfortunately, 15–30% of alloimmunized patients do not achieve good increments even with HLA-matched platelets. In these cases, one should search for a better HLA match and, if possible, avoid major ABO incompatibility; antibodies to platelet-specific antigens also need to be considered. Importantly, non-immune causes of platelet refractoriness may coexist with the immune ones, and must not be overlooked.[7]

Transfusion prior to bone marrow transplantation (BMT)

In the early days of BMT for aplastic anaemia, the risk of graft rejection was high, increasing with the number of transfusions received prior to transplant.[8] Patients who proceeded to a transplant without transfusions had a significantly better survival.[9] More recently there has been a decline in graft rejection to 5–10% in HLA-identical siblings, due to improved conditioning and post-transplant immunosuppression.[10] Still, judicious use of transfusions is advisable if transplantation is contemplated. Transfusion of platelets or red cells from potential bone marrow donors and other family members should be avoided prior to a BMT. Experiments in dogs showed a large increase in graft rejection (possibly due to immunization to non-HLA antigens) when bone marrow recipients received blood transfusions from the marrow donor, although evidence for a similar phenomenon in humans is scarce.[11] This policy has to be abandoned when a patient is already refractory to random-donor platelets, and the only HLA-matched platelet donor available is the prospective bone marrow donor.

Despite the data suggesting that leukodepletion of blood products effectively prevents cytomegalovirus (CMV) transmission,[12] many BMT centres continue to give CMV-negative blood products to CMV-negative recipients of cells from CMV-negative donors, prior to and after haematopoietic cell transplantation.

Alternative treatments

Myelodysplastic syndromes (MDS)

MDS is a heterogenous group of clonal disorders of haematopoiesis, characterized by a variable degree of ineffective haematopoiesis, morphologic myelodysplasia, and a tendency to evolve into acute leukaemia. Anaemia is present in a vast majority of patients, and thrombocytopenia in about 25–50% of cases. As the disease progresses, the majority of patients reach the stage of transfusion dependence. For patients with no excess of blasts and without karyotype abnormalities (with the exception of lone deletions 5q and 20q, which do not confer worse prognosis than the normal karyotype), the projected median survival is 3–5 years.[13] These patients generally fall into the clinical categories of acquired sideroblastic anaemia, refractory anaemia (cytopenia), and refractory anaemia with excess blasts.

The overall incidence of MDS in the UK is estimated at 2 cases per 100 000 per annum, rising sharply with age to attain nearly 22 per 100 000 per annum in people over the age of 75 years.[14] The median age in MDS is around 70 years.[15] Conceivably, 'greying' of the population in the Western world will result in a further increase in the prevalence of MDS.

Haematopoietic stem cell transplantation

Presently the only curative treatment for MDS, allogeneic haematopoietic stem cell transplantation (HSCT) is limited to a minority of patients because of advanced patient age and the lack of compatible donors. In addition, wider use of HSCT has been retarded due to the high transplant-related mortality rate (30–50% in several series),[16] and the uncertainty of the prognosis of low-risk cases. Nevertheless, the European group for Blood and Marrow Transplantation (EBMT) data show the best results for the low-risk patients, with a 3-year actuarial survival rate of 53%.[17] It is from this group of patients that most candidates for long-term transfusion support are recruited, unless they proceed to a transplant. Given the advanced age of patients and the high procedural toxicity, HSCT with non-myeloablative conditioning represents an attractive option. In a series of 20 patients

who received this form of transplant, the day-100 mortality rate was 5%; patients had fewer days with fever, less mucositis and received less antibiotic support than patients with conventional transplants.[18] In addition, transfusion requirements are decreased in patients receiving non-myeloablative transplants.

Pharmacological treatment

Antilymphocyte globulin (ALG) has been found to be effective in about 40% of patients with low/intermediate-grade MDS.[20] An update of this study reported that 76% of the responders remained transfusion-independent for a median of 32 months.[21] Encouraging results have also been reported with cyclosporin A.[22]

Of the numerous drugs with proliferative, differentiating, and anti-apoptotic properties that have been used in MDS, only erythropoietin (EPO) may be considered to have an impact on transfusion requirements in MDS, either on its own or together with granulocyte colony-stimulating factor (G-CSF). An Italian study reported 37% responses when EPO was given for 8 weeks at 150 units/kg/day, with about one-third of the responders achieving transfusion independence.[23] The addition of G-CSF to EPO appears to have a synergistic effect: Hellstrom-Lindberg et al[24] reported a response rate of 46% in the frequently resilient acquired sideroblastic anaemia. However, 72% of responders required 70 000 units/week of EPO.

Factors predicting response are a serum EPO level of less than 200–500 milliunits/l and a requirement of less than 2 units of red cells/month.[23,25] Clearly, the benefits of reducing transfusion requirements in a subset of moderately anaemic patients must be weighed against the significant cost of the treatment.

Aplastic anaemia (AA)

The prognosis of AA has significantly improved in the last 15 years, owing to the therapeutic success of immunosuppressive regimes and allogeneic HSCT. However, about 15% of patients fail to respond to one or two courses of immunosuppression, and a similar proportion of non-transplanted patients are at risk of developing paroxysmal nocturnal haemoglobinuria or MDS after several years.[26,27] Thus, even with improved management, up to 20% of patients may require long-term red cell and/or platelet transfusion support at some stage of the disease.

Haematopoietic stem cell transplantation

The use of BMT for AA began in the early 1970s, and by the 1990s it became the standard treatment for patients with a suitable family donor. EBMT data show a long-term survival rate of over 70% for those transplanted from HLA-matched siblings after 1990. The advantage of BMT over immunosuppression is particularly evident in young patients (less than 20 years) and those with a very low neutrophil count.[28]

Pharmacological therapies

ALG, alone or in combination with cyclosporin A and/or G-CSF, induces a response rate of about 70–80% in AA. It is the preferred therapeutic option for patients above the age of 40 years.[28]

A breakthrough in the pharmacological management of chronic thrombocytopenia due to bone marrow failure is still awaited. Preliminary results with low-dose interleukin-11 (IL-11) showed a response in platelet counts in 38% of patients with bone marrow failure (AA and MDS).[29] Currently there are no published studies of thrombopoietin in this setting.

Other diseases

EPO has eliminated the transfusion of an estimated 250 000–500 000 units of red cells in the USA annually, owing to its effect in anaemia of renal disease.[30] It is occasionally efficacious in anaemia caused by inflammatory disease (rheumatoid arthritis or Crohn's disease), HIV infection, or following BMT. *Splenectomy* may reduce transfusion requirements in patients with MDS and primary myelofibrosis who have an enlarged spleen. It is rarely of benefit in cold haemagglutinin disease and paroxysmal nocturnal haemoglobinuria.

CONGENITAL DISEASES REQUIRING LONG-TERM TRANSFUSION SUPPORT

Sickle cell disease

Sickle cell disease (SCD) is a family of disorders, in which the mutated gene coding for haemoglobin S exists in the homozygous state (SS disease), or in a compound heterozygous state with genes that code for other abnormal haemoglobins (C, E, etc), or mutations giving rise to β-thalassaemia. Haemoglobin S (HbS) differs from the normal adult haemoglobin A (HbA) in a single amino acid (Glu → Val) at position 6 of the β-globin chain. The mutation induces profound physicochemical changes in the haemoglobin molecule, resulting in a tendency of HbS to polymerize in deoxygenated state. Formation of polymers distorts the shape of the red cell and reduces its deformability, with ensuing membrane alterations and an increase in intracellular haemoglobin concentration. These events, together with the increased adherence of sickle cells to the endothelium, cause rheological changes responsible for most of the manifestations of SCD.

In practice, two major factors define the blood viscosity in SCD: the HbS concentration (as a percentage of total haemoglobin), and the total blood haematocrit. When the proportion of SS cells in mixtures of AA (normal) and SS (homozygous sickle) cells exceeds 40%, a sharp increase in viscosity occurs.[31] This finding concurs with clinical experience, acute sickle cell crises being rare when HbS is less than 40–50% of total haemoglobin. The impact of haematocrit on the blood viscosity in SCD was demonstrated by Schmalzer et al,[32] who showed that, at fixed mixtures of sickle and normal red cells, an increase in blood viscosity followed a rise in total haematocrit, with the increase being steeper at higher relative HbS values and low oxygen pressure (Figure 3.1); blood viscosity at a haematocrit over 0.40 (approximately haemoglobin 13.5 g/dl) increases significantly even with HbS as low as 20%. Eventually, at higher haematocrit, oxygen delivery to tissues is impaired as the effects of increased blood viscosity predominate over the increased oxygen-carrying capacity. These considerations are of paramount practical importance when planning transfusion in SCD.

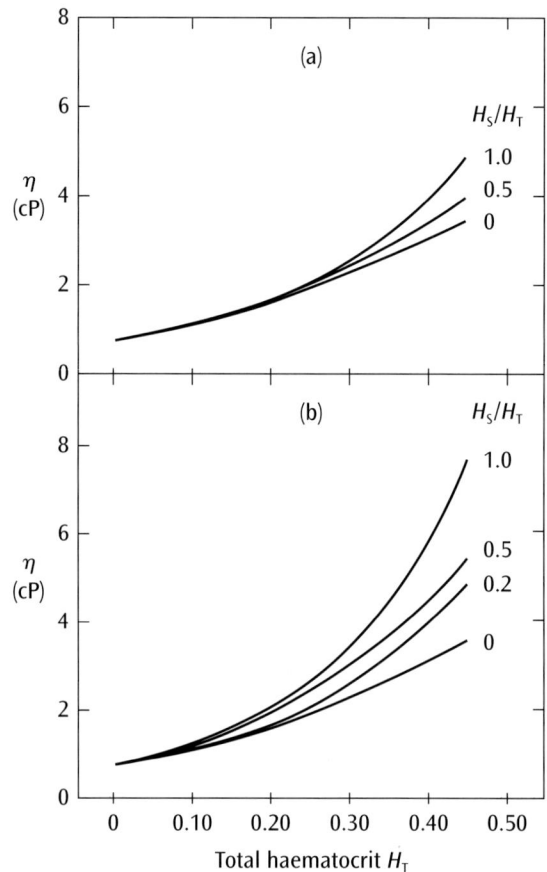

Figure 3.1
The rise in blood viscosity η (in centipoise) with haematocrit H_T at various proportions of sickle cells to total cells in suspension: (a) oxygenated suspensions ($PO_2 = 150$ mmHg); (b) deoxygenated suspensions ($PO_2 = 37$ mmHg). Taken with permission from reference 32.

Indications and modalities of transfusion

The majority of patients with SS disease run haemoglobins of 6–10 g/dl.[33] Anaemia is generally well tolerated and is not an indication for blood transfusion per se. However, in situations such as aplastic crisis caused by parvovirus B19 infection, acute splenic or hepatic sequestration, or acute haemorrhage, worsening of anaemia may require rapid correction. Overtransfusion to normalize the haemoglobin is unnecessary and may be harmful: it suffices to restore the haemoglobin to the baseline value of the particular patient.

In most instances, however, the goal of

transfusion in SCD is to reduce microvascular 'sickling' and improve organ perfusion, by diluting or replacing the patient's sickle cells with normal cells. This may sometimes be achieved by additive transfusions, but is more readily achieved by exchange transfusion (ET). Common indications for transfusion in SCD are shown in Table 3.2.

The advantages of ET include more profound reduction of HbS with simultaneous avoidance of haematocrit increase; ET also has the advantage of limiting iron overload[34,35] (Figure 3.2), albeit at the expense of higher blood usage and donor exposure. An increase in blood usage of 50–77% was reported when patients were switched to a regular (automated) exchange programme, compared with the period prior to its commencement.[35,36]

ET may be performed manually, using two venous lines or a three-way stopcock on a single line to alternatively bleed and transfuse the patient.[37] It is important to ensure that isovolaemia is maintained throughout the procedure, by replacing removed blood and saline. A 'full' manual exchange, aiming at an

HbS of 25–30%, is a laborious procedure generally divided into two or three exchanges lasting 2–4 hours each. By contrast, automated ET allows the exchange of 6–10 units

Table 3.2 Indications for transfusion in sickle cell disease[a]
Acute conditions
• Aplastic crisis (A)
• Splenic/hepatic sequestration (A)
• Acute bleeding (A)
• Acute chest syndrome (E)
• Stroke, transient ischaemic attack, subdural haematoma (E)
• Priapism (E)
• Intractable pain crisis (E)
• Retinal artery occlusion (E)
• Avascular hip necrosis
• Multiorgan failure (E)
Elective transfusion
• Preoperative[b] (A, E)
• Prior to injection of contrast material (E)
• Pregnancy[b] (A, E)
Chronic transfusion programme (A or E)
• Stroke prevention
• Prevention of recurrence of sequestration crisis (in children)
• Chronic organ failure
• Non-healing leg ulcers
• Recurrent pain crises
[a]Preferred transfusion modality: A, additive; E, exchange. [b]In selected patients.

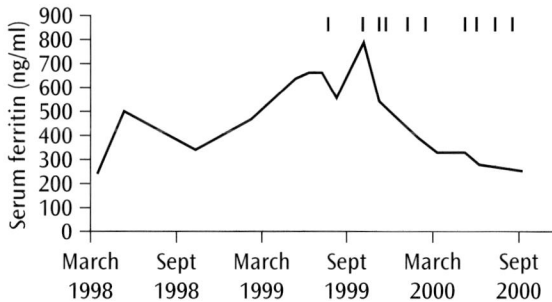

Figure 3.2
Serum ferritin value in a patient with sickle cell anaemia undergoing chronic exchange transfusions for leg ulcers. Despite regular exchanges of 6–8 units (bars), the ferritin declines owing to subsiding inflammation.

of red cells in 1.5–2 hours; continuous-flow separators are very efficacious in avoiding hypovolaemia; calculation of end-hematocrit and end-HbS percent are accurate and reliable. Therefore, automated ET has clear advantages over manual ET, especially in emergencies. The higher cost of automated ET is offset by the more rational use of resources. It is worth noting that automated ET is difficult to perform in small children, due to relatively large extracorporeal fluid volume, limited anticoagulant infusion rate, and inadequate venous access. Table 3.3 lists some useful hints for automated red cell exchange.

Endpoints of transfusion in sickle cell disease

In an acute sickling episode, the aim of transfusion is to bring the HbS below 30%, while maintaining the haematocrit. It is important not to raise the haematocrit excessively when transfusing a patient with SCD. In concordance with experimental data, clinical studies have shown that the risk of acute chest syndrome increases at higher haemoglobin levels;[38] similarly, high steady-state haemoglobin has been incriminated in the pathogenesis

of the 'acute multiorgan failure syndrome',[39] a dramatic form of sickle cell crisis. In some patients with HbSS, and particularly those with HbS/C disease or HbS/β+-thalassaemia, who have haematocrits of 0.28–0.42,[40] exchange transfusion with a lower end-haematocrit, or even phlebotomy alone are useful in the management of acute complications.[41]

There is less agreement as to what is an adequate HbS reduction in elective situations; surgery and pregnancy are discussed below.

Surgery
Preoperative transfusion or exchange designed to reduce HbS levels is frequently, even if at times indiscriminately, used in the management of SCD in developed countries. With progress in anaesthetic procedures and supportive care, indications for preoperative transfusions have become more restricted (Table 3.4). A review of children with SCD undergoing adenotonsillectomy showed that few needed transfusion prior to the procedure.[37] In a large randomized study,[42] a reduction of HbS to an average of 59%, achieved by additive transfusions to a mean

---

Table 3.3 Useful hints for automated red cell exchange

1. First obtain vascular access and a full blood count.
2. Blood must be warmed using a blood warmer and a coil extension before it is returned to the patient.
3. Bear in mind that the starting HbS may already be lowered by previous transfusions. Recalculate the end-HbS as in the following example: start HbS 65%, desired HbS 25%. Enter 'endpoint HbS' 25/65 = 0.38 (38%).
4. If another abnormal haemoglobin is present (e.g. HbC), calculate endpoints using 'fraction of sickleable cells'. For example, if a desired endpoint in SS disease is an HbS of 30%, this should be interpreted as HbS + HbC of 30% in HbSC disease.

Table 3.4 Indications for preoperative transfusions in sickle cell disease

No transfusion
- Tonsillectomy
- Hernia repair
- Circumcision
- Other minor surgery (e.g. tissue biopsy)

Additive/exchange transfusion to HbS of 30–60%
- Cholecystectomy
- Splenectomy
- Orthopaedic surgery
- Genitourinary surgery

Exchange transfusion to HbS < 20%
- Surgery in acutely ill patients
- Neurosurgery
- Cardiac surgery
- Eye surgery

haemoglobin of 10.6 g/dl, resulted in the same rate of serious postoperative complications (including acute chest syndrome) and 50% fewer transfusion-related complications as a more aggressive reduction of HbS to around 30%. The majority of surgical procedures that the patients in the study underwent were cholecystectomies, orthopaedic, and ear, nose, and throat operations. However, in major cardiac or neurosurgery, or prior to cerebral angiography, a reduction of HbS to less than 20% is warranted.[43] In a study of patients with SCD undergoing abdominal surgery, the incidence of sickle-cell-related complications was significantly higher in those who were not transfused prior to surgery (35% versus 0%).[44]

Pregnancy

Pregnant women with SCD have an increased risk of infections, organ infarction (including placenta), toxaemia, and heart failure, especially in the third trimester or post partum. Anaemia is often exacerbated by folate deficiency. The fetal survival rate is about 58%, and prematurity is more common than in the general population.[45] Koshy et al[46] conducted a randomized study in which pregnant women with SCD were assigned to prophylactic or 'as-required' transfusions: maternal and fetal outcomes were not different, except that the women in the prophylactic transfusion group had fewer painful episodes. These findings suggest that prophylactic transfusions in pregnancy may be unnecessary; however, the study did not answer if a subgroup of women with high-risk for fetal loss could benefit from regular transfusions.

Chronic transfusion programmes

Regular red cell transfusions are used to prevent particularly dangerous and crippling complications of SCD, such as stroke, recurrent chest syndrome, and splenic sequestrations; to halt progressive deterioration of organ (especially renal and cardiac) function; or alleviate frequent, intractable painful crises (Table 3.2).

Stroke

About 5–10% children with SS disease suffer a stroke before adolescence; if untreated, two out of three will have a recurrence, usually within 3 years.[47] Regular transfusion therapy reduces the recurrence rate to 10%,[48] but it increases again after cessation of regular transfusions.[49] The optimal duration of a chronic transfusion programme initiated for secondary stroke prevention is not known. Whereas most paediatricians advocate indefinite continuation of the programme, others stop regular transfusions at the age of 18 years, provided that no strokes have occurred in the previous 3 years.[50] Primary stroke prevention also seems possible: a randomized trial in children at high risk for stroke, based on cerebral artery flow velocity, found a much lower incidence of stroke in children on regular transfusions compared with the control group.[51]

Chronic transfusion programmes in children with sickle cell disease aim at maintaining the HbS at less than 25–30%, with the haemoglobin level between 10 and 14 g/dl ('hypertransfusion'), in a bid to suppress endogenous erythropoiesis.[37] There is evidence that after 3–5 years of regular transfusion, the endpoints may be relaxed to maintain HbS below 50%.[52]

Somewhat less ambitious goals may be set for adult patients who have regular exchanges for non-life-threatening conditions, such as chronic leg ulcers, painful crises, or congestive heart failure. At King's College Hospital, London we usually perform an automated red cell exchange aiming at an end-haematocrit of 0.28–0.30 (an approximate haemoglobin level of 9.5–10 g/dl) and a HbS of 30–40%. Besides preventing an untoward rise in blood viscosity, blood usage and donor exposure are reduced, and the duration of the procedure is shortened. Additive transfusions may also be used in chronic transfusion programmes to maintain HbS between 30% and 50%. This can be accomplished by transfusing one or two units of red cells every 2–4 weeks.[53]

The thalassaemias

The advent of nucleic acid-based molecular techniques has revealed the incredible variety of these disorders of globin chain synthesis. From a purely transfusion-related viewpoint, the clinically severe form, named *thalassaemia major*, deserves special attention. It is caused by inheritance of two β-thalassaemia genes, either in homozygous or compound heterozygous form. Thalassaemia major is characterized by gross ineffective erythropoiesis, as well as haemolysis, leading to severe anaemia.[54]

The survival and quality of life of patients with thalassaemia major have changed dramatically since the introduction of regular transfusion regimes. Most patients start transfusions in the first year of life, in the presence of symptoms and signs of severe anaemia, usually when haemoglobin drops below 7 g/dl; however, some children may not require blood until the age of 3–4 years. Current standards recommend the maintenance of a pretransfusion haemoglobin level of 9.5 g/dl and a *mean* haemoglobin level of 12 g/dl. Such regimes result in normal growth and development, as well as suppression of endogenous erythropoiesis, which prevents bone marrow expansion and skeletal deformities. Delay in the development of splenomegaly and improved cardiac reserve are also achieved by regular transfusions; furthermore, despite an overall increase in the number of blood units transfused, iron overloading is not accelerated, because of the suppression of intestinal iron absorption.[55] In practice, the 'hypertransfusion' regime translates into transfusing 1–3 units of red cells every 3–4 weeks, with non-splenectomized patients having about 30% higher requirements than splenectomized ones.[56]

Even more aggressive transfusion programmes, aiming to maintain haemoglobin above 11–12 g/dl, have been used ('super-transfusion'). These schedules almost completely suppress endogenous haematopoiesis; the ensuing reduction of total bone marrow mass and blood volume is anticipated to counterbalance the excess blood used to maintain the haemoglobin level. These programmes are very demanding and are associated with substantial iron overload, and have largely been abandoned.[57]

Use of blood components in haemoglobinopathies

It is desirable to transfuse red cells that are less than one week old. The UK National Blood Service issues tested HbS-negative red cells for patients with SCD. Leukodepletion is expected to benefit patients by reducing the frequency of non-haemolytic febrile reactions and HLA alloimmunization; the latter becomes particularly important if a haematopoietic stem cell or kidney transplant is contemplated. In countries where pre-storage leukodepletion is not feasible, bedside filtering of blood is recommended.

Although leukodepletion confers a high level of protection against transmission of CMV,[12] it is currently advisable to give CMV-negative children screened CMV-negative blood products, since they may be candidates for HSCT at a later stage.

Transfusion of young red cells in thalassaemia has been anticipated to result in prolonged transfused red cell survival and reduction of transfusion requirements; on centrifugation, these 'neocytes' segregate in the least dense fraction of red cells, just under the 'buffy coat' made up of leukocytes. Use of

neocytes has resulted in a modest reduction in blood requirement (extension of transfusion interval by 13–25%), at the expense of increased costs and donor exposure.[57] Therefore, neocyte transfusion is not recommended for routine use in thalassaemic patients. An elegant approach was described by Berdoukas et al,[58] who performed automated red cell exchange, removing the dense, old red cell fraction and replacing them with standard donor cells. They reported a 42% increase in transfusion interval and a 29% reduction in red cell consumption, but increased donor exposure and procedure cost.

Adjuvant and alternative treatments for haemoglobinopathies

An active search for methods that reduce transfusion requirements, mitigate organ damage, and ultimately cure the underlying disease is constantly ongoing. Adequate iron chelation has had a huge impact on the lives of patients with thalassaemia and SCD; vaccination programmes have greatly helped reduce the incidence of hepatitis B infection in these patients; and, in patients with thalassaemia whose annual transfusion requirement exceeds 200 ml red cells per kilogram body weight, splenectomy reduces transfusion requirements and iron overload. However, two major areas of research include pharmacological modification of abnormalities in haemoglobinopathies, and HSCT.

Pharmacological interventions

Fetal haemoglobin inducers

Patients with SCD and a high fetal haemoglobin (HbF) level generally have milder clinical picture; if hereditary persistence of HbF, a variant of δβ-thalassaemia, and sickle cell trait coexist in compound heterozygosity, the resulting clinical picture is very mild.[44] Observations of increased numbers of red cells containing HbF during recovery from aplastic anaemia or chemotherapy-induced pancytopenia led to the attempts of induction of HbF synthesis in SCD: in 1995, a multicentre trial showed unequivocally that adult SCD patients treated with hydroxyurea (HU) had significantly fewer painful crises and decreased transfusion requirements.[59] HU has also been found to be effective in HbS/β-thalassaemia, and the clinical improvement correlated with the HbF increase.[60] It appears that the favourable effects of HU are not brought about solely by HbF induction, but also by a reduction of white cell counts and interference with blood cell–endothelial interactions in SCD.[61] An analysis of cost-effectiveness of HU in SCD suggested its superiority over placebo.[62]

Although HU is relatively well tolerated, compliance is often a problem. Furthermore, long-term effects are still not defined; a modest increase in leukaemia risk may be difficult to detect in low-powered studies. Another matter of concern for patients on HU is its effect on fertility and outcome of pregnancy. 5-Azacytidine and its analogue 2'-deoxy-5-azacytidine have been used to enhance γ-globin chain synthesis in SCD and thalassaemia. Trials of 5-azacytidine have been stopped because of evidence of a carcinogenic effect in animals; 2'-deoxy-5-azacytidine has not been shown to be carcinogenic, and has resulted in increases of HbF in a phase I/II study in SCD.[63] Similarly, intermittent treatment with arginine butyrate has been reported to cause a sustained rise in HbF levels in SCD.[64]

Haematopoietic stem cell transplantation

Thalassaemia major

The ultimately poor prognosis of thalassaemia major and the intensity of medical care necessary to maintain the quality of life have spurred interest in BMT. The outcome is excellent in adequately chelated patients without hepatomegaly and liver fibrosis:[65] these patients (mainly children) have over 90% long-term event-free survival rate, equating in practical terms with cure. In patients younger than 17 years with all three risk factors, as well as in most adults, the long-term event-free survival rate is around 60%.[66]

Sickle cell disease

Advances in the management of SCD and the unpredictability of its clinical course have precluded wider use of HSCT in this disease. A Belgian group reported 50 transplanted patients,[67] with a median age of 7.5 years at transplant, and overall and disease-free survival rates of 93% and 85% respectively. Similar results have been reported by Walters et al.[68] No significant deteriorations in neurological and pulmonary function were observed after a median follow-up of nearly 5 years,[68] but gonadal function was frequently affected.[67,68]

At the centre of the dilemma of transplantation in SCD is the fact that the best outcomes would be expected if HSCT were performed early in life, before significant organ damage occurs. However, this would mean subjecting many patients with clinically mild disease to a potentially life-threatening procedure; conversely, if significant organ damage has occurred, the transplant-related mortality and morbidity may be unacceptably high. To help resolve this dilemma, a set of eligibility criteria for HSCT in SCD has been put forward.[69]

Novel transplantation techniques are currently being explored in haemoglobinopathies: non-myeloablative transplants have been successfully used in SCD;[70] the use of cord blood from healthy siblings or unrelated donors has the potential to expand the donor pool; and intrauterine transplantation with fetal liver cells, or paternal or maternal T-cell-depleted haematopoietic stem cells is under investigation.[71]

COMPLICATIONS OF LONG-TERM RED CELL TRANSFUSIONS

Immune complications

Alloimmunization to red cell antigens

Immunization to red cell antigens has been found in 8.3% of surgical patients transfused on average with 3 units of blood.[72] In a study of over 500 patients with haematological malignancies,[73] alloimmunization to red cell antigens occurred in 14.3% of MDS patients, requiring an average of 12 units of red cells to the formation of the first antibody. By contrast, in chronic lymphocytic leukaemia, the incidence of alloimmunization was 3.2%, with 53 units required to induce antibody formation. These variations reflect biological differences between diseases and the treatments received. The most commonly detected antibodies were anti-c, -E, -K, -D, and anti-Fy[a]. Whereas red cell alloimmunization in patients with bone marrow failure and MDS is an important, but not overwhelming, problem, it is a more serious problem in haemoglobinopathies. Formation of alloantibodies to red cell antigens occurs in around 25% (range 8–35%) of patients with SCD.[74] In part, this is due to the number of transfusions that these patients receive.[75] However, the main cause of red cell alloimmunization is the fact that Caucasians far outnumber other racial groups as blood donors in European and North American countries; thus, patients with SCD are frequently exposed to antigens less commonly expressed in individuals of Black race (Table 3.5). Antibodies usually appear early in the course of transfusion therapy, generally in a subset of 'responders', whereas the majority of patients do not form antibodies despite repeated exposure to foreign blood. Over half of the antibodies are directed against antigens of the Rh system (notably anti-C, -D, and -E), followed by antibodies against Kell, Kidd, MNS, and Duffy antigens.

The rate of alloimmunization to red cell antigens is generally lower in thalassaemia, with rates of 3.17%[78] and 5.2%[79] reported in ethnically more homogenous areas such as Italy. In Western Europe and North America, most thalassaemia patients are of Caucasian/Mediterranean descent, and thus have similar red cell antigen frequencies to the majority of blood donors. The importance of the donor/recipient ethnicity is exemplified by the alloimmunization rate of 20.8% reported in Asian thalassaemia patients living in California, who received blood from a donor pool with only 6% Asian donors.[80]

Other factors also contribute to red cell alloimmunization: in Greece, about 20% of thalassaemic patients developed alloantibodies when transfused with blood matched only for ABO/RhD.[81,82] In addition, factors related to the host immune system play a role; transfusions in patients with thalassaemia are commonly started in the first year of life, which may induce immune tolerance,[81] and

Table 3.5 Frequency (percentage of population positive) of red cell antigens and some phenotypes in different racial groups (compiled from references 76 and 77)

Antigen	Caucasian	African	Oriental
D	85	94	>99
CDe haplotype (R_1)	42	6–17	73
cDe haplotype (R_0)	2–4	44–59	3
cde haplotype (r)	39	20–26	2–3
K	9	1–2	0.02
Jk^a	77	92	25–40
Jk^b	74	49	—
s	89	97	—
S − s − U−	0	0.2–1	—
Fy (a − b−)	<0.01	68	<0.01

splenectomized patients were found to have a higher rate of alloimmunization.[80]

In order to prevent alloimmunization in susceptible patient populations, various phenotype matching schemes have been recommended. Extended prophylactic antigen matching may delay transfusion in critical situations, and cause depletion of the resources of rare blood phenotypes; moreover, in one institution, even matching for ABO, D, C, c, E, e, K, S, Fy^a, Fy^b, Jk^a, and Jk^b antigens would have failed to prevent alloimmunization in 27% of patients.[50] Alternative approaches include providing ABO/RhD/Kell-matched blood where anti-K is common,[80] or giving ABO/RhCcEeD/Kell-matched blood to thalassaemic children who start transfusions beyond the age of 12 months.[81] Alternatively, no prophylactic matching may be done until the appearance of the first antibody as an indicator of immune responsiveness. The policy for blood selection in SCD at King's College Hospital is presented in Table 3.6.

Haemolytic reactions

Usually, the only consequence of alloimmunization is a shorter lifespan of transfused red cells. However, delayed haemolytic transfusion reactions (DHTR) are particularly common in SCD, and are often associated with unusual clinical and serological findings; a DHTR may mimic sickle cell pain crisis; haemoglobinuria is more common; the direct antiglobulin test may be negative in as many as 26% of cases, and new antibodies are often undetectable.[74] The most perplexing condition is the development of a more severe anaemia following transfusion than was previously present, sometimes with evidence of the destruction of patient's own cells. The mechanism of this 'hyperhaemolysis' is not entirely clear: it has been suggested that recipient's cells are lysed by complement activated in the initial antigen–antibody reaction ('bystander haemolysis'), or by preformed autoantibodies boosted by the reaction;[74] however, Petz et al[83] observed reticulocytope-

---

Table 3.6 Blood selection for transfusion in patients on long-term support at King's College Hospital, London

Sickle cell disease
An extended red cell phenotype (ABO, Rh, Kell, Kidd, Duffy, MNS) is performed at diagnosis. Blood is selected to avoid exposure to Kell (K1) and RhCcEeD antigens. Patients with R_0 (cDe) phenotype will receive R_0 or rr (cde) red cells. When an alloantibody appears, an attempt is made to match as closely as possible to the patient's phenotype.

Other conditions
Blood is matched for ABO, RhD, and K1 antigens.

---

nia (relative to the patient's usual reticulocyte count) during these anaemic crises and argued that suppression of endogenous erythropoiesis may play a role in the worsening of anaemia. If 'hyperhaemolysis' is suspected, further transfusions should be withheld in spite of the falling haemoglobin, since they may exacerbate anaemia and haemolysis. Steroids or intravenous immunoglobulins can be useful.[84] In life-threatening anaemia, red cell transfusions have been given under immunoglobulin and steroid cover, without exacerbation of haemolysis.[85] It is not clear what preventive measures, if any, should be taken if blood is to be given to a patient who has had a 'hyperhaemolysis crisis' in the past.

Other immunological complications of transfusion

Non-haemolytic febrile transfusion reactions (NHFTR) used to be common in patients on long-term red cell or platelet support. Although they usually only result in discomfort, NHFTR may very occasionally be life-threatening.[53] The frequency of NHFTR is expected to decrease since the introduction of universal leukodepletion in several countries, and the recommendation to use filtered blood products for patients with long-term requirements. NHFTR may not be completely abrogated by filtration of platelet products (especially filtration at the bedside), since cytokines released from leukocytes and platelets during storage may play a role in its pathogenesis.[86]

Non-immune complications

Major non-immune complications affecting patients on long-term transfusion support are transfusion-transmitted infections, iron overload, and complications arising from vascular access devices. The impact of these complications on the survival and quality of life of patients, as well as their financial implications, far outweigh the impact of immunological complications of transfusion.

Transfusion-transmitted infections
Bacterial infections
A survey of transfusion-transmitted bacterial infections blood products in the USA showed a doubling of the number of deaths due to

contaminated blood components between 1986 and 1991 compared with the previous 10-year period.[87] Of these deaths, 55% were due to contaminated red cells, and a half of the cases of clinical sepsis due to red cell contamination were caused by *Yersinia enterocolitica*, with the overall mortality rate of 61% *Yersinia* grows at temperatures below 37°C in calcium-free media, which makes it a potential contaminant of red cell concentrates, especially when stored for longer than 20 days. There is some evidence that pre-storage leukodepletion reduces the risk of *Yersinia* contamination.[87]

Other bacteria transmitted by transfusion of blood products are *Staphylococcus*, *Pseudomonas aeruginosa*, *Escherichia coli*, *Serratia*, and *Klebsiella*. Contamination may originate from the donor's blood or skin, or from the environment.

Viral infections

The risks of acquiring a transfusion-transmitted viral disease are steadily diminishing in industrialized countries, owing to a combination of efficient donor exclusion systems, pre-donation testing, and viral inactivation of some blood products. Current estimates for the risk of acquiring hepatitis B or C viruses (HBV, HCV) or human immunodeficiency virus (HIV) by transfusion in the UK are shown in Table 3.7. Conceivably, patients with lifelong transfusion dependence, especially in countries with a high frequency of virus carriers, have been the most affected prior to introduction of routine testing. Previously common, HBV infection is now very rare in thalassaemia patients, as a result of efficacy of donor testing as well as regular vaccination of recipients.[56] By contrast, 85% of Italian thalassaemia patients now older than 10 years are infected with HCV (testing for antibodies against HCV was introduced in the early 1990s.[88] Infection with HCV, together with iron overload, is a major factor in the development of liver fibrosis and cirrhosis, leading to a high incidence of liver failure and hepatocellular carcinoma.[89] The multifactorial pathogenesis of liver disease in chronically transfused patients may preclude the effects of a successful antiviral treatment with interferon-α.[57] The prevalence of HIV infection in thalassaemia patients, which peaked in the mid-1980s, subsequently decreased owing to efficient donation screening, and the high mortality among infected patients. Seroconversion is now rare.[56]

Two more recently described viruses have been linked with post-transfusion hepatitis, namely hepatitis G virus (HGV) and the 'transfusion-transmitted' (TT) virus. For neither agent could infection be related to liver disease in thalassaemia patients.[56]

The leukocyte-associated viruses CMV and human T-cell leukaemia/lymphoma viruses I and II (human T-lymphotropic viruses, HTLV-I and -II) may also contribute to morbidity in long-term transfusion recipients. CMV infection used to be common in thalassaemic patients[90] but may be expected to decline as the practice of blood product leukodepletion gains popularity.

In Greece, 1.4% of thalassaemia patients tested positive for antibodies to HTLV-I/II.[91] HTLV-I-positive carriers have a 1–5% lifelong risk of developing T-cell lymphoma and a 2% risk of tropical spastic paraparesis; very few cases of transfusion-transmitted disease have been reported to date.[92] In contrast to the low incidence among the general donor popu-

Table 3.7 Estimated risks (per donation of blood) of viral transmission by blood transfusion[a]	
Human immunodeficiency viruses 1 and 2	1 in 5.26 million
Hepatitis C virus	1 in 1.66 million
Hepatitis B virus	1 in 50–200 thousand

[a]Calculations for England and Wales in year 2000.
Source: Blood Transfusion Task Force, British Committee for Standards in Haematology.

lation,[93] 1.5% of Black Caribbean women in a London antenatal clinic tested positive for HTLV-I antibodies.[94] These findings call for caution, especially in view of the efforts to recruit more non-Caucasian donors.

The effect of filtration on HTLV-I transmission is unclear. Although Okochi and Sato[95] reported that filtration of blood products effectively prevents transmission, an in vitro study indicated that filtering may not completely remove HTLV-I if the virus load is high.[96]

Iron overload

No regulated mechanism of iron excretion exists in humans: 1–2 mg iron per day is lost through bleeding and sloughing of the small-bowel mucosa.[97] Considering that a unit of blood contains 200–250 mg iron, it is easy to see that repeated transfusions lead to rapid iron loading. Being derived from ageing red cells, this iron is primarily deposited in the reticuloendothelial system, but subsequently also in the parenchyma of various organs, notably the heart, liver, and endocrine glands. Abnormal iron absorption caused by expansion of erythropoiesis also increases the iron burden.[53]

The extent of iron deposition depends on the number of transfusions received. There-fore the risk of iron overload is highest in thalassaemia major, patients with SCD on chronic transfusion programmes, some patients with MDS, and patients with rare disorders such as congenital dyserythropoietic anaemia. Another major determinant of iron balance is iron-chelation therapy. With availability and compliance to desferrioxamine treatment, survival of patients with thalassaemia major in developed countries has extended into the fourth decade of life; in countries where iron chelators are not available, or in cases of poor compliance, only 30–40% of patients survive over 25 years.[98,99] Heart disease is the major determinant of survival in thalassaemia, but liver disease becomes a major cause of death in older patients, with iron overload being aggravated by infections (hepatitis C) and alcohol abuse. However, in the absence of adequate chelation, liver fibrosis and cirrhosis may develop in the first decade of life.[54]

As the survival of patients with thalassaemia increased, endocrine dysfunction received more attention: with inadequate iron chelation, growth retardation and hypothyroidism occur around the age of 10 years.[98] In the second decade of life, diabetes mellitus, hypoparathyroidism, delayed puberty, and secondary hypogonadism supervene. Many of these complications may be prevented or alleviated by early commencement of iron chelation. However, established abnormalities are usually not reversible.[54] Commencement of desferrioxamine treatment by subcutaneous infusion is recommended after the first 10–20 units of transfused red cells, or when serum ferritin reaches 1000 ng/ml. This generally occurs at about 3 years of age. The treatment is continued for life, unless the natural course of the disease is reversed by BMT.

Vascular access

Good venous access is necessary for a long-term transfusion programme, requiring central venous line insertion in about 15–20% of patients. A range of catheters are in use: tunnelled subclavian or jugular vein catheters may remain in situ for weeks or months; femoral vein catheters are usually maintained for 5–6 days;[100] non-collapsible catheters are available if repeated apheresis procedures are envisaged. All types of venous catheters are associated with a 10–15% risk of sepsis[101] and a smaller risk of vessel thrombosis. Subclavian catheter insertion carries a small but finite risk of pneumothorax (about 1%) and bleeding. At King's College Hospital, we have found that a double-lumen femoral Vascath (6.5F for children and 10.8F for adults), or a femoral sheath (8–9F) with an inner catheter (6F) ending in the inferior vena cava, provides satisfactory temporary access, associated with few complications (unpublished data).

TRANSFUSION IN DEVELOPING COUNTRIES

The two haemoglobin disorders with a life-long transfusion requirement, β-thalassaemia and SCD, are very common diseases: about 3% of the world population (approximately 200 million people) carry β-thalassaemia genes;[55] around 8% of the Black population in the Americas carry the sickle gene, whereas in parts of central Africa up to 45% of the population are carriers.[45] Migrations of population have contributed to the spread of the haemoglobinopathy genes into Western countries.

Even in the developed countries of Southern Europe with large concentrations of β-thalassaemia and SCD (Italy and Greece), these diseases are a large medical and social problem. The demand of around 100 000 units of red cells annually for the treatment of haemoglobinopathies in Greece required the importing of up to 50 000 units.[91] The magnitude of the problem prompted large-scale prenatal diagnosis programmes in Sardinia and Greece, which led to a significant drop in the birth of β-thalassaemia and SCD homozygotes.[91,102]

The countries of the 'Third World', much more populous and economically deprived, face numerous problems in the management of their transfusion-dependent population. Blood collection does not match demand; the prevalence of viral infection and often inadequate donation testing make transfusion unsafe; and supportive care and adjuvant treatments, desferrioxamine in particular, remain beyond the reach of the vast majority of the population. The lack of facilities that are taken for granted in the developed world (although not always on the basis of hard evidence) may be an incentive to explore alternative approaches.[103] Production and use of virally inactivated blood products, introduction of prenatal diagnosis (depending on the cultural and religious background), and facilitation of the use of cheaper drugs with proven efficacy (e.g. deferiprone licensing in India), are examples of measures needed to improve medical care of the transfusion-dependent patients in the 'Third World'.

CONCLUSIONS

Long-term transfusion programmes continue to be an important modality in the management of various congenital and acquired conditions, improving the patient's quality of life and prolonging survival. Despite considerable improvements in blood safety and the general level of medical care, these programmes are cumbersome, costly, and have associated risks. It is hoped that with the advances in disease prevention, pharmacotherapy, and haemopoietic cell transplantation, the need for regular blood transfusion in these patients will be reduced, and perhaps ultimately abolished.

REFERENCES

1. Platt OS, Brambilla DJ, Rosse WF et al. Mortality in sickle cell disease. Life expectancy and risk factors for early death. *N Engl J Med* 1994; **330**: 1639–44.
2. Olivieri NF, Nathan DG, MacMillan JH et al. Survival in medically treated patients with homozygous β-thalassemia. *N Engl J Med* 1994; **331**: 574–8.
3. Sagmeister M, Oec L, Gmur J. A restrictive platelet transfusion policy allowing long-term support of outpatients with severe aplastic anemia. *Blood* 1999; **93**: 3124–6.
4. Slichter SJ, Harker LA. Thrombocytopenia: mechanisms and management of defects in platelet production. *Clin Haematol* 1978; **7**: 523–39.
5. Van Marwijk Kooy M, van Prooijen HC, Moes M et al. Use of leukocyte-depleted platelet concentrates for the prevention of refractoriness and primary HLA-alloimmunisation: a prospective, randomised trial. *Blood* 1991; **77**: 201–5.
6. The Trial to Reduce Alloimmunisation to Platelets Study Group. Leukocyte reduction and ultraviolet B irradiation of platelets to prevent alloimmunization and refractoriness to platelet transfusions. *N Engl J Med* 1997; **337**: 1861–9.
7. Novotny VMJ. Prevention and management of platelet transfusion refractoriness. *Vox Sang* 1999; **76**: 1–13.
8. Champlin RE, Horowitz MM, van Bekkum DW et al. Graft failure following bone marrow transplantation for severe aplastic anemia: risk factors and treatment results. *Blood* 1989; **73**: 606–13.
9. Storb R, Thomas ED, Buckner CD et al. Marrow transplantation in thirty 'untransfused' patients with severe aplastic anemia. *Ann Intern Med* 1980; **92**: 30–6.
10. Gordon-Smith EC, Marsh JCW. Management of acquired aplastic anemia. *Rev Clin Exp Hematol* 2000; **4**: 260–78.
11. Slichter SJ. Transfusion support in bone marrow transplantation. In: *Principles of Transfusion Medicine*, 2nd edn (Rossi EC, Simon TL, Moss GS et al, eds). Baltimore: Williams & Wilkins, 1996: 521–36
12. Bowden RA, Slichter SJ, Sayers MH et al. Use of leukocyte-depleted platelets and cytomegalovirus-seronegative red blood cells for prevention of primary cytomegalovirus infection after bone marrow transplantation. *Blood* 1991; **78**: 246–50.
13. Greenberg P, Cox C, LeBeau MM et al. International scoring system for evaluating prognosis in myelodysplastic syndromes. *Blood* 1997; **89**: 2079–88.
14. Cartwright RA. Incidence and epidemiology of the myelodysplastic syndromes. In: *The Myelodysplastic Syndromes* (Mufti GJ, Galton DAG, eds). Edinburgh: Churchill Livingstone, 1992: 23–32.

15. Aul C, Gattermann N, Schneider W. Epidemiological and etiological aspects of myelodysplastic syndromes. *Leuk Lymphoma* 1995; **16**: 247–62.

16. Anderson JE. Bone marrow transplantation for myelodysplasia. *Blood Rev* 2000; **14**: 63–77.

17. de Witte T, Hermans J, Vossen J et al. Haematopoietic stem cell transplantation for patients with myelodysplastic syndromes and secondary acute myeloid leukaemias. *Br J Haematol* 2000; **110**: 620–30.

18. Parker JE, Shafi T, Mijovic A et al. Allogeneic stem cell transplantation in MDS: interim results of outcome following non-myeloablative conditioning compared to standard preparative regimes. *Blood* 2000; **96**: 554a.

19. Weisinger F, Sandmaier BM, Maloney DG et al. Decreased transfusion requirements for patients receiving non-myeloablative compared with conventional peripheral blood stem cell transplants from HLA-identical siblings. *Blood* 2001; **98**: 3584–8.

20. Molldrem JJ, Caples M, Mavrovdis D et al. Antithymocyte globulin for patients with myelodysplastic syndromes. *Br J Haematol* 1997; **99**: 699–705.

21. Barrett AJ, Saunthararajah Y. Immune mechanisms and modulation in MDS. In: *Hematology 2000, American Society of Hematology Education Program Book*, 2000: 117–22.

22. Jonasova A, Neuwirtova R, Cermak J et al. Cyclosporin A therapy in hypoplastic MDS patients and certain refractory anaemias without hypoplastic bone marrow. *Br J Haematol* 1998; **100**: 304–9.

23. Italian Cooperative Study Group. A randomized double-blind placebo controlled study with subcutaneous recombinant human erythropoietin in patients with low-risk myelodysplastic syndromes. *Br J Haematol* 1998; **101**: 1070–4.

24. Hellstrom-Lindberg E, Ahlgren T, Beguin Y et al. Treatment of anemia in myelodysplastic syndromes with granulocyte colony-stimulating factor plus erythropoietin. Results from a randomized phase II study and long-term follow-up in 71 patients. *Blood* 1998; **92**: 68–75.

25. Hellstrom-Lindberg E, Negrin R, Stein R et al. Erythroid response to treatment with G-CSF plus erythropoietin for the anaemia of patients with myelodysplastic syndromes: proposal for a predictive model. *Br J Haematol* 1997; **99**: 344–51.

26. Socie G, Henry-Amar M, Bacigalupo A et al. Malignant tumors occurring after treatment of aplastic anemia. *N Engl J Med* 1993; **329**: 1152–7.

27. Najean Y, Hagenauer O. Long term (5 to 20 years) evolution of nongrafted aplastic anaemia. *Blood* 1990; **76**: 2222–8.

28. Bacigalupo A, Brand R, Oneto R et al. Treatment of acquired severe aplastic anemia: bone marrow transplantation compared with immunosuppressive therapy – the European Group for Blood and Bone Marrow Transplantation experience. *Semin Hematol* 2000; **37**: 69–80.

29. Kurtzrock R, Cortes J, Thomas D et al. Low dose interleukin-11 is well tolerated and induces platelet responses in myelodysplasia and other bone marrow failure states. *Blood* 2000; **96**: 147a.

30. Miller YM, Klein HG. Growth factors and their impact on transfusion medicine. *Vox Sang* 1996; **71**: 196–204.

31. Lessin LS, Kurantsin-Mills J, Klug PP et al. Determination of rheologically optimal mixtures of AA and SS erythrocytes for transfusion. *Prog Clin Biol Res* 1978; **20**: 123–37.

32. Schmalzer EA, Lee JO, Brown AK et al. Viscosity of mixtures of sickle and normal red cells at varying hematocrit levels. *Transfusion* 1987; **27**: 228–33.

33. Hayes RJ, Beckford M, Grandison Y et al. The haematology of steady state homozygous sickle cell disease: frequency distributions, variations with age and sex, longitudinal observations. *Br J Haematol* 1985; **59**: 369–82.

34. Kim HC, Dugan NP, Silber JH et al. Erythrocytapheresis therapy to reduce iron overload in chronically transfused patients with sickle cell disease. *Blood* 1994; **83**: 1136–42.

35. Hilliard LM, Williams BF, Lounsbury AE, Howard TH. Erythrocytopheresis limits iron accumulation in chronically transfused sickle cell patients. *Am J Hematol* 1998; **59**: 28–35.

36. Singer ST, Quirolo K, Nishi K et al. Erythrocytapheresis for chronically transfused children with sickle cell disease: an effective method for maintaining a low hemoglobin S level and reducing iron overload. *Am J Hematol* 1999; **14**: 122–5.

37. Davies SC, Roberts-Harewood M. Blood transfusion in sickle cell disease. *Blood Rev* 1997; **11**: 57–71.

38. Castro O, Brambilla DJ, Thorington B et al. The acute chest syndrome in sickle cell disease: incidence and risk factors. *Blood* 1994; **84**: 643–9.

39. Hassell KL, Eckman JR, Lane PA. Acute multiorgan failure syndrome: a potentially catastrophic complication of severe sickle cell pain episodes. *Am J Med* 1994; **96**: 155–62.

40. West MS, Wethers D, Smith J et al. Laboratory profile of sickle cell disease: a cross-sectional analysis. *J Clin Epidemiol* 1992; **45**: 893–909.

41. Rosse, WF. Blood viscosity in sickle cell disease. In: *Hematology 2000, American Society of Hematology Education Program Book*, 2000: 3–6.

42. Vichinsky EP, Haberkern CM, Neumayr L et al. A comparison of conservative and aggressive transfusion regimens in the preoperative management of sickle cell disease. *N Engl J Med* 1995; **333**: 206–13.

43. Sharon BI, Honig GR. Management of congenital hemolytic anemias. In: *Principles of Transfusion Medicine*, 2nd edn (Rossi EC, Simon TL, Moss GS et al, eds). Baltimore: Williams & Wilkins, 1996: 141–59.

44. Neumayr L, Koshy M, Haberkern C et al. Surgery in patients with hemoglobin SC disease. *Am J Hematol* 1998; **57**: 101–8.

45. Wang WC, Lukens JN. Sickle cell anemia and other sickling syndromes. In: *Wintrobe's Clinical Hematology*, 10th edn (Lee GR, Foerster J, Lukens JN et al, eds). Baltimore: Williams & Wilkins, 1999: 1346–97.

46. Koshy M, Burd L, Wallace D et al. Prophylactic red cell transfusions in pregnant patients with sickle cell disease: a randomised cooperative study. *N Engl J Med* 1988; **319**: 1447–52.

47. Powars D, Wilson B, Imbus C et al. The natural history of stroke in sickle cell disease. *Am J Med* 1978; **65**: 461–71.

48. Pegelow CH, Adams RJ, McKie V et al. Risk of recurrent stroke in patients with sickle cell disease treated with erythrocyte transfusions. *J Pediatr* 1995; **126**: 896–9.

49. Wang WC, Kovnar EH, Tonkin IL et al. High risk of recurrent stroke after discontinuance of five to twelve years of transfusion therapy in patients with sickle cell disease. *J Pediatr* 1991; **118**: 377–82.

50. Castro O. Management of sickle cell disease: recent advances and controversies. *Br J Haematol* 1999; **107**: 2–11.

51. Adams RJ, McKie VC, Hsu L et al. Prevention of a first stroke by transfusion in children with sickle cell anemia and abnormal results on transcranial Doppler ultrasonography. *N Engl J Med* 1998; **339**: 5–11.

52. Cohen AR, Martin MB, Silber JH et al. A modified transfusion program for prevention of stroke in sickle cell disease. *Blood* 1992; **79**: 1657–61.

53. McCullough J. *Transfusion Medicine*. New York: McGraw Hill, 1998.

54. Olivieri NF. The β-thalassemias. *Blood* 1999; **341**: 99–109.

55. Lukens JN. The thalassemias and related disorders. In: *Wintrobe's Clinical Hematology*, 10th edn (Lee GR, Foerster J, Lukens JN et al, eds). Baltimore: Williams & Wilkins, 1999: 1405–48.

56. Prati D. Benefits and complications of regular blood transfusions in patients with beta-

thalassemia major. *Vox Sang* 2000; **79**: 129–37.

57. Olivieri NF, Brittenham GM. Iron-chelating therapy and the treatment of thalassemia. *Blood* 1997; **89**: 739–61.

58. Berdoukas VA, Kwan YL, Sansotta ML. A study on the value of red cell exchange transfusion in transfusion dependent anemias. *Clin Lab Haematol* 1986; **8**: 209–20.

59. Charache S, Terrin MN, Moore RD et al. Effects of hydroxyurea on the frequency of painful crisis in sickle cell anemia. Investigators of the Multicentre Study of Hydroxyurea in Sickle Cell Anemia. *N Engl J Med* 1995; **18**: 1317–22.

60. Voskaridou E, Kalotychou V, Loukopoulos D. Clinical and laboratory effects of long-term administration of hydroxyurea to patients with sickle-cell/β-thalassemia. *Br J Haematol* 1995; **89**: 479–84.

61. Loukopoulos D. Management of the haemoglobinopathies. In: *European Hematology Association (EHA-5) Educational Book*, 2000: 141–5.

62. Moore RD, Charache S, Terrin ML et al. Cost effectiveness of hydroxyurea in sickle cell anemia. Investigators of the Multicenter Study of Hydroxyurea in Sickle Cell Anemia. *Am J Hematol* 2000; **64**: 26–31.

63. Koshy M, Dorn L, Bressler L et al. 2-Deoxy-5-azacytidine and fetal hemoglobin induction in sickle cell anemia. *Blood* 2000; **96**: 2379–84.

64. Atweh GF, Sutton M, Nassif I et al. Sustained induction of fetal hemoglobin by pulse butyrate therapy in sickle cell disease. *Blood* 1999; **93**: 1790–7.

65. Lucarelli G, Galimberti M, Polchi P et al. Bone marrow transplantation in patients with thalassemia. *N Engl J Med* 1990; **322**: 417–21.

66. Giardini C, Lucarelli G. Bone marrow transplantation for beta-thalassemia. *Hematol Oncol Clin North Am* 1999; **13**: 1059–64.

67. Vermylen C, Cornu G, Ferster A et al. Hematopoietic stem cell transplantation for sickle cell anaemia: the first 50 patients transplanted in Belgium. *Bone Marrow Transplant* 1998; **22**: 1–6.

68. Walters MC, Storb R, Patience M et al. Impact of bone marrow transplantation for symptomatic sickle cell disease: an interim report. *Blood* 2000; **95**: 1918–24.

69. Davies SC, Roberts IAE. Bone marrow transplant for sickle cell disease – an update. *Arch Dis Child* 1996; **75**: 3–6.

70. Krishnamurti L, Blazar BR, Wagner JE. Bone marrow transplantation without myeloablation for sickle cell disease. *N Engl J Med* 2001; **344**: 68.

71. Pixley JS, MacKintosh FR, Zanjani ED. Experimental and clinical basis of intrauterine stem cell transplantation. *Rev Clin Exp Hematol* 1999; **8**: 11–32.

72. Redman M, Regan F, Contreras M. A prospective study of the incidence of red cell alloimmunisation following transfusion. *Vox Sang* 1996; **71**: 216–20.

73. Schonewille H, Haak HL, van Zijl AM. Alloimmunisation after blood transfusion in patients with haematological and oncologic diseases. *Transfusion* 1999; **39**: 763–71.

74. Garratty G. Severe reactions associated with transfusion of patients with sickle cell disease. *Transfusion* 1997; **37**: 357–61.

75. Rosse WF, Gallagher D, Kinney TR et al. Transfusion and alloimmunisation in sickle cell disease. *Blood* 1990; **76**: 1431–7.

76. Mollison PL, Engelfriet CP, Contreras M. *Blood Transfusion in Clinical Medicine*. Oxford: Blackwell Science, 1997.

77. Isitt PD, Anstee DJ. *Applied Blood Group Serology*. Durham, NC: Montgomery Scientific Publications, 1998.

78. Rebulla P, Modell B. Transfusion requirements and effects in patients with thalassaemia major. *Lancet* 1991; **337**: 277–80.

79. Sirchia G, Zanella A, Parravicini A et al. Red cell alloantibodies in thalassemia major: results of an Italian cooperative study. *Transfusion* 1985: **25**: 110–12.

80. Singer ST, Wu V, Mignacca R et al. Alloim-

munisation and erythrocyte autoimmunisation in transfusion-dependent thalassemia patients of predominantly Asian descent. *Blood* 2000; **96**: 3369–73.

81. Michail-Merianou V, Pamphil-Panousopoulou L, Piperi-Lowes L et al. Alloimmunisation to red cell antigens in thalassemia: comparative study of usual versus better-match transfusion programmes. *Vox Sang* 1987; **52**: 95–8.

82. Spanos T, Karageorga M, Ladis V et al. Red cell alloantibodies in patients with thalassemia. *Vox Sang* 1990; **58**: 50–5.

83. Petz LD, Calhoun L, Shulman IA et al. The sickle cell hemolytic transfusion reaction syndrome. *Transfusion* 1997; **37**: 382–92.

84. Cullis JO, Win N, Dudley JM et al. Post-transfusion hyperhaemolysis in a patient with sickle cell disease: use of steroids and intravenous immunoglobulin to prevent further red cell destruction. *Vox Sang* 1995; **69**: 355–7.

85. Win N, Doughty H, Telfer P et al. Hyperhemolytic transfusion reaction in sickle cell disease. *Transfusion* 2001; **41**: 323–8.

86. Webb IJ, Anderson KC. Risks, costs, and alternatives to platelet transfusions. *Leuk Lymphoma* 1999; **34**: 71–84.

87. Klein HG, Dodd RY, Ness PM et al. Current status of microbial contamination of blood components: summary of a conference. *Transfusion* 1997; **37**: 95–101.

88. Prati D, Zanella A, Farma E et al. A multicenter prospective study on the risk of acquiring liver disease in anti-HCV negative patients affected from homozygous beta-thalassemia. *Blood* 1998; **92**: 3460–4.

89. Tong MJ, El-Farra NS, Reikas AR et al. Clinical outcomes after transfusion-associated hepatitis C. *N Engl J Med* 1995; **332**: 1463–6.

90. Nigro G, Lionetti P, Digilio G et al. Viral infections in transfusion-dependent patients with beta-thalassemia major: the predominant role of cytomegalovirus. *Transfusion* 1990; **30**: 808–13.

91. Loukopoulos D. Current status of thalassemia and the sickle cell syndromes in Greece. *Semin Hematol* 1996; **33**: 76–86.

92. Manns A, Hisada M, La Grenade L. Human T-lymphotrophic virus type I infection. *Lancet* 1999; **353**: 1951–8.

93. Brennan M, Runganga J, Barbara JA et al. Prevalence of antibodies to human T cell leukaemia/lymphoma virus in blood donors in north London. *BMJ* 1993; **307**: 1235–9.

94. Donati M, Seyedzadeh H, Leung T et al. Prevalence of antibody to human T cell leukaemia/lymphoma virus in women attending antenatal clinic in southeast London: a retrospective study. *BMJ* 2000; **320**: 92–3.

95. Okochi K, Sato H. Transmission of adult T-cell leukemia virus (HTLV-I) through blood transfusion and its prevention. *AIDS Res* 1986; **3**: 3157–61.

96. Pennington J, Sutherland J, Allain JP et al. Human T-cell leukaemia virus I (HTLV-I) removal from blood and platelets by leukocyte-depleting filters using real-time quantitative PCR. *Blood* 2000; **96**: 451a.

97. Andrews NC. Disorders of iron metabolism. *N Engl J Med* 1999; **341**: 1986–95.

98. Wonke B, De Sanctis V. Clinical aspects of transfusional iron overload. *Rev Clin Exp Hematol* 2000; **4**: 322–36.

99. Brittenham GM, Griffith PM, Nienhuis AW et al. Efficacy of deferroxamine in preventing complications of iron overload in patients with thalassemia major. *N Engl J Med* 1994; **331**: 567–73.

100. Guidelines for the clinical use of blood cell separators. *Clin Lab Haematol* 1998; **20**: 265–78.

101. Rizvi MA, Vesely SK, George JN et al. Complications of plasma exchange in 71 consecutive patients treated for clinically suspected thrombotic thrombocytopenic purpura–haemolytic–uremic syndrome. *Transfusion* 2000; **40**: 896–901.

102. Cao A, Galanello R, Rosatelli MC et al.

Clinical experience of management of tha-lassemia: the Sardinian experience. *Semin Hematol* 1996; **33**: 66–75.

103. Serjeant GR. Chronic transfusion pro-grammes in sickle cell disease: problem or panacea? *Br J Haematol* 1997; **97**: 253–5.

4 Transfusion support in transplantation

Darrell J Triulzi, Ileana López-Plaza

INTRODUCTION

The transfusion service plays an important supporting role in hematopoietic stem cell transplantation (HSCT) and solid organ transplantation by providing blood components and guidance on optimal blood component therapy during the peritransplantation period. Transplantation imposes demands on the transfusion service not only quantitatively in terms of blood product support but also qualitatively with respect to consultation for increasingly complex clinical issues. Transplant recipients present unique challenges in terms of requirements for specialized blood components, serologic problems, and immunologic effects of transfusion on both the allograft and the recipient. The laboratory and clinical issues involved in transfusion support of HSCT and solid-organ transplantation will be presented in this chapter.

TRANSFUSION SUPPORT IN HEMATOPOIETIC STEM CELL TRANSPLANTATION

Blood component requirements depend on donor and/or recipient factors[1] – i.e. donor–recipient human leukocyte antigen (HLA) matching and ABO compatibility, cytomegalovirus (CMV) status, the patient's pretransplantation conditioning regimen, the source of stem cells, the use of growth factors, and post-transplantation immunosuppressive therapy – all of which influence hematologic

engraftment and immune reconstitution. Table 4.1 summarizes the transfusion requirements in autologous and allogeneic recipients at the University of Pittsburgh. The introduction of recombinant hematopoietic growth factors has substantially reduced transfusion requirements, largely by augmenting peripheral blood progenitor cell (PBPC) collections quantitatively and qualitatively. The infusion of these products enriched for hematopoietic stem cells has significantly shortened the period of the neutropenia,[2–4] shortened the time to platelet engraftment, and decreased platelet transfusion requirements.[3–5]

Prophylactic platelet transfusions and management of platelet refractoriness

As with malignancy/chemotherapy-induced thrombocytopenia,[6–10] prophylactic platelet transfusion is the standard of care for the peritransplant period. A prophylactic platelet transfusion threshold of less than 10 000/mm^3 is used for otherwise clinically stable patients.[11,12] For patients presenting with complications such as fever, sepsis, or other clinical conditions in which the risk of bleeding is increased, a threshold of 20 000/mm^3 may be used.[11] In less common circumstances, such as during the immediate postoperative period or for clinically significant (intracranial, gastrointestinal, pulmonary, or retroperitoneal) hemorrhages, a higher threshold may be necessary. The recommended platelet transfu-

Table 4.1 Blood use in stem cell transplantation[a]

Diagnosis[b]	No.	Type[c]	Source[d]	Red cells (units)	Platelets (doses)
Breast	40	Auto	PBPC	8 ± 4	5 ± 4
	14	Auto	Marrow	17 ± 17	17 ± 16
Lymphoma	40	Auto	PBPC	10 ± 10	11 ± 16
AML	17	Auto	Marrow[e]	65 ± 58	80 ± 76
	27	Allo	Marrow	28 ± 23	30 ± 25
CML	33	Allo	Marrow	33 ± 25	39 ± 35
ALL	15	Allo	Marrow	36 ± 33	55 ± 56

[a]Consecutive transplants performed between July 1991 and December 1995. Includes transfusions leading up to and post-transplantation. [b]AML, acute myeloid leukemia; CML, chronic myeloid leukemia; ALL, acute lymphoblastic leukemia. [c]Allo, allogeneic; Auto, autologous. [d]PBPC – peripheral blood stem cell. [e]Monoclonal antibody-purged.

sion dose is one unit per 10 kilograms of body weight when using random pooled platelets or one unit of single-donor platelets per transfusion episode.[13] Clinical factors such as fever, sepsis, splenomegaly, bleeding, use of amphotericin,[14] veno-occlusive disease, disseminated intravascular coagulation, and early post-transplant period[15] are associated with decreased survival of transfused platelets.[16–18] Immune refractoriness, caused by allo- or autoantibodies with specificities to the HLA (25–50% of patients)[19,20] or platelet-specific antigens (2–9% of patients)[18,21] can also complicate platelet transfusion support in the peritransplant period. Platelet ABO incompatibility can also cause a reduction in platelet recovery.[22] Transient platelet autoantibodies may develop in 50% of HSCT recipients, but are rarely associated with refractoriness.[18,23] In preparation for transplant, previous platelet transfusion response should be evaluated. A past history of platelet transfusion refractoriness needs to be investigated. A patient with previous immune refractoriness generally needs HLA-matched or crossmatched platelet support during the peritransplant period.[22,24–31] An HLA antibody screen should be obtained as part of the pretransplant evaluation. If ABO incompatibility has been identified in prior platelet transfusions, ABO-compatible platelets should be used. The success of an HLA-matched platelet transfusion, however, still depends on the patient's clinical factors.[32] The management of clinical refractoriness to platelet transfusion depends on the clinical situation. Increasing the dose and/or frequency of transfusion is recommended until the underlying clinical problems have resolved. In our experience, HLA-matched products have not provided any additional benefit to patients with clinical refractoriness unless alloimmunization has also been present. Some alloimmunized patients do not achieve adequate increments with either HLA-matched or crossmatched platelets. Numerous strategies have been used to treat these patients, with conflicting results.[33–36] ε-Aminocaproic acid appears to be useful in controlling bleeding in patients with thrombocytopenia due to bone marrow hypoplasia.[37–39] For this infrequent clinical occurrence, our recommendations for such a thrombocytopenic patient in the setting of life-threatening bleeding or undergoing a major invasive procedure are as follows: Try to obtain the best HLA match possible[25] or initiate platelet transfusion support with 1.5–2 times the dose indicated for patient weight. Continue platelet transfusions support every 6–8 hours until bleeding is controlled. If more intensive platelet support is unsuccessful, intravenous immunoglobulin (IVIG) (1 g/kg × 2 days) may be given when short-term control of bleeding is required.[35,36] If necessary, the correction of abnormalities in the other components of the coagulation system should be pursued. If not contraindicated, the patient may be started on an antifibrinolytic agent (i.e. ε-aminocaproic acid). The goal of this therapeutic approach is not to increase the platelet count but to prevent, decrease, or stop the bleeding.

Prevention of alloimmunization

The primary mechanism of transfusion-induced alloimmunization has been summarized elsewhere.[10,40,41] Primary alloimmunization can be delayed or avoided when cellular blood components in the final container have a residual white blood cell (WBC) content of less than 5×10^6 as a result of leukoreduction.[42] The effectiveness of leukoreduction in the prevention of primary alloimmunization in patients with acute leukemia has been demonstrated.[43] The residual alloimmunization rate of 5–15% is most likely due to undetected previously alloimmunized patients and less frequently to filter failure. Platelets filtered at the bedside may not be as effective in reducing the risk of alloimmunization.[44] At the University of Pittsburgh, the standard of practice is to provide leukoreduced cellular blood products for all potential HSCT patients and continue after transplant.

Transfusion-associated graft-versus-host disease

Transfusion-associated graft-versus-host disease (TA-GvHD) results from the passive transfer of donor immunocompetent T cells capable of engrafting and initiating an immune response against the recipient.[45–48] All HSCT recipients are presumed to be at risk for TA-GvHD because they may experience transplant-associated GvHD, even in the autologous setting.[48–51] Like transplant-associated GvHD, the gastrointestinal tract, liver, and skin are involved, but to a more severe degree. The key feature that differentiates TA-GvHD from transplant-associated GvHD is a profound pancytopenia caused by the donor T-lymphocyte-derived destruction of the bone marrow. The TA-GvHD syndrome is characterized by high fever and an erythematous skin rash occurring 3–30 days after transfusion of a non-irradiated cellular blood component. This syndrome is typically refractory to all current therapies for transplant-associated GvHD and has an associated mortality rate of over 90%. The cellular blood components associated with this syndrome include red blood cells, platelets, and granulocytes. Plasma components such as fresh-frozen plasma, cryoprecipitate, and coagulation factor concentrates have not been associated with TA-GvHD. Because no successful treatment is currently available, the best option is to prevent the syndrome. TA-GvHD is prevented by gamma-irradiation[52–55] of cellular blood components prior to transfusion for patients who are at risk. The function of the red blood cells,[56,57] platelets,[58–60] or granulocytes[61] is not affected; however, the ability of red blood cells to tolerate storage is slightly decreased.[62] Gamma-irradiated cellular blood products should be provided for all HSCT patients.

Transfusion-associated cytomegalovirus infection

HSCT patients are at risk of significant morbidity and mortality from CMV infection. A pre-existent latent CMV infection may become reactivated. Primary CMV infection may be acquired from the community, the hematopoietic stem cell graft, or blood transfusions.[63,64] Cellular blood components (whole blood, red blood cells, platelets, or granuocytes) may contain latently infected leukocytes capable of transmitting CMV to recipients. Plasma blood components (fresh-frozen plasma or cryoprecipitate) do not transmit CMV, but may passively transfer antibodies to CMV. Risk factors for seroconversion include the number of units transfused[65,66] as well as the immunologic status of the host.[67] Although cellular blood components from CMV-seronegative blood donors carry a very low risk for CMV transmission compared with components from a CMV-seropositive donor,[65] this risk is not eliminated completely. Leukoreduction also significantly reduces the risk of transmission by removing more than 99.9% of the leukocytes harboring CMV.[65,68–71] The probability of acquiring a primary CMV infection from red cells and platelets in CMV-seronegative HSCT recipients has been shown to be similar between the CMV-seronegative and the leukoreduced blood components.[72–79] These data support the use of blood rendered CMV-safe by filtration as an alternative to CMV-seronegative blood. At the University of Pittsburgh, CMV-safe (leukoreduced) blood components are provided to CMV-negative autologous transplant recipients. CMV-negative HSCT recipients of seronegative allogeneic donors (CMV-negative pairs) receive leukoreduced and seronegative blood components when available and CMV-safe (leukoreduced) components when the latter are not available.

Immunohematologic consequences of ABO-mismatched bone marrow transplants

Because ABO and HLA genes are inherited independently, providing the best HLA match during allogeneic HSCT results in recipient/donor ABO/Rh mismatching in up to 15–20% of recipients.[80] Although ABO mismatching may adversely affect erythroid engraftment, ABO incompatibility does not affect engraftment of myeloid or megakaryocytic elements[81] or increase the risk of graft rejection[82] or GvHD.[83] ABO compatibility between donor and recipient in allogeneic HSCT can be subdivided into four categories: ABO-identical, minor ABO incompatibility, major ABO incompatibility, and minor and major ABO incompatibility. Depending on the type of incompatibility, manipulation of the donor marrow or PBPC and alteration of component ABO selection may be required to minimize the risk of acute hemolysis. Appropriate component selection during the peritransplant period can minimize delayed adverse effects of ABO mismatching (Table 4.2), which include delayed hemolysis and delayed red blood cell engraftment.[84–87] Red blood cells should be compatible with both donor and recipient plasma. Plasma components should be compatible with both donor and recipient red blood cells. Transfusion of

Table 4.2 Component selection in ABO-incompatible stem cell transplantation						
Donor	Recipient	Erythrocytes	Granulocytes	Plasma	Platelets (first choice)	Platelets (second choice)
ABO-identical						
A	A	A	A	A, AB	A, AB	B, O[a]
B	B	B	B	B, AB	B, AB	A, O[a]
O	O	O	O	O	O	A, B, AB
AB	AB	AB	AB	AB	AB	A, B, O
Minor ABO incompatibility						
O	A	O	O	A, AB	A, AB	B, O[a]
O	B	O	O	B, AB	B, AB	A, O[a]
A	AB	A	A	AB	AB	A, B, O[a]
B	AB	B	B	AB	AB	A, B, O[a]
O	AB	O	O	AB	AB	A, B, O[a]
Major ABO incompatibility						
A	O	O	O	A, AB	A, AB	B, O[a]
B	O	O	O	B, AB	B, AB	A, O[a]
AB	O	O	O	AB	AB	A, B, O[a]
AB	A	A	A	AB	AB	A, B, O[a]
AB	B	B	B	AB	AB	A, B, O[a]
Major and minor ABO incompatibility						
A	B	O	O	AB	AB	A, B, O[a]
B	A	O	O	AB	AB	A, B, O[a]

[a]Concentrate second-choice platelets to remove incompatible plasma if possible, especially for single-donor platelets.

incompatible plasma in cellular components (i.e. red blood cells, or platelets) should be minimized. Immune hemolysis has also been associated with major and minor non-ABO red cell antigen incompatibilities in HSCT recipients.[88–92]

Minor ABO incompatibility

Minor ABO incompatibility occurs when donor plasma is incompatible with recipient erythrocytes (e.g. O to A or A to AB). Complications from this type of incompatibility may include acute or delayed hemolysis. Acute immune hemolysis can occur during bone marrow or PBPC infusion because of the presence of isohemagglutinins in the donor plasma. By removing the donor plasma from the graft prior to the infusion, acute hemolysis can be prevented.[81] ABO component selection is intended to minimize the transfusion of plasma incompatible with recipient red blood cells (Table 4.2). Delayed immune hemolysis has occurred 1–3 weeks after transplantation owing to the production of isohemagglutinins by the immunocompetent passenger donor lymphocytes infused with the bone marrow or PBPC.[85,93–98] The diagnosis is made by demonstrating a positive direct antiglobulin test result due to ABO antibodies with laboratory and/or clinical evidence of hemolysis. The diagnosis may be complicated when the patient has received components that contain incompatible plasma. Detectable donor-derived isohemagglutinins are found in as many as 25%[81] to 57%[96] of patients receiving an ABO minor-mismatched bone marrow transplant, although hemolysis occurs in only 13–29%[81,96] of these patients. Hemolysis is generally mild and can be adequately treated

with transfusions. In patients with severe hemolysis and end-organ damage, red cell exchange may be indicated. Delayed hemolysis after bone marrow transplantation in the setting of minor ABO incompatibility appears to be limited to situations in which cyclosporine,[93] tacrolimus (FK506),[85] and/or T-cell depletion[96] is used. Studies have suggested that the profound inhibition/depletion of T-cell regulatory function may facilitate unopposed B-cell proliferation, with consequent antibody production.[93] Similarly, it has been shown that if other immunosuppressive agents that are cytotoxic to B cells are used in combination with T-cell depletion or T-cell inhibitory agents, the delayed hemolysis does not occur.[85,96] Although the frequency of this type of hemolysis in association with PBPC transplants is still unknown, the cases reported have involved severe hemolysis.[97–100] The lymphocyte yield in a PBPC collection has been reported to be 10 times higher than in a bone marrow harvest.[101] The severe hemolysis observed in these cases may be associated with the greater B-cell content passively infused at the time of the transplantation. B-cell immunosuppressive therapy (i.e. methotrexate) could potentially diminish the frequency and severity of this complication.

Major ABO incompatibility

Major ABO incompatibility occurs when the donor erythrocytes are incompatible with recipient plasma (e.g. A to O or AB to A). Complications expected from this type of incompatibility may include acute or delayed hemolysis and delayed red blood cell engraftment.[102,103] There are sufficient incompatible red blood cells in the harvested bone marrow to cause acute immune hemolysis when infused.[83] Several management options can be used to prevent this complication. Most frequently, the harvested marrow is processed prior to infusion to remove red blood cells.[80,81,104] Alternatively, recipient isohemagglutinins can be depleted by intensive plasma exchange and/or in vivo antibody adsorption or by extracorporeal (ex vivo) immunoadsorption.[105–108] These techniques have been used when the recipient isohemagglutinin titers are greater than or equal to 1 : 128.[109,110] Studies have shown that a delay in erythroid engraftment (reticulocyte count < 1% for more than 40 days) occurs in 15–40% of recipients. Limited hemolysis at the time of red blood cell engraftment is associated with the persistence of recipient isohemagglutinins.[80,111] Blood components should be selected by ABO group to minimize hemolysis at the time of engraftment (Table 4.2). Hemolysis occurs in 11–50% of patients, and is associated with increased red blood cell transfusion requirements (20 units versus 6 units in ABO-compatible HSCT).[80,81] The diagnosis is made by demonstrating a positive direct antiglobulin test due to ABO antibodies with laboratory and/or clinical evidence of hemolysis. Generally, no treatment is necessary except to transfuse with red blood cells compatible with recipient and donor isohemagglutinins (Table 4.2).

ABO major and minor mismatch

Recipients of a major and minor ABO-incompatible marrow (i.e. A to B or B to A) are at risk for the hematologic complications of both types of incompatibility (i.e. hemolysis during infusion, hemolysis 7–10 days post transplantation, delayed red blood cell engraftment, and hemolysis when donor red blood cells engraft). The marrow should be processed to remove both plasma and red blood cells. Component ABO selection is limited to O cells and AB plasma (Table 4.2).

Allogeneic hematopoietic stem cell donor blood component requirements

The amount of allogeneic marrow harvested for transplantation depends on the patient's body weight. For most marrow donors, red blood cell requirements can be met by pre-harvest autologous blood donation. When both the recipient and the donor are CMV-seronegative, allogeneic transfusions should be with CMV-seronegative or filtered (CMV-safe) components. Allogeneic transfusions for the stem cell donor should be irradiated to avoid the theoretical risk of TA-GvHD by the passive transfer of immunocompetent lymphocytes from a third person at the time of transplantation to the recipient.[112] Leukoreduction of cellular blood products for the donor is not routinely necessary unless filtered products are being used as a substitute for CMV-seronegative products. Donors from whom the hematopoietic stem cells are harvested by PBPC collection rarely if ever require transfusion support. If transfusion support were needed, the guidelines already described for marrow donors would apply.

Granulocyte transfusions

Because of the profound neutropenia that develops post transplantation, HSCT recipients are at risk for life-threatening bacterial and fungal infections. Results obtained from both controlled and uncontrolled studies of granulocyte transfusions have shown that there is a clinical benefit in a selected group of transplant recipients.[113–115] These are patients with the following characteristics: absolute neutropenia (neutrophil count < 500/mm^3), documented sepsis, unresponsiveness to at least 48 hours of adequate antibiotic therapy, and an expected bone marrow recovery.[113,114] A daily therapeutic dose of greater than 1×10^{10} granulocytes is of critical importance for a beneficial clinical response.[113,114] In the past, donors have been treated with corticosteroids prior to leukapheresis to increase the granulocyte yield per harvest, with limited success (average yield $1–2 \times 10^{10}$ WBC per collection). Clinical studies using granulocyte colony-stimulating factor (G-CSF) in volunteer donors have reported an increase in collection yields as much as four- or eightfold over unprimed donors.[116–120] In addition to the better collection achieved with G-CSF, the granulocytes have enhanced phagocytic and bactericidal activities.[121] Granulocyte transfusions are frequently accompanied by mild to severe side-effects. Mild reactions such as fever and chills can be controlled by treating the patient with antipyretics or short-acting steroids and meperidine. More severe reactions such as respiratory distress might require the discontinuation of the granulocyte transfusion therapy. Because of the synergistic effects on pulmonary function, simultaneous infusion of amphotericin and granulocytes should be avoided.[122] CMV infection and TA-GvHD can be complications of granulocyte transfusions. Therefore, the component should be irradiated for all HSCT recipients. If the patient is CMV-seronegative, a CMV-seronegative component is indicated. The risk of alloimmunization is higher for recipients of granulocytes. Special considerations for granulocyte transfusions include the following: never administer through a leukoreduction filter; transfuse as soon as possible after collection[123] (ideally within 6 hours of collection); if HLA antibodies are present, the component should be HLA-matched; and donor/recipient ABO compatibility is required because of red blood cell contamination. Granulocyte transfusion therapy is primarily indicated for the neutropenic patient with severe progressive bacterial infection who is already receiving G-CSF and proper antibiotic therapy. In such cases, a minimum of 4 days of therapy is recommended. Clinical benefits of granulocyte transfusion for fungal sepsis are controversial for the neutropenic patient.[124,125]

TRANSFUSION SUPPORT IN SOLID-ORGAN TRANSPLANTATION

Transplant volumes

Solid-organ transplantation continues to grow as a treatment modality in the USA. There are currently more than 74 000 patients waiting for an organ transplant. However in 1999 only 21 990 transplants were performed, limited primarily by the availability of organs. The total number of organ transplants performed was up 3.5% in 1999, with liver, lung, and kidney accounting for the majority of the increase (Table 4.3).

Blood component utilization

The typical requirements for blood components for each type of organ transplant in adults at the University of Pittsburgh are shown in Table 4.4. It is clear from the table

Table 4.3 Organ transplant volumes in the USA 1998–1999[a]

Year	Kidney	Liver	Heart	Lung	Heart–lung
1998	12 251	4463	2345	862	47
1999	12 529	4700	2185	901	48

[a]UNOS Scientific Registry, Research Department Richmond, VA (www.unos.com).

Table 4.4 Median blood use (Units) in organ transplantation procedures at the University of Pittsburgh Medical Center

Organ	Red cells	Plasma	Platelets	Cryoprecipitate
Liver (n = 118)	12	13	10	—
Heart (n = 51)	4	5	10	—
Lung:				
Single (n = 46)	0–2	—	—	—
Double (n = 30)	7	2	8	—
Heart–lung (n = 14)	4	7	20	4
Kidney	0–2	—	—	—

that liver transplant procedures use the most blood components, despite the fact that blood use in liver transplantation has declined dramatically over the last decade. In a study of 70 liver transplants performed between 1981 and 1983 at the University of Pittsburgh, the mean component usage was 43 units of red cells, 40 of fresh-frozen plasma (FFP), and 21 of platelets.[126] Eighty-six percent of patients required 10 or more units of red cells. Today, in the same center, the median component usage for an adult primary liver transplant procedure is 12 units of red cells, 13 of FFP, and 10 of platelets. Seventy-one percent of patients required 10 or more units of red cells. The factors contributing to the reduction in

blood usage are multiple, and include improvements in surgical technique, in organ preservation, and in anesthetic management, intraoperative cell salvage, and better intraoperative monitoring of coagulation status and pharmacologic treatment of fibrinolysis.[127] Heart–lung transplant surgery can also use substantial amounts of blood components, but remains an uncommon procedure, with only 48 transplants being performed in the USA in 1999. As compared with heart–lung transplantation, heart transplantation is associated with lower blood requirements that approximate blood usage observed in complex cardiopulmonary bypass procedures. Blood usage in lung transplantation varies by the type of lung transplant procedure. Over two-thirds of single-lung transplant recipients do not require any transfusions.[128] Double-lung transplant procedures typically require more red cells than heart or heart–lung transplant procedures, but slightly fewer plasma products. The majority of patients receiving kidney or kidney/pancreas transplants do not require blood.

Strategies for selection of compatible components

For solid-organ transplant procedures other than liver, transfusion requirements are generally not sufficient to require deviation from traditional selection criteria of ABO-identical/compatible red cells that are antigen-negative in patients with potentially clinically significant alloantibodies. However, in liver transplantation, the majority of cases still require a large number of transfusions and meet the accepted definition of massive transfusion: one blood volume transfused within a 24-hour period. Transfusion volumes in this range frequently exceed the available supply of ABO-identical red cells, antigen-negative red cells, or compatible plasma, and thus warrant the development of protocols to optimally use available resources in terms of components and blood bank staffing.

Group A patients
Group A patients are rarely switched to group O blood, since group A blood is generally plentiful and group O blood, the only alternative, is frequently in short supply. In patients who receive more than six to eight group O CPDA-1 red cells, a crossmatch with group A cells should be performed to ensure compatibility before switching back to group A red cells. A crossmatch does not appear to be necessary if group O additive red cells are used, since they contain less than half of the 60 ml of incompatible plasma found in CPDA-1 red cells.[129]

Group B patients
Group B patients may need to be switched to group O blood when their transfusion requirements exceed the available group B supply. Since only 10% of donors are group B, this occurs frequently when transfusion requirements exceed one to two blood volumes (10–20 units of red cells). The guidelines described above for group A red cells should be used to switch back to group B red cells.

Group AB patients
Since group AB patients can receive red cells of any ABO group, available outdating AB red cells should be used, and then the patient can be switched to group A cells since these are typically in greatest supply. Group A red cells and 10 units of AB FFP are routinely set up for liver transplantation procedures. The advantage of this approach is that after approximately 10 units of group A red cells have been transfused, the patient can be switched to group A FFP, thereby conserving group AB FFP. Group O cells are generally not required, but can be used if group A red cells are not available. Group AB patients who receive group A or O red cells can be switched back to group AB red cells following the guidelines outlined above.

Group O patients
Group O patients cannot be switched to other red cell groups, but can receive any ABO group FFP. The FFP ABO choice is mainly determined by inventory availability.

Rh$_0$ (D) selection

Rhesus-negative (D−) patients should be provided with D− red cells as supply allows. D− women over childbearing age and adult men may be switched to D+ red cells when their transfusion requirement exceeds one blood volume. Greater effort should be made to maintain D− women of childbearing age and children on D− blood, although the risk of D alloimmunization in liver transplantation is low. Casanueva et al[130] reported that none out of 17 patients developing anti-D. The major clinical significance of an anti-D is that it may limit the ability to switch to D+ red cells if retransplantation is required or massive bleeding is encountered postoperatively. Hemolytic disease of the newborn is less of a concern, although pregnancy has been reported following liver transplantation.[131]

Patients with clinically significant alloantibodies

Pre-existing potentially clinically significant red cell alloantibodies are found in approximately 6% of liver transplant candidates.[132] Usually at least 8–10 units of antigen-compatible blood can be found for surgery. In order to minimize the risk of hemolysis, these patients are ideally managed by using antigen-negative units for the first 5–10 units, switching to antigen-unscreened units in the middle of the case, and then switching back to antigen-negative units for the last 5–10 units transfused. This strategy requires close cooperation between the anesthesiologist and the blood bank, and has been used successfully in the University of Pittsburgh numerous times; only rarely is it complicated by delayed hemolysis.[132,133]

Indications for specialized blood components

Patients undergoing solid-organ transplantation receive immunosuppressive agents to prevent allograft rejection. One complication of immmunosuppressive therapy is that the patient may be more susceptible to infectious or immunologic complications of transfusion, such as CMV infection or TA-GvHD. Other immunologic consequences of transfusion, such as alloimmunization, may also be severe, resulting in acute or chronic graft rejection. The transfusion specialist must recommend the optimal approach to reducing the risk of these complications in organ transplant recipients.

CMV-negative/safe blood components

CMV infection is the most frequent infectious complication following solid-organ transplantation.[134] In seropositive solid-organ recipients, reactivation of latent virus represents the major risk for CMV infection.[135] Although superinfection with a second strain of CMV has been reported from an organ donor,[136] this has not been reported from a blood component. Thus, there is no documented benefit to providing blood components that have reduced risk for transmitting CMV to patients who are CMV-seropositive. In seronegative patients, the major source for primary CMV infection is the seropositive transplanted organ and, to a lesser extent, transfused blood components. The most severe infections are seen in CMV-negative recipients of a CMV-positive organ.[134] The magnitude of the risk of CMV transmission by transfusion can be determined by studying CMV-negative recipients of a CMV-negative organ who receive unscreened blood components. A summary of

Table 4.5 Incidence of transfusion-transmitted CMV infections in seronegative recipients of seronegative organs

Organ	Total no. of patients	Patients with infection
Kidney[136–138]	289	18 (6%)
Heart[137,139–141]	87	13 (15%)
Lung[141]	3	0 (0%)
Heart–lung[137,142]	40	5 (13%)
Liver[137,143,144]	34	3 (9%)

published data[137–144] is shown in Table 4.5. Although the overall rate of CMV transmission is low (5–15%), the morbidity associated with this complication would support the use of methods to prevent CMV transmission from blood components.

Historically, this was accomplished by using blood components from donors who lack antibodies to CMV. Data in allogeneic bone marrow transplant recipients suggest that leukocyte reduction by filtration is equally effective in reducing the risk of CMV transmission from a blood component.[74–79] It is likely that this method would also be effective in solid-organ transplant recipients. A small study by Lopez et al[145] in heart or lung transplant recipients support this assertion. The volumes of blood used in organ transplant procedures other than liver transplantation generally do not pose supply problems when restricted to CMV-negative pairs.

Irradiated blood components

GvHD occurs much less commonly following solid-organ transplantation compared with bone marrow transplantation, and has a much lower mortality rate (47% versus >90%).[146] This is a function of a smaller dose of lympho-

cytes in the lymphoid tissue accompanying the allograft and the less intense recipient immunosuppression. GvHD has been reported following liver (43 cases), small-bowel (6 cases), kidney (4 cases), pancreas–spleen–duodenum (4 cases), heart (1 case), and heart–lung (1 case) transplantation, and has been extensively reviewed elsewhere.[146] The organ donor was suspected or proven to be the source of cytotoxic T cells in all but four cases: one liver,[147] one heart,[148] and two kidney[149,150] (Table 4.6). The two purported transfusion-related cases in kidney transplant recipients did not have confirmation of foreign lymphocytes in peripheral blood or affected tissues by HLA or DNA typing of the lymphocytes.[149,150] There is only a single report of GvHD in a liver transplant recipient. Foreign lymphocytes were convincingly demonstrated by DNA analysis to be from a transfusion.[147] The recipient was a 14-month-old male with fulminant hepatic failure of unknown etiology and pancytopenia with marrow hypoplasia. This case should not, however, be used to extrapolate risk to all liver transplant recipients, because of the patient's age and a preexisting hematologic abnormality that may have placed the patient at increased risk for GvHD. A single case with supportive

Table 4.6 Reported TA-GvHD in solid-organ transplant recipients[147–150]				
Organ	Age/Sex	Primary disease	Outcome	Evidence for GvHD of transfusion origin
Liver	1 yr/M	Fulminant hepatic failure	Died, day 119	HLA/DNA typing
Kidney	54 yr/M	Polycystic kidney	Survived	Clinical diagnosis of GvHD; no DNA or HLA evidence in skin or blood.
Kidney	53 yr/M	Unknown etiology	Survived	GvHD by clinical and skin biopsy. No DNA or HLA evidence for transfusion
Heart	58 yr/F	Cardiomyopathy	Died, day 29	HLA typing peripheral blood leukocytes

HLA evidence has also been reported in a heart transplant recipient.[148] It is worth noting that there have now been two reports in the literature of living related-donor organ recipients (liver[151] and kidney[152]) who developed GvHD. In both cases, HLA and DNA testing revealed that peripheral blood lymphocytes were of donor origin and that the parental donor was homozygous for a shared HLA haplotype in the recipient. This situation is a well-recognized risk for TA-GvHD.[153] Based on these data, it would be prudent to determine the HLA type of a potential living related donor before organ donation and to eliminate donors who are homozygous for a shared HLA haplotype.

Although under-reporting may be occurring, GvHD is a rare complication, reported most frequently in liver transplantation, and is almost always due to the donor organ. Two cases of GvHD reported in recipients of organs from donors homozygous for a shared HLA haplotype would support a policy of avoiding the use of these donors. TA-GvHD is very rare in solid-organ transplant recipients, with only four published cases, only two of which have convincing supportive evidence – and one of these had an underlying hematologic abnormality. These few cases do not support a policy of routine irradiation of cellular blood components for solid-organ transplant recipients.

Leukocyte-reduced blood components: alloimmunization versus the transfusion effect on graft prolongation

Alloimmunization to HLA antigens is of considerable importance to patients considered for organ transplantation. A sensitized patient presents problems in identifying a cross-match-compatible donor, and, for some organs, the outcome of transplantation is inferior.[154] However, white cells in blood components may be beneficial in inducing tolerance and prolonging allograft survival.[155] Thus, the decision to provide leukocyte-reduced components must weigh the risks and benefits of these opposing effects.

Alloimmunization versus the transfusion effect in renal transplantation

It has been recognized for almost three decades that patients with preformed lymphocytotoxic antibodies are at risk for hyperacute kidney rejection.[156] Patients who become sensitized through transfusion, pregnancy, or previous transplantation are less likely to find a crossmatch-compatible donor. Although it is clearly desirable to avoid sensitization by leukocytes, these same leukocytes have been shown to prolong allograft survival.[157] Studies of renal transplant candidates receiving pretransplant non-leukocyte-reduced transfusions have reported alloimmunization rates of 29% with donor-specific transfusions (DST)[158] and 19% with random-donor transfusions.[159] These rates can be substantially reduced by giving concomitant azothiaprine[160] or cyclosporine[161] or by using HLA-haploidentical transfusions[159,162] In the 1980s, clinicians accordingly gave renal transplant candidates conditioning with azothiaprine or cyclosporine when giving non-leukocyte-reduced transfusions. By the early 1990s, the widespread use of cyclosporine largely removed any advantage to pretransplant transfusions,[163] and the concern over the residual risk of sensitization

from transfusion resulted in a decline in this practice. If the transfusion effect is not a concern, then leukocyte reduction makes sense as an attempt to reduce the risk of alloimmunization. There is a substantial body of data showing that HLA alloimmunization results in decreased renal allograft graft survival.[154] Christiaans et al[164] reported a 5-year survival rate of 34% versus 76% in the non-alloimmunized recipient. The efficacy of leukocyte reduction in preventing alloimmunization in this setting has not been established, but supportive data do exist.[165] More recently, pretransplant transfusions have regained some favor as longer-term follow-up has revealed a survival advantage.[166] Additionally, the transfusion effect appears to be enhanced and alloimmunization minimized by using blood from HLA-haplo-identical donors.[159,162,167] The transfusion service must therefore determine how transfusions are used for renal transplant candidates/patients in their institution. If they are used to prolong allograft survival, then filtration is contraindicated. If they are not used for this purpose, then filtration is indicated to reduce the risk of alloimmunization.

Alloimmunization versus the transfusion effect in cardiac transplantation

Humoral alloimmunization in cardiac transplant candidates has been shown to correlate with lower cardiac allograft survival.[168-171] Patients with lymphocytotoxicity panel reactive antibodies (PRA) had a threefold higher risk of acute rejection[170,171] and a modestly lower 5-year survival rate of 91% versus 78%.[172] These data indicate that HLA alloimmunization is a risk factor for acute and/or chronic cardiac allograft rejection. HLA antibodies do not appear to be associated with hyperacute rejection.[168]

The transfusion effect and the role of DST in cardiac transplantation have not been well documented in human studies, although animal studies have demonstrated a graft-prolongation effect.[173] Retrospective single-center clinical data have demonstrated a transfusion effect;[174–178] however, the Collaborative Transplant Study Group reported no cardiac graft survival advantage in 419 transfused versus 2195 untransfused cardiac allograft recipients.[179] An explanation for this discrepancy may be found in two small studies looking at the effect of random pretransplant transfusions.[162,180] Patients who had received blood matched for one HLA-DR antigen had a lower rate of alloimmunization and fewer rejection episodes and a trend toward better survival than those receiving blood mismatched for both DR antigens. Thus, unless a clinical protocol using HLA-DR-matched blood donors is used, the risk of alloimmunization seems to be of greater clinical concern. Although data on the efficacy of leukoreduction in this setting are not available, it would seem prudent to provide leukocyte-reduced blood components to cardiac transplant candidates/recipients.

Alloimmunization versus the transfusion effect in lung transplantation

Hyperacute rejection after lung transplantation is rare; it was suspected in only 2 cases among 359 lung transplants performed at the University of Pittsburgh and was felt to be the result of pre-existing alloantibodies to vascular endothelium.[181] However, a limited amount of data have implicated HLA antibodies in mediating acute rejection[182] and chronic rejection characterized by obliterative bronchiolitis.[183,184] There are no published clinical data demonstrating a transfusion effect in lung transplantation. Therefore, providing leukocyte-reduced blood components to lung transplant patients appears to be warranted, given the potential serious clinical consequences of HLA alloimmunization in lung transplant recipients.

Alloimmunization versus the transfusion effect in liver transplantation

The role of humoral alloimmunization in liver transplantation is unclear. Hyperacute rejection in a patient with donor-specific lymphocytotoxic antibodies has been described, but is uncommon.[185] There are conflicting data regarding the long-term effects of liver transplantation in the presence of lymphocytotoxic antibodies. Data from the University of Pittsburgh showed a lower 1-year graft survival rate of 56% in patients with donor-specifc antibody, compared with 82% in patients without antibody.[186] In contrast, Lobo et al[187] reported that pre-existing donor-specific lymphocytotoxic antibodies had no effect on 1-year graft survival. The deleterious effect of pretransplant alloimmunization on liver allograft survival appears to be less than that observed in renal or cardiac transplantation. Initial studies suggested that alloimmunized patients require more transfusions during their liver transplant procedure – presumably owing to shortened survival of transfused platelets and more bleeding.[188] This has not been found in a more recent study.[187] These data, along with the practical considerations (cost and logistics) of providing large numbers of transfusions to these patients, do not support the routine use of leukoreduced components in liver transplant patients. The role of pretransplant transfusions in mediating the transfusion effect in liver transplantation is poorly defined. Animal models have suggested that a transfusion effect exists,[189] but clinical data are sparse and equivocal.[190,191] The available data are insufficient to recommend intentional pretransplant transfusions in liver transplantation at this time.

ABO blood group system in organ transplantation

The ABO system is clinically important in two areas involving solid-organ transplantation: first as a transplantation antigen important in graft survival, and second as an antigen–antibody system implicated in immune hemolytic anemias in ABO non-identical organ transplant recipients.

ABO blood group system as a transplantation antigen

The importance of the ABO system in organ transplantation was recognized over 30 years ago when rapid rejection of ABO-incompatible kidney transplants was observed.[192] Preformed recipient isohemagglutinins bind to ABO antigens on endothelial surfaces in the organ, resulting in complement activation, endothelial damage, ischemic necrosis, and rapid (hyperacute) graft loss.[193] Transplantation across ABO lines will typically cause hyperacute rejection of kidney[194] and heart transplants,[195] although exceptions do exist.[196,197] Successful transplantation of kidneys and hearts across ABO lines has been accomplished by removing ABO antibodies in the recipient[196,198] or by taking advantage of the variable expression of ABO antigens on endothelial surfaces such as in A2

individuals.[199] For the most part, ABO-incompatible organs are avoided in kidney and heart transplantation.

ABO-incompatible (major mismatch) liver allografts are used in 6.9% of pediatric and 2.4% of adult liver recipients because of organ shortages.[200] Liver allografts are felt to be resistant to hyperacute rejection when transplanted across ABO barriers;[201] however, reports of hyperacute rejection do exist.[202,203] ABO-incompatible liver transplants are commonly associated with acute graft failure, with a 46% graft failure rate reported within 30 days of transplant.[203] Long-term results in adults demonstrate that the 1-year graft survival rate is lower compared with ABO-compatible transplants (30%[203] versus 80%[200]); however, the 1-year patient survival rate (52%) did not differ from that of recipients of ABO-compatible grafts matched for medical urgency and indication.[203] Pediatric recipients of ABO-incompatible livers appear to fare better, with reported 1- and 3-year patient and graft survival rates comparable to those of recipients of ABO-identical livers.[204] A combination of plasmapheresis (to remove recipient isohemagglutinins) and B-cell immunosuppression may be of benefit.[205,206] Currently, ABO-incompatible liver allografts are reserved for patients with fulminant liver failure in whom death is imminent without transplantation and when an ABO-compatible organ is not available.[207]

ABO-compatible but non-identical (minor mismatch) liver transplants are associated with a modest reductions in 1- and 3-year survival; however, the factor of urgency may account for some of the observed difference.[208] Approximately 15% of liver transplants performed at the University of Pittsburgh are

ABO minor mismatches and are also at risk for the immunohematologic complications described below.

Immunohematologic complications of ABO minor mismatch organ transplants

Unexpected antibodies of A and B specificity have been reported in adult[209] and pediatric[210] recipients of ABO minor mismatch (O donors to non-O recipients, or A or B donors to AB recipients) solid organs. Isohemagglutinins are produced by the viable donor lymphocytes passively transferred with the organ at the time of transplantation. The donor origin of the antibody has been confirmed using immunoglobulin allotyping.[211] Over 100 cases have been described involving transplantation of the liver,[209,212] kidney,[209,213] pancreas,[209] spleen,[209] heart,[209] lung,[209,214,215] and heart–lung.[209,216,217] A review[209] of reported cases found that the frequencies of antibodies and hemolysis were 70% (for both) in heart–lung transplant recipients, 40% and 29% respectively in liver transplant recipients, and 17% and 9% respectively in kidney transplant recipients. It has been suggested that the amount of lymphoid tissue transplanted with the organ accounts for these differences. Rarely, antibodies to red cell antigens outside the ABO system (i.e. anti-D and Kell) have been reported in association with transplanted kidney,[209] liver,[209] and heart–lung.[217]

Donor-derived ABO antibody (DDAb) typically develops 7–14 days after transplantation, with a time-course independent of the type of organ transplanted. The appearance of DDAb in the serum and the development of a positive direct antiglobulin test (DAT) are generally concurrent. Serum antibody is predominantly IgG, but may also be IgM. Red cell eluates contain anti-A, anti-B, or anti-A,B. DDAbs are short-lived antibodies that persist for a median of 5 weeks in kidney transplant recipients and 2–3 weeks in liver transplant recipients. It is not clear why the antibody disappears, nor whether it is related to elimination or downregulation of donor lymphocytes.

DDAbs are associated with hemolysis in a variable proportion of ABO minor mismatched organ transplant recipients. Among kidney transplant recipients with DDAb, approximately 50% developed hemolysis, and most required transfusion of red cells.[209] Hemolysis was complicated by acute renal failure requiring hemodialysis in several patients, and one patient died.

In liver transplant recipients, the incidence of hemolysis in those with DDAb is higher than in renal transplantation. Between 68%[209] and 100%[212] of liver transplant patients with DDAbs develop hemolysis. Although the hemolysis is usually mild and self-limiting, substantial morbidity associated with hemolysis, including acute renal failure, disseminated intravascular coagulation, hypotension, and multiorgan failure, has been reported.[209,212]

Currently there are no reliable factors that can predict which recipients of ABO-unmatched organs will develop DDAb or hemolysis. However, it is more likely in group A recipients of group O organs who receive cyclosporine or tacrolimus immunosuppression.[209,210,212,218] In most cases, the hemolysis associated with DDAb is mild and can be treated with transfusions. Transfused red cells should be of *organ donor* ABO group to replace susceptible red cells with cells that will not be hemolyzed. Plasma products should be of *recipient* ABO group to reduce the risk of hemolysis by providing soluble

ABO antigen capable of neutralizing DDAb. Patients who develop severe hemolysis can be treated with plasmapheresis or red cell exchange with donor-type red cells. Although there are anecdotal reports of success with these therapies,[209,212] their efficacy remains unproven. Steroids have not been shown to be of benefit in treating hemolysis in this setting.

CONCLUSIONS AND FUTURE CONSIDERATIONS

Transplant recipients are among the most complex patients requiring transfusion support. The immunosuppression required for successful transplantation requires specialized blood components to minimize the risk of transfusion-related complications. These requirements are summarized in Table 4.7. Clinical and technological advances in transfusion medicine are sure to play a role in future support of transplant recipients. Currently available growth factors for clinical use,[219] such as granulocyte–macrophage and

granulocyte colony-stimulating factors (GM-CSF and G-CSF), interleukin-11(IL-11), and erythropoietin, and those under clinical investigation, such as thrombopoietin,[220] shorten but do not eliminate pancytopenia in HSCT patients. Studies with these growth factors, however, have led to ex vivo expansion of hematopoietic stem cells, and transfusion of expanded hematopoietic progenitors during the early post-transplantation period may reduce or eliminate the duration of pancytopenia.[221] Apheresis technology has a key role to play in the development of adoptive immunotherapy. This investigational therapeutic intervention has been used in the treatment of some solid tumors, myeloid leukemias, and viral infections.[222] Donor lymphocyte transfusions collected by apheresis have also been used in solid-organ transplant recipients to treat hematopoietic malignancies.[223] Lastly, blood substitutes currently under study, including platelet[224] and red cell substitutes,[225] may find a niche in transplant recipients.

Table 4.7 Recommendations for use of specialized blood components in CMV seronegative hematopoietic stem cell transplant (HSCT) and solid-organ transplant recipients

Type	CMV negative/safe	Filtered	Irradiated
Autologous HSCT	Yes	Yes	Yes
Allogeneic HSCT	Yes[a]	Yes	Yes
Kidney	Yes[a]	Yes	No
Heart	Yes[a]	Yes	No
Lung	Yes[a]	Yes	No
Liver	Yes[a]	No	No

[a]CMV-negative pairs only. Components rendered CMV-safe by filtration are a reasonable substitute.

REFERENCES

1. McCullough J. Collection and use of stem cells: role of transfusion centers in bone marrow transplantation. *Vox Sang* 1994; **67** (suppl 3): 35–42.
2. Siena S, Bregni M, Brando B et al. Circulation of CD34+ hematopoietic stem cells in the peripheral blood of high-dose cyclophosphamide-treated patients: enhancement by intravenous recombinant human granulocyte–macrophage colony-stimulating factor. *Blood* 1989; **74**: 1905–14.
3. Applebaum FR. Allogeneic marrow transplantation and the use of hematopoietic growth factors. *Stem Cells* 1995; **13**: 344–50.
4. Besinger WI, Weaver CH, Applebaum FR et al. Transplantation of allogeneic peripheral blood stem cells mobilized by recombinant human granulocyte colony stimulating factor. *Blood* 1995; **85**: 1655–8.
5. Sheridan WP, Begley CG, Juttner CA et al. Effect of peripheral blood progenitor cell mobilized by filgrastin (G-CSF) on platelet recovery after high dose chemotherapy. *Lancet* 1992; **339**: 640–4.
6. Baer MR, Bloomfield CD. Controversies in transfusion medicine: prophylactic platelet transfusion therapy: pro. *Transfusion* 1992; **266**: 377–80.
7. Gaydos LA, Freireich EJ, Mantel N. The quantitative relation between platelet count and hemorrhage in patients with acute leukemia. *N Engl J Med* 1962; **266**: 905 9.
8. Gmur J, Burger J, Schanz U et al. Safety of stringent prophylactic platelet transfusion policy for patients with acute leukaemia. *Lancet* 1991; **338**: 1223–6.
9. Bishop JF, McGrath K, Wolf MM et al. Clinical factors influencing the efficacy of pooled platelet transfusion. *Blood* 1988; **71**: 383–7.
10. Slichter SJ. Platelet transfusion *therapy Hematol Oncol Clin North Am* 1991; **4**: 291–311.
11. Platelet Transfusion Therapy Consensus Conference. *JAMA* 1987; **257**: 1777–80.
12. Ancliff PJ, Machin SJ. Trigger factors for prophylactic platelet transfusion. *Blood Rev* 1998; **12**: 234–8.
13. Vengelen-Tyler V (ed). *AABB Technical Manual*, 13th edn. Bethesda MD: American Association of Blood Banks, 1999.
14. Hussein MA, Fletcher R, Long TJ et al. Transfusing platelets 2 h after the completion of amphotericin-B decreases its detrimental effect on transfused platelet recovery and survival. *Transfus Med* 1998; **8**: 43–7.
15. Bernstein SH, Nademanee AP, Vose JM et al. A multi-center study of platelet recovery and utilization in patients after myeloablative therapy and hematopoietic stem cell transplantation. *Blood* 1998; **91**: 3509–17.
16. McFarland JG, Anderson AJ, Slichter SJ. Factors influencing the transfusion response to HLA-selected apheresis donor platelets in patient's refractory to random platelet concentrates. *Br J Hematol* 1989; **73**: 380–6.
17. Gordon B, Tarantolo S, Ruby E et al. Increased platelet transfusion requirements is associated with multiple organ dysfunctions in patients undergoing hematopoietic stem cell transplantation. *Bone Marrow Transplant* 1998; **22**: 999–1003.
18. Delaflor-Weiss E, Mintz PD. The evaluation and management of platelet refractoriness and alloimmunization. *Transfus Med Rev* 2000; **14**: 180–96.
19. Murphy MF, Waters AH. Platelet transfusions: the problem of refractoriness. *Blood Rev* 1990; **4(1)**: 16–24.
20. Kickler TS. The challenge of platelet alloimmunization: management and prevention. *Transfus Med Rev* 1990; **4**: 8–18.
21. Kickler T, Kennedy SD, Braine HG. Alloimmunization to platelet specific antigens on glycoproteins IIb/IIIa and Ib/IX in multiply transfused thrombocytopenic patients. *Transfusion* 1990; **30**: 622–5.
22. Heal JM, Blumberg N, Masel D. An evaluation of crossmatching, HLA, and ABO

matching for platelet transfusions to refractory patients. *Blood* 1987; **70**: 23–30.

23. Murphy MF, Waters AH. Platelet transfusions: the problem of refractoriness. *Blood Rev* 1990; **4**: 16–24.

24. Daly PA, Schiffer CA, Aisner J, Wiemik PH. Platelet transfusion therapy: one-hour post-transfusion increments are valuable in predicting the need for HI-A-matched preparations. *JAMA* 1980; **243**: 435–8.

25. Duquesnoy RJ, Filip DJ, Rodey GE et al. Successful transfusion of platelets 'mismatched' for HLA antigens to alloimmunized thrombocytopenic patients. *Am J Hematol* 1977; **2**: 219–26.

26. Freedman J, Gafni A, Garvey MB, Blanchette V. A cost-effectiveness evaluation of platelet crossrnatching and HLA matching in the management of alloimmunized thrombocytopenic patients. *Transfusion* 1989; **29**: 201–7.

27. Kakaiya RM, Gudino MD, Miller VN et al. Four crossmatch methods to select platelet donors. *Transfusion* 1984; **24**: 35–41.

28. Kickler TS, Ness PM, Brame HG. Platelet crossmatching: a direct approach to the selection of platelet transfusions for the alloimmunized thrombocytopenic patient. *Am J Clin Pract* 1988; **90**: 69–72.

29. O'Connell BA, Lee EJ, Rothko K et al. Selection of histocompatible apheresis platelet donors by cross-matching random donor platelet concentrate. *Blood* 1992; **79**: 527–31.

30. Rachel JM, Sinor LT, Tawfik OW et al. A solid-phase red cell adherence test for platelet crossmatching. *Med Lab Sci* 1985; **42**: 194–5.

31. Petz LD, Garratty G, Calhoun L et al. Selecting donors of platelets for refractory patients on the basis of HLA antibody specificity. *Transfusion* 2000; **40**: 1446–56.

32. Friedberg RC, Donnelly SF, Boyd JC et al. Clinical and blood bank factors in the management of platelet refractoriness and alloimmunization. *Blood* 1993; **81**: 3428–34.

33. Besinger WI, Buckner CD, Clift RA et al. Plasma exchange for platelet alloimmunisation. *Transplantation* 1986; **41**: 602–5.

34. Zeigler ZR, Shadduck RK, Rosenfeld CS et al. Intravenous gamma globulin decreases platelet-associated IgG and improves transfusion responses in platelet refractory states. *Am J Hematol* 1991; **38**: 15–23.

35. Kickler T, Brame HG, Piantadosi S et al. A randomized, placebo controlled trial of intravenous gammaglobulin in alloimmunized thrombocytopenic patients. *Blood* 1990; **75**: 313–16.

36. Nagasawa T, Kim BK, Baldini MG. Temporary suppression of circulating anti-platelet alloantibodies by the massive transfusion of fresh, stored or lyophilized platelets. *Transfusion* 1978; **18**: 429–35.

37. Gardner FH, Helmer RE. Aminocaproic acid: use in control of hemorrhage in patients with amegakaryocytic thrombocytopenia. *JAMA* 1980; **243**: 35–7.

38. Dean A, Tuffin P. Fibrinolytic inhibitors for cancer-associated bleeding problems. *J Pain Sympt Manage* 1997; **13**: 20–4.

39. Shpilberg O, Blumenthal R, Safer O et al. A controlled trial of tranexamic acid therapy for the reduction of bleeding during treatment of acute myeloid leukemia. *Leuk Lymphoma* 1995; **19**: 141–4.

40. Merryman HT. Transfusion-induced alloimmunization and immunosuppression and the effects of leukocyte depletion. *Transfus Med Rev* 1989; **3**: 180–93.

41. Blachjman MA, Bardossy L, Carmen RA et al. An animal model of allogeneic donor platelet refractoriness: the effect of the time of leukodepletion. *Blood* 1992; **79**: 1371–5.

42. Bordin JO, Heddle NM, Blajchman MA. Biologic effects of leukocytes present in transfused cellular blood products. *Blood* 1994; **84**: 1703–21.

43. The Trial to Reduce Alloimmunization to Platelets Study Group. Leukocyte reduction and ultraviolet B irradiation of platelets to prevent alloimmunization and refractoriness

to platelet transfusions. *N Engl J Med* 1997; **337**: 1861–9.

44. Williamson LM, Wimperis JZ, Williamson P et al. Bedside filtration of blood products in the prevention of HLA alloimmunization – a prospective randomized study. *Blood* 1994; **83**: 3028–35.

45. Leitman SF. Post-transfusion graft-versus-host disease. In: *Special Considerations in Transfusing the Immunocompromised Patient.* (Smith DM, Silvergleid AJ, eds). Arlington, VA: American Association of Blood Banks, 1985.

46. Linden JV, Pisciotto PT. Transfusion-associated graft-versus-host disease and blood irradiation. *Transfus Med Rev* 1992; **6**: 116–23.

47. Anderson KC, Weinstein HJ. Transfusion-associated graft-versus-host disease. *N Engl J Med* 1990; **323**: 315–21.

48. Brubaker DB. Immunopathogenic mechanisms of pos-transfusion graft-vs-host disease. *Proc Soc Exp Biol Med* 1993; **202**: 122–47.

49. Rappeport JM, Mehm N, Reinherz EL et al. Acute graft-vs-host disease in recipients of bone marrow transplants from identical twin donors. *Lancet* 1979; **ii**: 717–20.

50. Gluckman E, Devergie A, Sohler J, Sauret JH. Graft-versus-host disease in recipients of syngeneic bone marrow. *Lancet* 1980; **1**: 253–4.

51. Vogelsang GB, Jones RJ, Hess AD et al. Induction of autologous graft-versus-host disease. *Transplant Proc* 1989; **21**: 2997–8.

52. Pelszynski MM, Moroff G, Luban NLC et al. Effect of γ-irradiation of red blood cell units on T-cell inactivation as assessed by limiting dilution analysis: implications for preventing transfusion-associated graft-versus-host disease. *Blood* 1994; **83**: 1683–9.

53. *Standards for Blood Banks and Transfusion Services*, 20th edn. Bethesda, MD: American Association of Blood Banks, 2000.

54. Draft guidance for irradiation of blood products. AABB Blood Bank Week. 1993; **10**: 1–2.

55. Rosen NR, Weidner JG, Boldt HD, Rosen DS. Prevention of transfusion-associated graft-versus-host disease: selection of an adequate dose of gamma radiation. *Transfusion* 1993; **33**: 125–7.

56. Moore GL, Ledford ME. Effects of 4000 rad irradiation on the in vitro storage properties of packed red cells. *Transfusion* 1985; **25**: 583–5.

57. Brugnara C, Churchill WH. Effect of irradiation on red cell cation content and transport. *Transfusion* 1992; **32**: 246–52.

58. Read EJ, Kodis C, Carter CS, Leitman SF: Viability of platelets following storage in the irradiated state: a pair controlled study. *Transfusion* 1988; **28**: 446–50.

59. Rock G, Adams A, Labow PS. The effects of irradiation on platelet function. *Transfusion* 1988; **28**: 451–5.

60. Moroff G, George VM, Siegl AM, Luban NLC. The influence of irradiation on stored platelets. *Transfusion* 1986; **26**: 453–6.

61. Valerius NH, Johansen KS, Nielsen OS et al. Effect of in vitro X-irradiation on lymphocyte and granulocyte function. *Scand J Haematol* 1981; **27**: 9–18.

62. Davey RJ, McCoy NC, Yu M et al. The effect of pre-storage irradiation on post-transfusion red cell survival. *Transfusion* 1992; **32**: 525–8.

63. Tegtmeier G. Posttransfusion cytomegalovirus infections. *Arch Pathol Lab Med* 1989; **113**: 236–45.

64. Smith KL, Kulski JK, Cobain T, Dunstan RA. Detection of cytomegalovirus in blood donors by polymerase chain reaction. *Transfusion* 1993; **33**: 497–503.

65. Hillyer CD, Emmiens RK, Zago-Novaretti M, Berkman EM. Methods for the reduction of transfusion-transmitted cytomegalovirus infection: filtration versus the use of seronegative donor units. *Transfusion* 1994; **34**: 929–34.

66. Hillyer CD, Lankford KV, Roback JD et al. Transfusion of the HIV-seropositive patient; immunomodulation, viral reactivation, and limiting exposure to EBV (HHV-4), CMV

(HHV-5), and HVV-6,7,8. *Transfus Med Rev* 1999; **13**: 1–17.

67. Preiksaitis JK, Brown L, McKenzie M. The risk of cytomegalovirus infection in seronegative transfusion recipients not receiving exogenous immunosuppression. *J Infect Dis* 1988; **157**: 523–9.

68. Sayers MH, Anderson KC, Goodnough LT et al. Reducing the risk for transfusion-transmitted cytomegalovirus infection. *Ann Intern Med* 1992; **116**: 55–62.

69. Smith KL, Cobain T, Dunstan RA. Removal of cytomegalovirus DNA from donor blood by filtration. *Br J Haematol* 1993; **83**: 640–2.

70. De Graan-Hentzen YC, Gratama JW, Mudde GC et al. Prevention of primary cytomegalovirus infection in patients with hematologic malignancies by intensive white cell depletion of blood products. *Transfusion* 1989; **29**: 757–60.

71. Preiksaitis JK. The cytomegalovirus-'safe' blood product: is leukoreduction equivalent to antibody screening? *Transfus Med Rev* 2000; **14**: 112–36.

72. Bowden RA, Slichter SJ, Sayers MH et al. Use of leukocyte-depleted platelets and cytomegalovirus-seronegative red blood cells for the prevention of primary cytomegalovirus infection after marrow transplant. *Blood* 1991; **78**: 246–50.

73. De Witte T, Schattenberg A, Van Dijk BA et al. Prevention of primary cytomegalovirus infection after allogeneic bone marrow transplantation by using leukocyte-poor random blood products from cytomegalovirus-unscreened blood bank donors. *Transplantation* 1990; **50**: 964–8.

74. Bowden RA, Slichter SJ, Sayers M et al. A comparison of filtered leukocyte-reduced and cytomegalovirus (CMV) seronegative blood products for the prevention of transfusion-associated CMV infection after marrow transplant. *Blood* 1995; **86**: 3598–603.

75. Van Prooijen HC, Visser JJ, Van Oostendorp WR et al. Prevention of primary transfusion associated cytomegalovirus infection in bone marrow transplant recipients by the removal of white cells from blood components with high affinity filters. *Br J Haematol* 1994; **87**: 144–7.

76. Pamphilon DH, Rider JR, Barbara JAJ, Williamson LM. Prevention of transfusion-transmitted cytomegalovirus infection. *Transfus Med* 1999; **9**: 115–23.

77. Center for Disease Control and Prevention, Infectious Disease Society of America, and the American Society of Blood and Marrow Transplantation. Guidelines for preventing opportunistic infections among hematopoietic stem cell transplant recipients. *Morb Mort Weekly Rep* 2000; **49**: (suppl) 11–14.

78. Narvios AB, Przepiorka D, Tarrand J et al. Transfusion support using filtered unscreened blood products for cytomegalovirus-negative allogeneic marrow transplant recipients. *Bone Marrow Transplant* 1998; **22**; 575–7

79. Blajchman MA, Goldman M, Freedman JJ, Sher GD. Proceedings of a Consensus Conference: Prevention of Post-transfusion CMV in the Era of Universal Leukoreduction. *Transfus Med Rev* 2001; **15**: 1–20.

80. Sniecinsky IJ, Petz LD, Oien L, Blume KG. Immunohematologic problems arising from ABO incompatible bone marrow transplantation. *Transplant Proc* 1987; **19**: 4609–11.

81. Lasky LC, Warkenin PI, Kersey JH et al. Hemotherapy in patients undergoing blood group incompatible bone marrow transplantation. *Transfusion* 1983; **23**: 277–85.

82. Hershko C, Gale RP, Ho W, Fitchen J. ABH antigens and bone marrow transplantation. *Br J Haematol* 1980; 44: 65–73.

83. Buckner CD, Clift RA, Sanders JE et al. ABO-incompatible marrow transplants. *Transplantation* 1978; **26**: 233–8.

84. Benjamin RJ, McGurk S, Ralston MS et al. ABO incompatibility as an adverse risk factor for survival after allogeneic bone marrow transplantation. *Transfusion* 1999; **39**: 179–87.

85. Greeno EW, Perry EH, Ilstrup SJ, Weisdorf DJ. Exchange transfusion the hard way: massive hemolysis following transplantation of bone marrow with minor ABO incompatibility. *Transfusion* 1996; **36**: 71–4.

86. Petz LD. Immunohematologic problems associated with bone marrow transplantation. *Transfusion Med Rev* 1987; **1**: 85–100.

87. Benjamin RJ, Antin JH. ABO-incompatible bone marrow transplantation: the transfusion of incompatible plasma may exacerbate regimen-related toxicity. *Transfusion* 1999; **39**: 1273–4.

88. Leo A, Mytilineos J, Voso MT et al. Passenger lymphocyte syndrome with severe hemolytic anemia due to an anti-Jka after allogeneic PBPC transplantation. *Transfusion* 2000; **40**: 632–6.

89. Lopez A, De la Rubia J, Arriaga F et al. Severe hemolytic anemia due to multiple red cell alloantibodies after an ABO-incompatible allogeneic bone marrow transplant. *Transfusion* 1998; **38**: 247–51.

90. De la Rubia J, Arriaga F, Andreu R et al. Development of non-ABO RBC alloantibodies in patients undergoing allogeneic HPC transplantation. Is ABO incompatibility a predisposing factor? *Transfusion* 2001; **41**: 106–10.

91. Franchini M, De Gironcoli M, Gandini G et al. Transmission of an anti-RhD alloantibody from donor to recipient after ABO-incompatible BMT. *Bone Marrow Transplant* 1998; **21**: 1071–3.

92. Chen FE, Owen I, Savage D et al. Late onset haemolysis and red cell autoimmunisation after allogeneic bone marrow transplant. *Bone Marrow Transplant* 1997; **19**: 491–5.

93. Gajewski JL, Petz LD, Calhoun L et al. Hemolysis of transfused group O red blood cells in minor ABO-incompatible unrelated donor bone marrow transplants in patients receiving cyclosporine without posttransplant methotrexate. *Blood* 1992; **79**: 3076–85.

94. Hows J, Beddow K, Gordon-Smith E et al. Donor-derived red blood cell antibodies and immune hemolysis after allogenic bone marrow transplantation. *Blood* 1986; **67**: 177–81.

95. Hazlehurst GRP, Brenner MK, Wimperis JZ et al. Haemolysis after T-cell depleted bone marrow transplantation involving minor ABO incompatibility. *Scand J Haematol* 1986; **37**: 1–3.

96. Robertson VM, Henslee PJ, Jennings CD et al. Early appearance of anti-A isohemagglutinin after allogeneic, ABO minor incompatible, T cell depleted bone marrow transplant. *Transplant Proc* 1989; **29**: 4612.

97. Broketa G, Simpson JK, Hammett L et al. Delayed hemolysis after minor ABO mismatched peripheral blood stem cell transplantation. *Transfusion* 1997; **37**: 37S (abst).

98. Oziel-Taieb S, Faucher-Barbey C, Chabannon C et al. Early and fatal immune haemolysis after so-called 'minor' ABO-incompatible peripheral blood stem cell allotransplantation. *Bone Marrow Transplant* 1997; **19**: 1155–6.

99. Salmon JP, Michaux S, Hermanne JP et al. Delayed massive immune hemolysis mediated by minor ABO incompatibility after allogeneic peripheral blood progenitor cell transplantation. *Transfusion* 1999; **30**: 824–7.

100. Laurencet FM, Sanii K, Bressoud A et al. Massive delayed hemolysis following PBPCT with minor ABO incompatibility. *Hematol Cell Ther* 1997; **39**: 159–62.

101. Weaver CH, Longin K, Buckner CD, Besinger W. Lymphocyte content in peripheral blood mononuclear cells collected after the administration of recombinant human granulocyte colony-stimulating factor. *Bone Marrow Transplant* 1994; **13**: 411–15.

102. Worel N, Greinix WT, Schneider B et al. Regeneration of erythropoiesis after related- and unrelated-donor BMT or peripheral blood HPC transplantation: a major ABO mismatch means problems. *Transfusion* 2000; **40**: 543–50.

103. Lee JH, Lee KH, Kim S et al. Anti-A isoagglu-

tinin as a risk factor for the development of pure red cell aplasia after major ABO-incompatible allogeneic bone marrow transplantation. *Bone Marrow Transplant* 2000; **25**: 179–84.

104. Blacklock HA, Gilmore MJML, Prentice HG et al. ABO-incompatible bone-marrow transplantation: removal of red blood cells from donor marrow avoiding recipient antibody depletion. *Lancet* 1982; **ii**: 1061–4.

105. Tichelli A, Gratwohl A, Wenger R et al. ABO-incompatible bone marrow transplantation: in vivo adsorption, an old forgotten method. *Transplant Proc* 1987; **19**: 4632–7.

106. Bensinger WI, Buckner CD, Clift RA et al. Comparison of techniques for dealing with major ABO-incompatible marrow transplants. *Transplantation* 1987; **19**: 4605–8.

107. Anderson KC. The role of the blood bank in hematopoietic stem cell transplantation. *Transfusion* 1992; **32**: 272–85.

108. Petz LD: Bone marrow transplantation. In: *Clinical Practice of Transfusion Medicine*, 3rd edn (Petz LD, Swisher SN, Kleinman S et al eds). New York: Churchill Livingstone, 1996: 757–82.

109. Hows JM, Chipping PM, Palmer S, Gordon-Smith EC. Regeneration of peripheral blood cells following ABO incompatible allogeneic bone marrow transplantation for severe aplastic anemia. *Br J Haematol* 1983; **53**: 145–51.

110. Gmur JP, Burger J, Schaffner A et al. Pure red cell aplasia of long duration complicating major ABO-incompatible bone marrow transplantation. *Blood* 1990; **75**: 290–5.

111. Braine HG, Sensenbrenner LL, Wright SK et al. Bone marrow transplantation with major ABO blood group incompatibility using erythrocyte depletion of marrow prior to infusion. *Blood* 1982; **60**: 420–5.

112. Drobyski W, Thibodeau S, Truitt RL et al. Third party mediated graft rejection and graft-versus-host disease after T-cell depleted bone marrow transplantation as demonstra-

ted by hypervariable DNA probes and HLA-DR polymorphism. *Blood* 1989; **74**: 2285–94.

113. Strauss RG. Granulocyte transfusion. In: *Principles of Transfusion Medicine*: (Rossi EC, Simon TL, Moss GS, Gould SA eds). Baltimore: Williams & Wilkins, 1996: 321–8.

114. McCullough J. Granulocyte transfusion. In: *Clinical Practice of Transfusion Medicine*, 3rd ed (Petz LD, Swisher SN, Kleinman S et al, eds). New York: Churchill Livingstone, 1996: 413–32.

115. Hubel K, Dale DC, Engert A, Liles WC. Current status of granulocyte (neutrophil) transfusion therapy for infectious diseases. *J Infect Dis* 2001; **183**: 321–8.

116. Bensinger WI, Price TH, Dale DC et al. The effects of daily recombinant human granulocyte colony stimulating factor administration on normal granulocyte donors undergoing leukapheresis. *Blood* 1993; **81**: 1883–7.

117. Dale DC, Liles WC, Llewellyn C et al. Neutrophil transfusions: kinetics and function of neutrophils mobilized with granulocyte-colony-stimulating factor and dexamethasone. *Transfusion* 1998; **38**: 713–21.

118. Liles WC, Huang JE, Llewellyn C et al. A comparative trial of granulocyte colony-stimulating factor and dexamethasone, separately and in combination, for the mobilization of neutrophils in the peripheral blood of normal volunteers. *Transfusion* 1997; **37**: 182–7.

119. Leitman SF, Oblitas JM. Optimization of granulocytapheresis mobilization regimens using granulocyte colony stimulating factor (G-CSF) and dexamathasone (dexa). *Transfusion* 1997; **37**(Suppl): 67S (abstr).

120. Liles WC, Rodger E, Dale DC. Combined administration of G-CSF and dexamethasone for the mobilization of granulocytes in normal donors: optimization of dosing. *Transfusion* 2000; **40**: 642–4.

121. Roilides E, Walsh TJ Pizzo PA, Rubin M. Granulocyte colony stimulating factor enhances the phagocytic and bactericidal

activity of normal and defective human neutrophils. *J Infect Dis* 1991; **163**: 579–83.

122. Wright DG, Robichaud KJ, Pizzo PA, Deisscroth AB. Lethal pulmonary reaction associated with the combined use of amphotericin B and leukocyte transfusions. *N Engl J Med* 1981; **304**: 1185–9.

123. Lightfoot T, Leitman SF, Stroncek DF. Storage of G-CSF-mobilized granulocyte concentrates. *Transfusion* 2000; **40**: 1104–10.

124. Bhatia S, McCullough J, Perry EH et al. Granulocyte transfusions: efficacy in treating fungal infections in neutropenic patients following bone marrow transplantation. *Transfusion* 1994; **34**: 226–32.

125. Hester JP, Dignani MC, Anaissie EJ, Kantarjian HM et al. Collection and transfusion of granulocyte concentrates from donors primed with granulocyte stimulating factor and response of myelosuppressed patients with established infection. *J Clin Apheresis* 1995; **10**: 188.

126. Bontempo FA, Lewis JH, Van Thiel DH et al. The relation of preoperative coagulation findings to diagnosis, blood usage, and survival in adult liver transplantation. *Transplantation* 1985; **39**: 532–6.

127. Kang Y, Lewis JH, Navalgund A et al. ε-Aminocaproic acid for treatment of fibrinolysis during liver transplantation. *Anesthesiology* 1987; **66**: 766–73.

128. Triulzi DJ, Griffith BJ. Blood usage in lung transplantation. *Transfusion* 1998; **38**: 12–15.

129. Nicol SL, Shirey RS, Banez-Sese GC, Ness PM. Significance of residual plasma from group O additive solution RBC transfusions. *Transfusion* 1995; **35**(Suppl): S247 (abst).

130. Casanueva M, Valdes MD, Ribera MC. Lack of allo-immunization to D antigen in D-negative immunosuppressed liver transplant recipients. *Transfusion* 1994; **34**: 570–2.

131. Jain A, Venkataramanan R, Lever J et al. FK506 and pregnancy in liver transplant patients. *Transplantation* 1993; **56**: 751.

132. Ramsey G, Cornell FW, Hahn LF et al. Red cell antibody problems in 1000 liver transplants. *Transfusion* 1989; **29**: 396–9.

133. Ramsey G, Cornell FW, Hahn LF et al. Incompatible blood transfusions in liver transplant patients with significant red cell alloantibodies. *Transplant Proc* 1989; **21**: 3531.

134. Rubin RH. Impact of cytomegalovirus infection on organ transplant recipients. *Rev Infect Dis* 1990; **12**(Suppl): S754–66.

135. Ho M. Epidemiology of cytomegalovirus infections. *Rev Infect Dis* 1990; **12**(Suppl): S701–10.

136. Grundy JE, Super M, Sweny P et al. Symptomatic cytomegalovirus infection in seropositive kidney recipients: reinfection with donor virus rather than reactivation of recipient virus. *Lancet* 1988; **371**: 132–5.

137. Preiksaitis JK. Indications for the use of cytomegalovirus seronegative blood products. *Transfus Med Rev* 1991; **5**: 1–17.

138. Fryd DS, Peterson PK, Ferguson RM et al. Cytomegalovirus as a risk factor in renal transplantation. *Transplantation* 1980; **30**: 436–9.

139. Laske A, Gallino A, Carrel T et al. Cytomegalovirus infection and prophylaxis in heart transplantation. *Transplant Proc* 1993; **25**: 1427–8.

140. Grossi P, Minoli L, Percivalle E et al. Clinical and virological monitoring of human cytomegalovirus infection in 294 heart transplant recipients. *Transplantation* 1995; **59**: 847–51.

141. Egan JJ, Barber L, Lomax J et al. Detection of human cytomegalovirus antigenaemia: a rapid diagnostic technique for predicting cytomegalovirus infection/pneumonitis in lung and heart transplant recipients. *Thorax* 1995; **50**: 9–13.

142. Smyth RL, Scott JP, Borysiewicz LK et al. Cytomegalovirus infection in heart–lung transplant recipients: risk factors, clinical associations, and response to treatment. *J Infect Dis* 1991; **164**: 1045–50.

143. Winston DJ, Wirin D, Shaked A, Busuttil RW. Randomised comparison of ganciclovir and high-dose acyclovir for long-term cytomegalovirus prophylaxis in liver-transplant recipients. *Lancet* 1995; **346**: 69–74.

144. Rakela J, Wiesner RH, Taswell HF et al. Incidence of cytomegalovirus infection and its relationship to donor-recipient serologic status in liver transplantation. *Transplant Proc* 1987; **19**: 2399–402.

145. Lopez-Plaza I, Triulzi DJ, Kusne S. Effectiveness of decreasing the risk of transfusion transmitted CMV infection in heart and lung transplant patients using CMV safe blood components. *Transfusion* 1999; **39**: S385 (abst).

146. Triulzi DT, Nalesnik M. Microchimerism, graft versus host disease, and tolerance in solid organ transplantation. *Transfusion* 2001; **41**: 419–26.

147. Wisecarver JL, Cattral MS, Langnas AN et al. Transfusion-induced graft-versus-host disease after liver transplantation. *Transplantation* 1994; **58**: 269–71.

148. Sola MA, Espana A, Redondo P et al. Transfusion-associated acute graft-versus-host disease in a heart transplant recipient. *Br J Dermatol* 1995; **132**: 626–30.

149. Andany MA, Martinez W, Arnal F et al. Transfusion-associated graft-versus-host disease in a renal transplant recipient. *Nephrol Dial Transplant* 1994; **9**: 196–8.

150. Andersen CB, Ladefoged SD, Taaning E. Transfusion-associated graft-versus-graft and potential graft-versus-host disease in a renal allotransplanted patient. *Hum Pathol* 1992; **23**: 831–4.

151. Whittington PF, Rubin CM, Alonso EM et al. Complete lymphoid chimerism and chronic graft-versus-host disease in an infant recipient of a hepatic allograft from an HLA-homozygous parental living donor. *Transplantation* 1996; **62**: 1516–19.

152. Ohtsuka Y, Sakemi T, Ichigi Y et al. A case of chronic graft-versus-host disease following living-related donor kidney transplantation. *Nephron* 1998; **78**: 215–17.

153. Shivdasani RA, Haluska FG, Dock NL et al. Graft-versus-host disease associated with transfusion of blood from unrelated HLA-homozygous donors. *N Engl J Med* 1993; **328**: 766–9.

154. McKenna RM, Takemoto SK, Terasaki PI. Anti-HLA antibodies after solid organ transplantation. *Transplantation* 2000; **69**: 319–26.

155. Opelz G, Sengar DPS, Mickey MR et al. Effect of blood transfusions on subsequent kidney transplants. *Transplant Proc* 1973; **5**: 253–9.

156. Kissmeyer-Nielsen F, Olsen S, Petersen VP, Fjeldborg O. Hyperacute rejection of kidney allografts, associated with pre-existing humoral antibodies against donor cells. *Lancet* 1966; **ii**: 662–5.

157. Horimi T, Terasaki PI, Chia D, Sasaki N. Factors influencing the paradoxical effect of transfusions on kidney transplants. *Transplantation* 1983; **35**: 320–3.

158. Colombe BW, Lou CD, Salvatierra O, Jr, Garovoy MR. Two patterns of sensitization demonstrated by recipients of donor-specific transfusion: limitations to control by Imuran. *Transplantation* 1987; **44**: 509.

159. Bayle F, Masson D, Zaoui P et al. Beneficial effect of one HLA haplo- or semi-identical transfusion versus three untyped blood units on alloimmunization and acute rejection episodes in first renal allograft recipients. *Transplantation* 1995; **59**: 719–23.

160. Radvany RM, Patel KM. Donor-specific transfusions. Donor–recipient HLA compatibility, recipient HLA haplotype, and antibody production. *Transfusion* 1988; **28**: 137–41.

161. Cheigh JS, Suthanthiran M, Fotino M et al. Minimal sensitization and excellent renal allograft outcome following donor-specific blood transfusion with a short course of cyclosporine. *Transplantation* 1991; **51**: 378–81.

162. Lagaaij EL, Hennemann IPH, Ruigrok M et al. Effect of one-HLA-DR antigen-matched

and completely HLA-DR-mismatched blood transfusions on survival of heart and kidney allografts. *N Engl J Med* 1989; **321**: 701–5.

163. Ahmed Z, Terasaki PI. Effect of transfusion. In: *Clinical Transplants* (Terasaki PI, ed). Los Angeles: UCLA Tissue Typing Laboratory, 1991: 305–12.

164. Christiaans MH, Overhof-de Roos R, Nieman F et al. Donor-specific antibodies after transplantation by flow cytometry: relative change in fluorescence ration most sensitive risk factor for graft survival. *Transplantation* 1998; **65**: 427.

165. Fisher M, Chapman JR, Ting A, Morris PJ. Alloimmunization to HLA antigens following transfusion with leukocyte-poor and purified platelet suspensions. *Vox Sang* 1985; **49**: 331–5.

166. Flye MW, Burton K, Mohanakumar T et al. Donor-specific transfusions have long-term beneficial effects for human renal allografts. *Transplantation* 1995; **60**: 1395–401.

167. Bayle F, Masson D, Zaoui P et al. One HLA haplo-identical transfusion in first renal allograft recipients: effect on alloimmunisation, acute rejection episodes, and graft survival. *Transplant Proc* 1995; **27**: 2457–8.

168. Lavee J, Kormos RL, Duquesnoy RJ et al. Influence of panel reactive antibody and positive lymphocytotoxic crossmatch on cardiac transplant survival. *J Heart Lung Transplant* 1991; **10**: 921–9.

169. Sucui-Foca N, Reed E, Marboe C. The role of anti-HLA antibodies in heart transplantation. *Transplantation* 1993; **51**: 716–24.

170. Smith JD, Danskine AJ, Rose ML, Yacoub MH. Specificity of lymphocyte antibodies formed after cardiac transplantation and correlation with rejection episodes. *Transplantation* 1992; **53**: 1358–62.

171. McCarthy JF, Cook DJ, Massad MG et al. Vascular rejection post heart transplantation is associated with positive flow cytometric cross-matching. *Eur J Cardiothorac Surg* 1998; **14**: 197–200.

172. Barr ML, Cohen DJ, Benvenisty AI et al. Effect of anti-HLA antibodies on the long term survival of heart and kidney allografts. *Transplant Proc* 1993; **25**(1 Pt 1): 262–4.

173. Johnson CP, Munda R, Alexander JW et al. The effect of donor-specific transfusions on rat heart allograft survival. *Transplantation* 1984; **38**: 575–8.

174. Dong E, Stinson EB, Griepp RB et al. Cardiac transplantation following failure of previous cardiac surgery. *Surg Forum* 1973; **24**: 150–2.

175. Cooper DKC, Boyd ST, Lanza RP, Barnard CN. Factors influencing survival following heart transplantation. *Heart Transplant* 1983; **3**: 86–91.

176. Katz MR, Barnhart GR, Goldman MH et al. Pretransplant transfusions in cardiac allograft recipients. *Transplantation* 1987; **43**: 499–501.

177. Kerman RH, Van Buren CT, Lewis RM et al. The impact of HLA A, B, and DR blood transfusions and immune responder status on cardiac allograft recipients treated with cyclosporine. *Transplantation* 1988; **45**: 333–7.

178. Keogh A, Baron D, Chang V. The effect of blood pretransfusion on orthotopic cardiac transplantation. *Transplant Proc* 1987; **19**: 2503.

179. Opelz G. Factors affecting the outcome of kidney and heart transplants today. 8th Scientific Meeting of the Transplantation Society of Australia and New Zealand, March 1990.

180. van der Mast BJ, Balk AHMM. Effect of HLA-Dr-shared blood transfusion on the clinical outcome of heart transplantation. *Transplantation* 1997; **63**: 1514–19.

181. Keenan RJ, Zeevi A. Immunologic consequences of transplantation. *Basic Biol Thorac Surg* 1995; **5**: 107–20.

182. Nelson KA, Albert RK, Davies C et al. Association of antibody to donor HLA class I antigens with early acute lung rejections in lung transplant recipients. *Am J Respir Crit Care Med* 1994; **149**: A1097.

183. Bando K, Paradis IL, Similo S et al. Obliterative bronchiolitis after lung and heart–lung transplantation. An analysis of risk factors and management. *J Thorac Cardiovasc Surg* 1995; **110**: 4–13.

184. Jaramillo A, Smith MA, Phelan D et al. Development of ELIS-detected anti-HLA antibodies precedes the development of bronchiolitis obliterans and correlates with progressive decline in pulmonary function after lung transplanatation. *Transplantation* 1999; **67**: 1155–61.

185. Bird G, Friend P, Donaldson P et al. Hyperacute rejection in liver transplantation: a case report. *Transplant Proc* 1989; **21**: 3742–4.

186. Takaya S, Bronsther O, Iwaki Y et al. The adverse impact on liver transplantation of using positive cytotoxic crossmatch donors. *Transplantation* 1992; **53**: 400–6.

187. Lobo PI, Spencer C, Douglas MT et al. The lack of long-term detrimental effects on liver allografts caused by donor-specific anti-HLA antibodies. *Transplantation* 1993; **55**: 1063–6.

188. Weber T, Marino IR, Kang YG et al. Intraoperative blood transfusions in highly alloimmunized patients undergoing orthotopic liver transplantation. *Transplantation* 1989; **47**: 797–801.

189. Yokoi Y, Yamaguchi A, Kimura H et al. Donor-specific transfusion: critical role of class I antigen presenting molecules in rat liver transplantation. *Transplant Proc* 1995; **27**: 1558–9.

190. Rouch DA, Thistlethwaite JR, Lichtor L et al. Effect of massive transfusion during liver transplantation on rejection and infection. *Transplant Proc* 1988; **20**: 1135–7.

191. Palomo JC, Jiminez C, Moreno E et al. Effects of intraoperative blood transfusion on rejection and survival after orthotopic liver transplantation. *Transplant Proc* 1995; **27**: 2326–7.

192. Starzl TE, Marchioro TL, Holmes JH, Waddell WR. The incidence, cause and significance of immediate and delayed oliguria or anuria after human renal transplantation. *Surg Gynecol Obstet* 1964; **188**: 819–27.

193. Demetris AJ, Murase N, Nakamura K et al. Immunopathology of antibodies as effectors of orthotopic liver allograft rejection. *Semin Liver Dis* 1992; **12**: 51–9.

194. Cook DJ, Graver B, Terasaki PI. ABO incompatibility in cadaver donor kidney allografts. *Transplant Proc* 1987; **19**: 4549–52.

195. Cooper DKC. Clinical survey of heart transplantation between ABO blood group incompatible recipients and donors. *J Heart Transplant* 1990; **9**: 376–81.

196. Alexandre GPJ, Squiffiet JP, De Bruyere M et al. Present experiences in a series of 26 ABO-incompatible living donor renal allografts. *Transplant Proc* 1987; **19**: 4538–42.

197. Carvana RJ, Zumbro GL Jr, Hoff RG et al. Successful cardiac transplantation across an ABO blood group barrier. *Transplantation* 1988; **46**: 472–4.

198. Cooper DKC, Ye Y, Kehoe M et al. A novel approach to 'neutralization' of preformed antibodies: cardiac allotransplantation across the ABO blood group barrier as a paradigm of discordant transplantation. *Transplant Proc* 1992; **24**: 566–71.

199. Nelson PW, Helling TS, Shield CF et al. Current experience with renal transplantation across the ABO barrier. *Am J Surg* 1992; **164**: 541–4.

200. Belle SH, Beringer KC, Murphy JB, Detre KM. The Pitt–UNOS liver transplant registry. In: *Clinical Transplants 1992* (Terasaki PI, Cecka JM, eds). Los Angeles, CA: UCLA Tissue Typing Laboratory, 1992: 7.

201. Demetris AJ, Jaffe R, Tzakis A et al. Antibody mediated rejection of human liver allografts: transplantation across ABO blood group barriers. *Transplant Proc* 1989; **21**: 2217–20.

202. Gugenheim J, Samuel D, Fabiani B et al. Rejection of ABO incompatible liver allografts in man. *Transplant Proc* 1989; **21**: 2223–4.

203. Farges O, Kalil AN, Samuel D et al. The use of ABO-incompatible grafts in liver transplanta-

tion: a lifesaving procedure in highly selected patients. *Transplantation* 1995; **59**: 1124–33.

204. Cacciarelli TV, So SKS, Lim J et al. A reassessment of ABO incompatibility in pediatric liver transplantation. *Transplantation* 1995; **60**: 757–68.

205. Mor E, Skerrett D, Manzarbeitia C et al. Successful use of an enhanced immunosuppressive protocol with plasmapheresis for ABO-incompatible mismatched grafts in liver transplant recipients. *Transplantation* 1995; **59**: 986–90.

206. Renard TH, Andrews WS. An approach to ABO-incompatible liver transplantation in children. *Transplantation* 1992; **53**: 116–21.

207. Conference of the Consensus on the Indications of Liver Transplantation. *Hepatology* 1994; **20**(1 pt 2).

208. Gordon RD, Iwatsuki S, Esquivel CO et al. Liver transplantation across ABO blood groups. *Surgery* 1986; **100**: 342–8.

209. Ramsey G. Red cell antibodies arising from solid organ transplants. *Transfusion* 1991; **31**: 77–86.

210. Manack L, Triulzi DJ, Lopez-Plaza I. Donor derived red cell antibodies in pediatric liver transplant recipients treated with FK-506. *Transfusion* 1999; **39**(Suppl): S507 (abst).

211. Swanson JL, Sastamoinen RM, Steeper TA, Sebring ES. Gm allotyping to determine the origin of red cell antibodies in recipients of solid organ transplants. *Vox Sang* 1987; **52**: 75–8.

212. Triulzi DJ, Shirey RS, Ness PM, Klein AS. Immunohematologic complications of ABO unmatched liver transplants. *Transfusion* 1992; **32**: 829–33.

213. Orchard J, Young NT, Smith C et al. Severe intravascular haemolysis in a renal transplant recipient due to anti-B of donor origin. *Vox Sang* 1990; **59**: 172–5.

214. Magrin GT, Street AM, Williams TJ, Esmore DS. Clinically significant anti-A derived from B lymphocytes after single lung transplantation. *Transplantation* 1993; **56**: 466–7.

215. Taaning E, Morling N, Mortensen SA et al. Hemolytic anemia due to graft-derived anti-B production after lung transplantation. *Transplant Proc* 1994; **26**: 1739.

216. Perlman EJ, Shirey RS, Farkosh M et al. Immune hemolytic anemia following heart–lung transplantation. *Immunohematology* 1992; **8**: 38–40.

217. Knoop C, Andrien M, Antoine M et al. Severe hemolysis due to a donor anti-D antibody after heart–lung transplantation. Association with lung and blood chimerism. *Am Rev Respir Dis* 1993; **148**: 504–6.

218. Bradley R, Triulzi DJ, Starzl TE. Donor derived red cell antibodies in liver transplant recipients treated with FK-506. *Transfusion* 1993; **33**(Suppl): S163 (abst).

219. Cottler-Fox M, Klein HG. Transfusion support of hematology and oncology patients: the role of recombinant hematopoietic growth factors. *Arch Pathol Lab Med* 1994; **118**: 417–20.

220. Kuter DJ. Thrombopoietins and thrombopoiesis: a clinical perspective. *Vox Sang* 1998; **74**: 75–85.

221. Bertolini F, Battaglia M, Pedrazzoli P et al. Megakaryocytic progenitors can be generated ex vivo and safely administered to autologous peripheral blood progenitor cell transplant recipients. *Blood* 1997; **89**: 2679–88.

222. Brenner M, Rossig C, Sili U et al. Transfusion medicine: new clinical applications of cellular immunotherapy. In: *American Society of Hematology Education Program Book*. 2000: 356–75.

223. Nalesnik MA, Rao AS, Zeevi A et al. Autologous lymphokine-activated killer cell therapy of lymphoproliferative disorders arising in organ transplant recipients. *Transplant Proc* 1997; **29**: 1905–6.

224. Lee DH, Blajchman MA. Novel treatment modalities. New platelet preparations and substitutes. *Br J Haematol* 2001; **114**: 496–505.

226. Stowell CP, Levin J, Spiess BO, Winslow RM. Progress in development of RBC substitutes. *Transfusion* 2001; **41**: 287–99

5 Blood and blood component use in cardiac surgery or 'why do cardiac surgical patients bleed?'

Robert R Jeffrey, Michael J Desmond

INTRODUCTION

Although blood and blood component transfusion requirements have steadily fallen since the introduction of improved techniques for cardiopulmonary bypass (CPB), such as membrane oxygenators, a significant proportion of patients still require to be transfused following cardiac surgical procedures. In some series,[1] up to 25% of patients have increased postoperative bleeding, necessitating re-operation in up to 5%,[2] which contributes to increased morbidity and perhaps mortality in less well patients.

Transfusion practises vary widely between institutions for first-time coronary artery bypass surgery,[3] and do not appear to be related to patient or surgical variables. In one audit study involving 18 institutions, the mean allogeneic red cell use per patient was 2.9 (range 0.4–6.3), with up to 97% of patients receiving plasma and 80% platelets in some institutions.[4]

MECHANISMS RESPONSIBLE FOR DISORDERED HAEMOSTASIS

Since up to one-third of patients who are re-explored for postoperative bleeding may not demonstrate a surgical cause, and the commonest indication for red cell transfusion is peri- and postoperative bleeding, it is pertinent to consider some of the mechanisms responsible for this excess bleeding that is uniformly associated with CPB.

The causes of non-surgical bleeding are complex and multifactorial, and may be attributed to the period of CPB. Coagulation factor XII is activated when blood contacts the artificial surface of the CPB circuit, and activated XIIa triggers amplifying mechanisms involving coagulation, fibrinolysis, and complement activation. Platelets and white cells are also activated when they come into contact with the synthetic surfaces of the extracorporeal circuit, and are important in the systemic inflammatory response (SIRS) associated with cardiac surgery.

As systemic heparinization is utilized for CPB, the factors responsible for bleeding must include heparin-induced effects – including anticoagulation, fibrinolysis, and complement activation related to XIIa – and (most importantly) disturbance of platelet function associated with CPB.[5] Heparin binds to the endothelial surface as a complex, and 'heparin rebound' is a term used to explain the later reappearance of heparin in the circulation following CPB. The duration of this effect may be temperature-related and may play a role in postoperative bleeding.

Cardiac surgeons usually attribute postoperative bleeding to an inadequate protamine dose for heparin reversal and to the heparin rebound effect. Despite the attraction of this belief (it would be reversed by protamine), there is unfortunately little evidence to support this widely held contention and additional doses of protamine are not without anticoagulant effect.

Heparin exerts its anticoagulant effect by binding with antithrombin III, and this complex inhibits several of the coagulation factors, including XIIa, X1a, and Xa. Heparin also induces platelet dysfunction prior to CPB and increases fibrinolysis.[6] At the termination of CPB, heparin is neutralized with protamine, but the residual effects on platelets and fibrinolysis may not be completely reversed. Early studies suggested that fibrinolysis, which is increased with hypothermia and prolonged CPB times, was the principal cause of postoperative bleeding. However, other factors are undoubtedly involved, and the role of platelet dysfunction cannot be underestimated.

Preoperative template bleeding time, which depends on platelet function,[7] fails to predict postoperative blood transfusion. However, prolonged bleeding time following CPB was associated with postoperative blood loss.[8] Following the administration of heparin and before the onset of CPB, platelet function is disturbed.[6] However, it would appear that CPB itself has further deleterious effects upon platelet function. Platelet dysfunction cannot be wholly attributed to thrombocytopenia induced by haemodilution.[9] The platelet membrane receptor GPIIIb/IIa is expressed following platelet activation during CPB, and reduced expression of this receptor was proposed as a potential cause of platelet dysfunction. However, Kestin et al[10] did not demonstrate during CBP any reduction in the expression of GPIIb/IIIa or of GPIb-Ix, the receptor involved in binding of the platelet to von Willebrand protein on exposed damaged sub-endothelium, which is the initial event in platelet aggregation.

Since these important membrane receptors seem to be preserved during CPB, other mechanisms must be acting upon the platelet, and it has been suggested that a primary fibrinolytic syndrome is triggered by mechanisms that remain unresolved but may be extrinsic to the platelet. These factors include hypothermia and heparin. Heparin affects platelet function through inhibition of thrombin, which is an important platelet agonist promoting aggregation and degranulation. Further, heparin inhibits platelet function through generation of plasmin, which may induce cleavage of GPIb-Ix, and one group has demonstrated that aprotonin, a serine protease inhibitor with potent antifibrinolytic activity, may protect this receptor during CPB and be responsible for this drug's significant antibleeding effects.[11]

Initial platelet reactions in the control of bleeding from an incision involve the interaction of the platelet with the exposed basement membrane and the von Willebrand receptor. Further platelets are attracted to the area by many stimuli, and the platelets at this stage reversibly aggregate. Following aggregation, the platelets degranulate, releasing further chemotactic factors, including serotonin, ADP, and thromboxane, from their granules. Following degranulation, the platelet plug has formed and this state is not reversible. Coagulation factors interact with the platelet, among which fibrin is one of the most important stimulating platelet aggregation.

WHAT CAN BE DONE TO REDUCE BLEEDING?

As the principal indication for postoperative red cell transfusion is continued postoperative bleeding, any intervention that reduces this will have a beneficial effect in reducing red cell transfusion. Preoperative evaluation of patients attending for cardiac surgery involving CPB therefore involves critical assessment to make sure that they do not have an underlying bleeding diathesis. A careful history may identify patients who have a bleeding tendency or known hepatic dysfunction, and further appropriate investigations can then be undertaken.

As preoperative anaemia is an important factor identifying those patients who will require postoperative transfusion, a full blood count is mandatory and identifies anaemic patients in whom appropriate investigations should be arranged. Similarly, thrombocytopenia may be found, and the advice of a haematologist is often valued in treating these patients in order to improve preoperative platelet counts. It is routine for patients attending for cardiac surgery to have a clotting screen performed, but this seldom identifies those with previously unknown bleeding problems. It is, however, of particular value in those patients who are on warfarin, and may help in the therapies adopted to reverse the

affects of this or other oral anticoagulant drugs. Bleeding times are not undertaken as a routine preoperative investigation and, as noted above, are of limited valve in identifying patients who will bleed excessively in the postoperative period.

A careful drug history is important, and particular attention should be paid to aspirin and other non-steroidal anti-inflammatory drugs (NSAIDs), which act by inhibiting cyclooxygenase, the enzyme that catalyses the first step in the synthesis from arachidonic acid of thromboxane (a powerful stimulus to further platelet aggregation and a vasoconstrictor) by the platelet and of prostacyclin (a potent inhibitor of platelet aggregation and a vasodilator) by the endothelium.

Other important drugs in this area include the recently introduced clopidogrel, a potent ADP antagonist. The antiplatelet effects of aspirin and clopidogrel appear to last for the lifespan of the platelet, reflecting its inability (unlike vascular endothelium) to manufacture further cyclooxygenase. It would therefore seem appropriate in elective stable angina patients to discontinue aspirin or clopidogrel for 7 days to allow replenishment of functioning platelets. However, withdrawal of aspirin therapy may precipitate myocardial ischaemia, and careful clinical consideration should be given to evaluating the balance between ischaemic vascular events and reduced postoperative bleeding and transfusion.

From a surgical point of view, haemostasis must be paramount in the operator's mind when undertaking surgery. Careful attention to haemostasis before administration of heparin is important in minimizing postoperative blood loss. Heparin should be administered after mobilization of the internal mammary if it is to be left attached until immediately prior to its use. However, if the internal mammary artery is to be divided then heparinization is mandatory prior to its division. Following the period of CPB, protamine should not be given to reverse the effects of the heparin until all major bleeding sites on the surface of the heart and major vessels have been surgically secured.

DRUGS TO REDUCE BLEEDING

Aprotinin is a non-specific serine protease inhibitor derived from bovine lung tissue. It possesses significant antifibrinolytic activity and appears to 'protect' the platelet from the deleterious effects of CPB. Aprotinin was first used in patients undergoing re-do cardiac operations or for cardiac surgery in the presence of infective endocarditis, where it has been conclusively demonstrated to reduce blood loss. Rich[12] reviewed 21 studies in approximately 5000 patients undergoing primary coronary artery bypass graft or valve operations. The reduction in blood loss varied from 33% to 66% with full-dose aprotinin therapy. In 15 of these studies, significant reductions in transfusion requirements were reported, ranging from 31% to 85%. Controversy has surrounded its more widespread use in first-time CABG surgery, since some authors have questioned whether this drug may predispose to early graft failure. Alderman and colleagues,[13] using data from the IMAGE trial, demonstrated significantly increased saphenous vein graft occlusion in those patients receiving aprotinin in first-time coronary revascularization (15.4% versus 10.9%; $p = 0.03$). When statistical allowance was made for other factors predisposing to

vein graft occlusion (e.g. female gender, no prior aspirin therapy, and small and poor distal vessels) the risk associated with aprotinin versus control became non-significant overall. In a subgroup of patients with more adverse characteristics predisposing to early saphenous graft failure, occlusions occurred in 23.0% of aprotinin-treated and 12.4% of placebo-treated patients ($p = 0.01$). The reduction in wound drainage and the reduction in allogeneic blood use were 43% and 49% respectively ($p < 0.0001$). It can be questioned whether the benefit of the savings in allogeneic transfusion is worth the increased risk of early graft occlusion.

Tranexamic acid is another antifibrinolytic drug, which shares many of the pharmacological properties of aprotinin, and indeed in the meta-analysis undertaken by Laupacis and Fergusson,[14] is also of similar benefit in reducing postoperative bleeding in cardiac surgery. There is a cost economy with the use of tranexamic acid compared with high-dose aprotinin.

In this same meta-analysis, desmopressin acetate (DDAVP) was not shown to reduce postoperative bleeding after cardiac surgery. Its use is therefore not recommended, except in the management of specific haemostatic defects known to be responsive to its use (e.g. Von Willebrand disease).

BLOOD COMPONENT THERAPY WITH FRESH-FROZEN PLASMA AND PLATELETS

Patients who attend for surgery on oral anticoagulation with warfarin (or similar drugs) and for whom there has been insufficient time to reduce their INR (international normalized ratio) to a satisfactory level in the immediate preoperative period will benefit from fresh-frozen plasma (FFP) given postoperatively to correct their clotting abnormality. There is no study that has examined the routine use of FFP in cardiac surgery in an attempt to reduce postoperative bleeding or transfusion.

There has been no randomized controlled study showing that routine platelet administration reduces postoperative bleeding or allogeneic blood requirements following cardiac surgery. However, the importance of appropriate platelet transfusion in those patients who attend on preoperative aspirin therapy cannot be underestimated. Aprotinin has been demonstrated to reduce the postoperative bleeding in such patients, and its use should be considered in aspirin-pretreated patients.

AUTOLOGOUS TECHNIQUES IN CARDIAC SURGERY

Autologous techniques potentially applicable to cardiac surgery include preoperative autologous donation (PAD), acute normovolaemic haemodilution (ANH), and peri/postoperative cell salvage (PCS).

Preoperative autologous donation

PAD has been demonstrated to be feasible, but the organization and administration of such a programme can be difficult. Patients who pre-donate must be guaranteed a date for operation, since pre-donated blood has a finite lifespan. In the UK, it is difficult to guarantee a date for cardiac surgery. Some transfusionists have been understandably reluctant to consider this 'high-risk' group for pre-donation in local donor clinics. Patients are then required to travel greater distances to attend the cardiac centre in order to predeposit blood, creating further logistical problems. If the PAD is to be effective, the patient should be able to make up the haemoglobin removed from them at venesection prior to attending for their surgery. They should also not suffer any adverse response to the donation itself. The risks avoided by the procedure are primarily those of viral transmission associated with allogeneic transfusion, and are relatively very small. If the patient fails to make up for the haemoglobin removed at PAD, they will attend for surgery in a relatively anaemic state and will be more at risk of needing a transfusion of some description to cover their surgery. The ISPOT group found in their meta-analysis of trials of PAD that the procedure decreased exposure to allogeneic blood but increased exposure to any transfusion (allogeneic and/or autologous).[15] Some of the risks of allogeneic transfusion (clerical error resulting in a unit being given to the wrong patient or a unit developing bacterial contamination during collection and storage) are also inherent in PAD, and would therefore be increased by anything that increases the overall transfusion rate. The risks of the donation procedure are likely to be higher in those patients awaiting cardiac surgery than in many other groups for several reasons. Patients on a variety of drugs (e.g. β-blockers, calcium-channel blockers, nitrates, angiotensin-converting enzyme (ACE) inhibitors, etc.) to control angina and/or hypertension will have an impaired response to the blood volume reduction associated with the procedure, and may have an increased incidence of vaso-vagal syncope. In patients with impaired ventricular function or significant left main stem disease, the hypotension associated with a faint may take longer to correct and may in extremes result in angina or even myocardial infarction. It can be argued that cardiac surgery patients have had their cardiac problems very well delineated prior to surgery, and, with appropriate selection procedures, a safe PAD programme can be run for many of them. Birkmeyer and colleagues[16] have put this particular issue into perspective in a cost-effectiveness analysis of PAD in cardiac surgery. They calculated that a fatality rate from the predeposit programme itself of greater than 1 in 101 000 donations would negate all likely benefit from the programme. Anyone wishing to set up such a programme in cardiac surgery has therefore to overcome considerable logistical difficulties and at the same time provide an impeccable level of safety. PAD may well have a place in other areas, but currently its use in cardiac surgery is limited and will remain so while allogeneic blood remains readily available and relatively safe.

Acute normovolaemic haemodilution

Haemodilution is an inevitable consequence of cardiopulmonary bypass with a crystalloid prime, and in some units additionally up to a litre of the patient's own blood is withdrawn prior to the onset of cardiopulmonary bypass and stored aside from the bypass machine for administration following the reversal of heparin. The logic behind the procedure is that the haemodilution, by causing a temporary anaemia, reduces the amount of red cells lost during the operation (assuming that the volume of surgical blood loss remains the same). A significant quantity of the patient's own fresh clotting factors and platelets have

also avoided exposure to the bypass circuit, and should theoretically be of value in reducing bleeding when they are reinfused after bypass and reversal of heparinization. If this is the case then it should be an easy matter to prove it. The evidence that ANH will reduce intraoperative red cell loss and thereby allogeneic requirements comes largely from mathematical modelling.[17,18] Weiskopf's most recent analysis[18] concluded that surgical blood loss should be 0.50 or more for ANH to begin to 'save' erythrocytes and 0.70 or more of the patient's blood volume for ANH to save 1 unit of erythrocytes, for the usual surgical patient with an initial hematocrit of 0.32–0.36 and a transfusion 'trigger' hematocrit (the value at which transfusion is initiated) of 0.18–0.21. There is a paucity of clinical data to show that this technique on its own actually reduces the need for allogeneic transfusion, and two UK consensus conferences at the Royal College of Physicians in Edinburgh have concluded as much.[19,20] There is no doubt that allowing patients to tolerate a degree of normovolaemic haemodilution after surgery (in other words, lowering one's transfusion target) will reduce the amount of allogeneic transfusion. It is possible that ANH has made its biggest contribution to reducing allogeneic transfusion by demonstrating that patients will tolerate lower haemoglobin levels than had previously been considered necessary.

Peri/postoperative cell salvage

PCS can be employed during surgery or postoperatively. It can also employ devices for processing and washing or can involve the use of whole-blood reinfusion without any processing. The intraoperative use of centrifugal cell separators for PCS in cardiac surgery has been shown to be beneficial in reducing allogeneic transfusion requirements.[21,22] The overall safety of PCS utilizing centrifugal cell separation would appear to be high when done with appropriate standard operating procedures.

During surgery, when the patient is not systemically anticoagulated, PCS entails the use of a locally anticoagulated collection system for spilt blood. After surgery, the mediastinal drainage blood is defibrinated and does not normally require anticoagulation. In either case, the blood can be reinfused whole or after concentrating and washing using centrifugal cell separators. During the period of heparinization for bypass, 'spilt blood' is normally returned to the cardiotomy reservoir (whole) and recirculated using the bypass machine. Significant blood loss can (and does) sometimes occur at the start of the operation, prior to heparinization, and can also occur following the administration of protamine. On these occasions, PCS is particularly useful. Off-bypass coronary artery grafting is a recent development made possible by advances in surgical equipment and techniques, but in the process the bypass machine is no longer available for recirculating blood loss, and PCS will be more important in reducing allogeneic blood use in these cases.

Debate continues as to whether salvaged blood should be washed or unwashed when returned to the patient. Unwashed techniques are simpler, but in cardiac surgery they have largely only been used in the postoperative period (with the exception of recirculation of shed blood by the bypass circuit). Also, it has been suggested that they may induce a coagulopathy (leading to increased postoperative bleeding), and that they confer little benefit in terms of overall allogeneic blood consumption.[23] The same authors also found that the use of cell washing (in the few control patients who actually bled sufficiently postoperatively to warrant such intervention) was not associated with evidence of coagulopathy, and was probably as effective overall. This was only a small study in itself; however, a recent meta analysis by Huet and colleagues[24] found the reinfusion of unwashed mediastinal drainage blood to be only marginally effective in reducing allogeneic blood use. Although washed techniques are more complicated and require more technical support, their advantage is that particulate debris, heparin, and activated clotting factors can be removed from the salvaged blood prior to its reinfusion. There is of course the theoretical disadvantage that any unactivated clotting factors are also washed from the red cells that are then returned to the patient in a saline suspension. In very two large published series that included cardiac patients, this has not proved to be a significant problem,[25,26] and indeed these two papers are a testimony to the relative safety of the technique. Both of these groups employed centrifugal cell separation for PCS with washing, and between them included approximately 46 000 multispecialty patients. In practice, where large volumes of autologous blood are salvaged in PCS in this way, a washout of clotting factors is as inevitable as it would be if a large haemorrhage were dealt with by allogeneic red cell transfusion alone. Eventually, if the volumes are large enough, the use of allogeneic clotting factors will become necessary.

Unlike the other modalities of autologous transfusion, PCS has the ability to make a source of blood available for a haemorrhaging patient in proportion to the rate at which haemorrhage is occurring. It does not entail any extra physiological disturbance for the patient, and (provided that the blood is kept with the patient) it avoids the risk of clerical error resulting in mismatched transfusion. Cardiac surgery, by its nature, can very occasionally result in sudden and massive blood loss. Having a PCS service available for cardiac patients improves their safety margin in this respect. Whether the overall savings in allogeneic blood offset the costs and effort involved depends on several factors. Firstly, the service must be deployed sufficiently often to be well run and not expose patients to further avoidable risks. Secondly, the service needs to be deployed in situations where significant blood loss can reasonably be expected, and it must be readily available in other situations where such loss is possible but less likely. If cost is the only consideration in deploying PCS then it will be deployed less frequently and only in those cases considered likely to bleed substantially. If patient safety (safety in the smooth running of the PCS service), avoidance of allogeneic transfusion, and conservation of the allogeneic blood supply are given greater weight then PCS will be deployed more frequently.

TARGET HAEMOGLOBIN FOLLOWING CARDIAC SURGERY

The patient's body weight and starting haemoglobin, together with the surgical/anaesthetic team's preferred target postoperative haemoglobin, determine the amount of blood loss the patient can sustain without the need for a blood transfusion (i.e. while receiving only crystalloid or colloid volume replacement). The nature of the cardiac operation,[27] together with the technique and skill of the team carrying it out, will determine the likely extent of blood loss sustained by the patient. There are therefore a limited number of data points that require collection in order to provide a database that would allow regular feedback to clinicians on their performance regarding blood conservation. Such data, as well as being an indicator of the quality of the cardiac surgical/anaesthetic service, would allow more effective targeting of the blood conservation measures listed above. The benefit of such data has been demonstrated in the sphere of orthopaedic surgery by Mercuriali and colleagues,[28] who developed an algorithm based on their own unit's transfusion data to predict when more aggressive blood conservation measures were necessary. Such principles are likely to be equally applicable to cardiac surgery.

Transfusion guidelines in the postoperative period are desirable, and the question arises of the haemoglobin level at which one should transfuse a stable patient. This has important implications for the quantities of red cells utilized in the postoperative period. The adoption of an 8.0 g/dl threshold compared with a 9.0 g/dl or even a 10.0 g/dl threshold can result in considerable blood savings. Stover and colleagues[4] demonstrated the importance of a liberal versus a conservative transfusion policy in terms of blood utilization. It would therefore seem reasonable to adopt a trigger for red cell transfusion of 8.0 g/dl in the postoperative period. The same group also looked at the effect of different initial haematocrits (haematocrits on arrival in the intensive care unit postoperatively) on outcomes following coronary artery bypass grafting. They found that, rather than being predictive of a good outcome, a high initial haematocrit was an independent predictor of myocardial infarction.[29] The decision to transfuse must be based on more factors than simply the patient's haemoglobin level in the immediate postoperative period. Some patients describe dizziness and faintness with low haemoglobin levels, and it is appropriate to transfuse these patients to alleviate these symptoms. Again, in the elderly (greater than 80 years of age) it is reasonable to consider a less conservative transfusion policy, whilst in the younger patient one may accept lower haemoglobin levels of 7.0 g/dl in the immediate postoperative period. A period of haemoconcentration follows any episode of CPB, assuming normal renal function, and typically patients appear to gain about 10 g/dl between day one and day five. The appropriate management of anaemia may in a number of patients therefore be to await the development of this haemoconcentration.

SUMMARY

Cardiac surgery is a large specialty and an expanding one. Currently it uses approximately 10–20% of the UK blood resource, with the proportion in the USA being similar.[29] As the safety of the allogeneic blood supply is now probably higher than at any time previously, the alternatives to allogeneic transfusion have themselves to offer a very high level of safety. Save for careful attention to surgical haemostasis, no one technique of blood conservation is necessarily applicable in all patients. It is possible to say, as we have done, that it is safe to lower target haemoglobin levels in comparison with the values aimed for in the past. It is not possible, however, to offer a single value for postoperative haemoglobin or haematocrit that will be suitable for all patients. Patients who are asymptomatic, stable, and recovering well from their surgery are unlikely to benefit from transfusion. Their initial anaemia will be due in part to haemodilution that will recover, and further recovery can be hastened by iron therapy. The other various methods of blood conservation outlined above will not be necessary in all patients, and are unlikely to be cost-effective if deployed in all patients. Ongoing audit of transfusion practice is essential, although currently poorly developed in the UK. The use of algorithms would allow the selective application of different techniques such as cell salvage and the use of aprotinin. The results of such audits would also allow clinicians to alter their transfusion practice in the light of good data. The wider deployment of the more expensive forms of blood conservation will become mandatory if we move from the present situation of viewing allogeneic blood as readily available and relatively safe. It should be noted that in the UK (and elsewhere) many millions of pounds have been spent to introduce universal leukodepletion of blood products because of a theoretical risk of transmission of the prion responsible for variant Creutzfeldt–Jakob disease (vCJD). Safety of the blood supply is therefore not an absolute concept but is very susceptible to public and political perception. The ready availability of allogeneic blood is something that in the developed world we have come to take for granted. This situation may not pertain indefinitely. Demographic changes will reduce the number of blood donors in relation to potential recipients, and also the introduction of screening tests for new diseases may also reduce the number of potential donors. The possible development of a screening test for vCJD has precipitated a major contingency planning exercise by the UK National Blood Service to examine how to cope with a reduction of 10–50% of the donor pool. If such circumstances were to arise, the arguments for restricting the use of allogeneic transfusion would increase considerably. We have argued for more conservative allogeneic transfusion strategies simply because the available evidence suggests that they represent good practice.

REFERENCES

1. Woodman RC, Harker LA. Bleeding complications associated with cardiopulmonary bypass. *Blood.* 1990; **76**: 1680–97.

2. Unsworth-White MJ, Herriot A, Valencia O et al. Resternotomy for bleeding after cardiac operation: a marker for increased morbidity and mortality. *Ann Thorac Surg* 1995; **59**: 664–7.

3. Goodnough LT, Johnston MFM, Toy PTCY et al. The variability of transfusion practice in coronary artery bypass surgery. *JAMA* 1991; **265**: 86–90.

4. Stover EP, Siege LC, Parks R et al. Variability in transfusion practice for coronary artery bypass surgery persists despite national consensus guidelines: a 24-institution study. *Anesthesiology* 1998; **88**: 327–33.

5. Kirklin JK, Westaby S, Blackstone EH. Complement and the damaging effects of cardiopulmonary bypass. *J Thorac Cardiovasc Surg* 1983; **86**: 845–57.

6. Khuri SF, Valeri R, Loscalzo J et al. Heparin causes platelet dysfunction and induces fibrinolysis before cardiopulmonary bypass. *Ann Thorac Surg* 1995; **60**: 1008–14.

7. Burns ER, Billett HH, Frater RWM. The preoperative bleeding time as a predictor of postoperative hemorrhage after cardiopulmonary bypass. *J Thorac Cardiovasc Surg* 1986; **92**: 310–12.

8. Harker LA. Bleeding after cardiopulmonary bypass. *N Engl J Med* 1986; **314**: 1446–8.

9. Khuri SF, Wolfe JA, Josa M. Haematologic changes during and following cardiopulmonary bypass and their relationship to the bleeding time and non-surgical blood loss. *J Thorac Cardiovasc Surg* 1992; **107**: 94–107.

10. Kestin AS, Valeri CR, Khuri SF. The platelet function defect of cardiopulmonary bypass *Blood* 1993; **82**: 107–11.

11. Van Oeveren W, Harder MP, Roozendaal K et al. Aprotonin protects platelets against the initial effect of cardiopulmonary bypass. *J Thorac Cardiovasc Surg* 1990; **99**: 788–97.

12. Rich JB. The efficacy and safety of aprotinin use in cardiac surgery. *Ann Thorac Surg* 1998; **66**(5 Suppl): S6–11; discussion S25–8.

13. Alderman EL, Levy JH, Rich JB et al. Analyses of coronary graft patency after aprotinin use: results from the International Multicenter Aprotinin Graft Patency Experience (IMAGE) trial. *J Thorac Cardiovasc Surg* 1998; **116**: 716–30.

14. Laupacis A, Fergusson D. Drugs to minimize perioperative blood loss in cardiac surgery: meta-analyses using perioperative blood transfusion as the outcome. The International Study of Peri-operative Transfusion (ISPOT) Investigators. *Anesthes Analges* 1997; **85**: 1258–67.

15. Forgie MA, Wells PS, Laupacis A, Fergusson D. Preoperative autologous donation decreases allogeneic transfusion but increases exposure to all red blood cell transfusion: results of a meta-analysis. International Study of Perioperative Transfusion (ISPOT) Investigators. *Arch Intern Med* 1998; **158**: 610–16.

16. Birkmeyer JD, AuBuchon JP, Littenberg B et al. Cost-effectiveness of preoperative autolo-

gous donation in coronary artery bypass grafting. *Ann Thorac Surg* 1994; **57**: 161–8; discussion 168–9.

17. Weiskopf RB. Mathematical analysis of isovolemic hemodilution indicates that it can decrease the need for allogeneic blood transfusion. *Transfusion* 1995; **35**: 37–41.

18. Weiskopf RB. Efficacy of acute normovolemic hemodilution assessed as a function of fraction of blood volume lost. *Anesthesiology* 2001; **94**: 439–46.

19. Final consensus statement of the Royal College of Physicians of Edinburgh Consensus Conference on Autologous Transfusion, 4–6 October 1995. *Br J Haematol* 1996; **92**: 766.

20. Update statement from the conference 'Autologous transfusion, 3 years on – What is new?' what has happened?" held at the Royal College of Physicians of Edinburgh, 10–11 November 1998. *Br J Haematol* 1999; **104**: 640.

21. Breyer RH, Engelman RM, Rousou JA, Lemeshow S. Blood conservation for myocardial revascularization. Is it cost effective? *J Thorac Cardiovasc Surg* 1987; **93**: 512–22.

22. Bell K, Stott K, Sinclair CJ et al. A controlled trial of intra-operative autologous transfusion in cardiothoracic surgery measuring effect on transfusion requirements and clinical outcome. *Transfus Med* 1992; **2**: 295–300.

23. Vertrees RA, Conti VR, Lick SD et al. Adverse effects of postoperative infusion of shed mediastinal blood. *Ann Thorac Surg* 1996; **62**: 717–23.

24. Huet C, Salmi LR, Fergusson D et al. A meta-analysis of the effectiveness of cell salvage to minimize perioperative allogeneic blood transfusion in cardiac and orthopedic surgery. International Study of Perioperative Transfusion (ISPOT) Investigators. *Anesthes Analges* 1999; **89**: 861–9.

25. Tawes RL Jr. Duvall TB. Is the 'salvaged-cell syndrome' myth or reality? *Am J Surg* 1996; **172**: 172–4.

26. Giordano GF, Giordano GM, Wallace BA et al. An analysis of 9,918 consecutive perioperative autotransfusions. *Surg Gynecol Obstet* 1993; **176**: 103–10.

27. Hardy JF, Perrault J, Tremblay N et al. The stratification of cardiac surgical procedures according to use of blood products: a retrospective analysis of 1480 cases. *Can J Anaesthes* 1991; **38**: 511–17.

28. Mercuriali F, Inghilleri G. Proposal of an algorithm to help the choice of the best transfusion strategy. *Curr Med Res Opin* 1996; **13**: 465–78.

29. Spiess BD, Ley C, Body SC et al. Haematocrit value on intensive care unit entry influences the frequency Q-wave myocardial infarction after coronary artery bypass grafting. The Institutions of the Multicentre Study of Perioperative Ischemia Research Group. *J Thorac Cardiovasc Surg* 1998; **116**: 460–7.

6 Surgical transfusions: Non-cardiac

Lawrence Tim Goodnough, Terri G Monk

THE BENEFIT OF TRANSFUSION

The therapeutic goal of a blood transfusion is to increase oxygen delivery according to the physiologic need of the recipient. To achieve this outcome, the decision to transfuse each unit of blood should be based on the physiologic mechanisms that may be causing the deficit in oxygen delivery. If a physiologic need exists, a transfusion should be given on a unit-by-unit basis. If no physiologic need is identified, there is no role for transfusion.

The usual response to an acute reduction in hemoglobin level in the normovolemic state is to increase cardiac output to maintain adequate oxygen delivery[1] (Figure 6.1). The heart is therefore the principal organ at risk in acute anemia. Myocardial anaerobic metabolism, indicating inadequate O_2 delivery, occurs when lactate metabolism in the heart converts from lactate uptake to lactate production. The normal whole-body oxygen-extraction ratio (the ratio of oxygen consumption to oxygen delivery) is 20–25%. The oxygen-extraction ratio approaches 50% when myocardial lactate production occurs, indicating anerobic metabolism. In a normal heart, this lactate production and an oxygen-extraction ratio of 50% occur at a hemoglobin level of approximately 3.5–4 g/dl.[2] In a model of coronary stenosis, the anerobic state occurs at a hemoglobin level of approximately 6–7 g/dl.[3] These values

also coincide with the onset of ventricular wall motion abnormalities.

The observations that the critical extraction ratio and anaerobic threshold occur at a different hemoglobin level in different physiologic states suggest that the oxygen-extraction ratio represents a reasonable indicator of the adequacy of oxygen delivery and, therefore, need for transfusion. No single number, either extraction ratio or hemoglobin level, can serve as an absolute indicator of transfusion need. However, the use of such a physiologic value in conjunction with clinical assessment of the patient status permits a rational decision

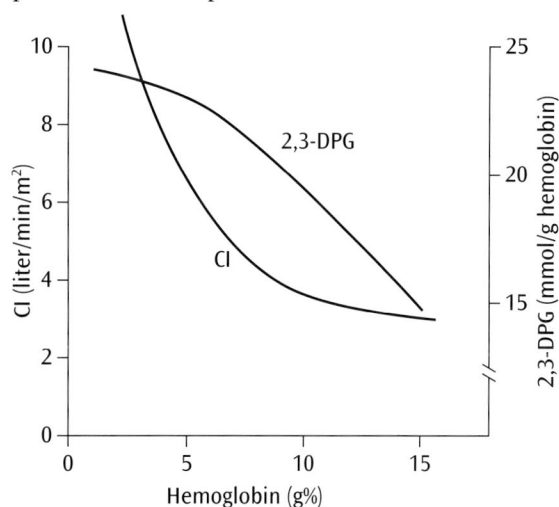

Figure 6.1
Effect of anemia on cardiac index (CI) and 2,3-diphosphoglycerate (2,3-DPG). Reprinted by permission of *The New England Journal of Medicine*, Finch CA, Lenfant C, Vol. **286**: 407–15, 1972; © 1972 Massachusetts Medical Society. All rights reserved.

regarding the appropriateness of transfusion prior to the onset of hypoxia or ischemia.[4]

If a transfusion is appropriate, then a benefit should occur. In a literature assessment of the benefit of transfusion, data on mortality are the clearest. In a review of 16 reports of the surgical outcomes in Jehovah's Witnesses who underwent major surgery without blood transfusion, mortality associated with anemia occurred in 1.4% of the 1404 operations.[5] In one large study, the risk of death was found to be higher in patients with cardiovascular disease than in those without.[6] These data suggest that in surgery-induced anemia, survival as an outcome may be improved with blood transfusion. In a study of patients undergoing repair of hip fracture, 84 patients were randomly assigned to receive transfusions either at a predetermined threshold (a hemoglobin level of 10.0 g/dl) or only if symptoms of anemia occurred (with the lower limit of hemoglobin set at 8.0 g/dl); the respective mortality rates at 60 days were 4.8% and 11.9%.[7] Because of the small numbers of patients in the study, one needs to be cautious about drawing definitive conclusions. In a large, retrospective study of elderly patients who underwent surgical repair of hip fracture, the use of perioperative transfusion in patients with hemoglobin levels as low as 8.0 g/dl did not appear to influence 30-day or 90-day mortality.[8]

In a multi-institutional Canadian study by Hebert et al,[9] 418 critical-care patients were to receive red cell transfusions when the hemoglobin level dropped below 7.0 g/dl, with hemoglobin maintenance in the range of 7.0–9.0 g/dl, and 420 patients were to receive transfusions when the hemoglobin level dropped below 10.0 g/dl, with levels maintained in the range of 10.0–12.0 g/dl. The 30-day mortality rates were not different in the two groups (18.7% versus 23%, $p = 0.11$), indicating that a transfusion threshold as low as 7.0 g/dl is as safe as a higher transfusion threshold of 10.0 g/dl in critical-care patients. A follow-up analysis found that the more restrictive strategy of red blood cell transfusion appeared to be safe in most patients with cardiovascular disease; but among a subgroup of patients with ischemic heart disease, there was a non significant ($p = 0.30$) decrease in overall survival among patients treated according to the restrictive transfusion strategy.[10] Clearly, more data are needed to determine when transfusion in this setting is beneficial, particularly in patients known to have risk factors for ischemic heart or cerebral disease.

Data on morbidity, on the other hand, are much less clear. Gore et al[11] hypothesized that a reduction in morbidity may be possible with transfusion in critically ill patients, especially those with hypoxia or sepsis, by optimizing oxygen delivery and minimizing the frequency of potential complications. In their study, hemodynamic and oxygen transport measurements were examined in five severely burned male patients who did not receive blood transfusions for 36–48 hours after the operative incision. The hemoglobin level was then raised by 3 g/dl with multiple transfusions. While transfusion raised the red cell mass significantly and increased oxygen delivery, the physiologic benefit seemed marginal. The O_2 extraction ratio, in particular, was not markedly deranged before the transfusion, which indicates that the compensation for the anemia was quite adequate. In addition, there was no change in oxygen consumption, which suggests that blood transfusion may not have benefited these critically ill patients.

In a report by Babineau et al,[12] the benefit of transfusion was examined in 30 surgical intensive care unit patients who were normovolemic and hemodynamically stable. Once again, transfusion increased the hemoglobin level and total oxygen delivery but had a negligible effect on oxygen consumption. There were no important hemodynamic benefits in this group of patients. One can conclude from these data that the assumed benefit of an increase in the red cell mass does not always translate into a true benefit in terms of oxygen transport in critically ill patients.

Silent perioperative myocardial ischemia has been observed in patients undergoing non-cardiac[13] as well as cardiac[14] surgery. Hemoglobin levels ranging from 6.0 to 10.0 g/dl (a range in which indicators other than hemoglobin may identify patients who may benefit from blood) therefore need to be the most closely scrutinized.[4,15] A study of elderly patients who were undergoing elective non-cardiac surgery found that intraoperative or postoperative myocardial ischemia was more likely to occur in patients with hematocrits below 28%, particularly in the presence of tachycardia.[16] In the absence of a physiologic need in a stable, non-bleeding patient, a decline in hemoglobin level alone is not a good reason to give a transfusion.[17]

Published data related to the benefit of transfusion on function are scant. Kim et al[18] did not find a relationship between hemoglobin level and length of hospital stay for 332 patients who underwent total hip arthroplasty. Johnson et al[19] did not identify any overall correlation between hematocrit value

and exercise capacity in a randomized prospective trial of two transfusion strategies in 39 patients undergoing elective myocardial revascularization. No significant differences in postoperative exercise endurance were found between patients who received transfusions in order to maintain a hematocrit of 32% and patients who received transfusions only if the hematocrit dropped below 25%. A study by Wu et al[20] analyzed the relationships among anemia blood transfusion and mortality in a retrospective analysis of nearly 80 000 elderly (>65 years) patients, hospitalized for acute myocardial infarction. In this study, lower hematocrit values on admission were associated with higher 30-day mortality rates. Secondly, anemia (defined as hemocrit <39%) was present on hospital admission in nearly half (43.7%) of patients and was clinically significant (i.e. 33% or lower) in 10.4% of patients. Finally, transfusion in patients with hematocrit levels ≤33% at admission was associated with significantly lower 30-day mortality.

There are no documented effects on terms of length of hospital stay, rehabilitation, return to work, or healthcare costs as a consequence of transfusion. Whether blood transfusion is associated with a clinically significant immunomodulatory effect (e.g. perioperative infections) is the subject of debate.[21,22]

TRANSFUSION PRACTICES

Utilization review

Audits of a facility's transfusion practices can improve the efficiency and appropriateness of transfusion if they are performed in a timely manner and if the results are communicated to physicians who order transfusions for their patients.[23] Audits of the use of plasma and platelet products are particularly amenable to this approach and can reduce the use of blood components by up to 50%.[24] However, a multihospital study found that a retrospective utilization review did not reduce the use of red cell transfusions.[25]

This lack of success may be a consequence of several factors. First, it is difficult to evaluate the appropriateness of the use of transfusion in patients with hemorrhage who are seen in emergency rooms and trauma units, operating rooms, and intensive care units. Second, some studies have found that fewer than 5% of red cell transfusions are unjustified.[26] One reason for this low rate may be that clinical indicators for transfusion appropriateness are too generous. It is difficult to improve transfusion practices if over 95% of transfusions are found to be justified. Third, there is often no clearly documented information in a medical chart that explains why a transfusion was administered. In only two-thirds of cases in which postoperative transfusions are administered on the day of surgery is blood loss or a change in vital signs noted in the medical record, and the rationale for transfusion is documented in fewer than one-third of cases.[27] This lack of success has raised questions regarding the overall value and effectiveness of retrospective utilization review.[26] Point-of-care testing and transfusion algorithms show promise in improving transfusion appropriateness.[28]

Surgery

The discharge hematocrit levels of patients who underwent orthopedic surgery ranged from 31% to 34% in the mid-1980s, suggesting that perisurgical anemia was being treated too aggressively with transfusion.[29] Subsequently however, the overall rate of transfusions for patients undergoing hip and knee arthroplasty has declined by 15–35%.[30] The patient's gender has been found to influence the outcome of transfusion in such patients,[31] and this has been attributed to the fact that physicians use the same hematocrit value as a threshold for transfusion for both women and men, without taking into account that women have lower hematocrit levels. Studies found substantial variability in the use of red cell transfusions for patients undergoing total hip and knee arthroplasty,[30] and the variability was attributed to the lack of clearly defined criteria for transfusion and to hospital-specific differences.

There is also considerable variation in transfusion practices among institutions with respect to patients who undergo cardiac surgery. A multicenter audit of 18 institutions demonstrated a wide range in the outcomes of allogeneic transfusions among patients who underwent primary coronary artery bypass gratting.[32] A subsequent study reported similar findings.[33] The variability in transfusion outcomes in these patients has also been attributed to differences in training that are specific to hospitals and physicians, rather than to differences in patient populations.[34]

Guidelines for transfusion

Guidelines for blood transfusion have been issued by several organizations, including a US National Institutes of Health consensus conference on perioperative transfusion of red cells,[35] the American College of Physicians,[36] the American Society of Anesthesiologists,[14] and the Canadian Medical Association.[37] These guidelines recommend that blood not be transfused prophylactically, and suggest that in patients who are not critically ill, the threshold for transfusion should be a hemoglobin level of 6.0–8.0 g/dl. A hemoglobin level of 8.0 g/dl seems to be an appropriate threshold for transfusion in surgical patients with no risk factors for ischemia, whereas a threshold of 10.0 g/dl can be justified for patients who are considered at risk. A recent mathematical analysis suggested that surgical blood losses that exceed 70–120% (e.g. 3500–6000 ml in a 70 kg patient with a 5 l blood volume) of patients' baseline estimated blood volumes are necessary before any blood transfusion, and therefore any blood conservation intervention, such as autologous blood procurement, is indicated;[38] however, this model assumes a perisurgical red cell transfusion trigger of a hematocrit of 18–21%.[14] With substantial improvements in blood safety,[39] concern has been expressed that patients are now at risk for undertransfusion.[40,41] The study by Wu[20] provides evidence for the first time that patients with a specific clinical presentation are affected adversely by the underuse of transfusion. On the basis of this study, hemocrit levels have been recommended to be maintained above 33% in patients who present with acute myocardial infarction.[42]

AUTOLOGOUS BLOOD PROCUREMENT

Interest in autologous blood procurement was stimulated in the 1980s by a renewed awareness that infectious diseases are transmissible by blood transfusion, including not only post-transfusion hepatitis but also human immunodeficiency virus (HIV). Preoperative

autologous blood donation (PAD), acute normovolemic hemodilution (ANH), and intraoperative/postoperative autologous blood cell recovery and reinfusion ('peri/postoperative cell salvage', PCS) are all techniques that have been promoted[43] in the surgical arena to minimize allogeneic blood exposure.

The role of autologous blood procurement in surgery remains in evolution, based on improving blood safety, increasing blood costs, and emerging pharmacologic alternatives to blood transfusion.[44] PAD became accepted as a standard practice in elective surgical settings such as total joint replacement surgery, so that in 1992 over 6% of the blood transfused in the USA was autologous.[39] In contrast, ANH was rarely practiced and published data regarding its merits were scant. Subsequently, substantial improvements in blood safety have been accompanied by a decline in PAD (Table 6.1)[39,45] as well as an interest in ANH as an alternative, lower-cost autologous blood procurement strategy.[46] A recent survey of hospitals in the USA found that 83% of respondents utilized PAD, 82% utilized cell salvage, and 33% utilized ANH.[47] Current applications of autologous blood procurement strategies and techniques in the surgical setting will be summarized here.

Preoperative autologous blood donation

Efficacy
Patients undergoing PAD may donate a unit (450 ± 45 ml, or up to 10.5 ml/kg body weight) of blood as often as twice weekly, until 72 hours before surgery. Under routine conditions, patients usually donate once weekly. Oral iron supplements are routinely

Table 6.1 Collection and transfusion of autologous blood in the USA[a]							
Source	1980	1986	1989	1992	1994	1997	1999
Transfused:							
Total	9 934	12 159	12 059	11 307	11 107	11 476	12 389
Autologous	NA	NA	369	566	482	421	367
(% of total)			(3.1%)	(5.0%)	(4.3%)	(3.7%)	(3.0%)
Collected:							
Total	11 174	13 807	13 554	13 169	12 908	12 550	13 649
Autologous	28	206	655	1 117	1 013	611	651
(% of total)	(0.25%)	(1.5%)	(4.8%)	(8.5%)	(7.8%)	(4.9%)	(4.7%)

[a]Modified by permission of *The New England Journal of Medicine*, Goodnough LT et al. 1999; **340**: 439–47. © 1999 Massachusetts Medical Society. All rights reserved; The National Blood Data Resource Center's comprehensive report on blood collection and transfusion in the USA, 1999.
NA, not available.

prescribed. This iatrogenic blood loss is accompanied by a response in endogenous erythropoietin levels that, while increased significantly over basal levels, remain within the range of normal. The erythropoietic response that occurs under these conditions is therefore modest.[48] A summary of prospective, controlled trials[49–54] of patients undergoing such blood loss via autologous phlebotomy is presented in Table 6.2, along with calculated estimates of red blood cell (RBC) volume expansion (erythropoiesis in excess of basal rates). With routine PAD, 220–351 ml (11–19% RBC expansion,[49,50] or the equivalent of 1–1.75 blood units) are produced in excess of basal erythropoiesis, defining the efficacy of this blood conservation practice.

For patients subjected to more aggressive (up to 2 units weekly) phlebotomy, the endogenous erythropoietin response is more substantial.[51–53] In one clinical trial,[52] a linear–logarithmic relationship was demonstrated between change in hemoglobin level and the endogenous erythropoietin response.[55] Erythropoietin-mediated erythropoiesis in this setting is 397–568 ml (19–26% RBC expansion,[51–54] or the equivalent of 2–3 blood units).

Selection of patients

PAD is most beneficial for patients at risk for blood transfusion who are undergoing procedures with substantial blood loss, such as orthopedic joint replacement, vascular surgery, cardiac or thoracic surgery, and radical prostatectomy. Autologous blood is unnecessary for procedures that seldom require transfusion, such as transurethral resection of the prostate, cholecystectomy, herniorrhaphy, vaginal hysterectomy, and uncomplicated obstetric delivery.[56]

It is important to establish guidelines for the appropriate number of units to be collected, so that patient exposure to allogeneic blood in minimized. A hospital's maximal surgical blood order schedule (MSBOS) for blood

Table 6.2 Erythropoiesis during autologous blood donation (data expressed as means)[a]

No. of patients	Blood removed (donated)			Blood produced				
	Baseline RBC volume (ml)	Requested/donated units	RBC volume (ml)	RBC volume (ml)	Expansion (%)	Iron therapy	Ref	
'Standard phlebotomy'								
108	1884	3/2.7	522	351	19	p.o.	49	
22	1936	3/2.8	590	220	11	None	50	
45	1881	3/2.9	621	331	17	p.o.	50	
41	1918	3/2.9	603	315	16	p.o. + i.v.	50	
'Aggressive phlebotomy'								
30	2075	≥3/3.0	540	397	19	None	51	
30	2024	≥3/3.1	558	473	23	p.o.	51	
30	2057	≥3/2.9	522	436	21	i.v.	51	
24	2157	6/4.1	683	568	26	p.o.	52,53	
23	2257	6/4.6	757	440	19	p.o.	54	

[a]Modified by permission from Goodnough LT et al. *Blood* 2000; 96: 823–33. © American Society of Hematology.
[b]p.o., oral; i.v., intravenous

crossmatch can provide estimates of transfusion needs for specific procedures; the generally accepted cut-off at which transfusion is 'unlikely' and autologous blood procurement should not be recommended is 10%.[57] Collection of units should be scheduled as far in advance of surgery as possible for liquid blood storage (up to 42 days), in order to allow compensatory erythropoiesis[48] to correct the induced anemia. A recent study demonstrated that compensatory erythropoiesis to PAD was greatly enhanced by increasing the interval between the last donation and the preadmission screening visit before surgery[58] (Figure 6.2). If the erythropoietic response to autologous blood phlebotomy is not able to maintain the patient's level of hematocrit during the donation interval, the pre-deposit of autologous blood may actually be harmful. A study of patients undergoing hysterectomy[59] demonstrated that preoperative autologous blood donation resulted in perioperative anemia and an increased likelihood of any blood transfusion. Table 6.3 summarizes the rates of allogeneic blood exposure in patients undergoing total joint replacement, with or without PAD, in the USA in 1996–97.[60]

While the most important indicator for PAD is the effectiveness in reduced allogeneic transfusions, the 'wastage' rate of autologous units is an index of its efficiency. Even for procedures such as total joint replacement surgery, discard rates of up to 50% of collected units are common.[59,60] The additional costs associated with the collection of autologous units and the inherent 'wastage' of these units, along with advances in the safety of allogeneic blood, now make the predonation of autologous blood poorly cost-effective.[61] Some suggestions that have been made to make autologous blood programs less costly include abbreviating the donor interview for autologous collection, utilizing only whole blood and discontinuing component production, limiting the use of frozen autologous blood, applying the same transfusion guidelines for autologous and allogeneic blood, and testing only the first donated autologous blood unit for infectious disease markers. Attempts to stratify patients into groups at high and low risk for transfusion based on the baseline level of hemoglobin and on the type of procedure show some promise. In a study using a point score system, 80% of patients undergoing total joint replacement procedures were identified to be at low risk (less than 10%) for transfusion, so that autologous blood procurement for these patients would not be recommended.[62]

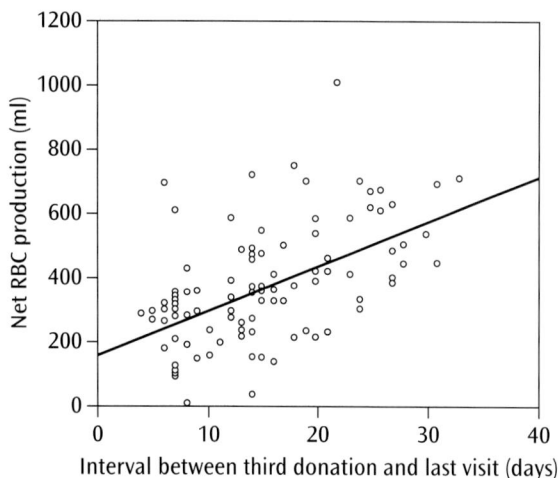

Figure 6.2
Scatterplot of all patients' net red blood cell (RBC) production with the interval between the third donation and the last (i.e. preoperative) visit. Reprinted by permission from Weisbach V et al. *Transfusion* 2001; **41**: 179–83. © 2001 Blackwell Science Ltd.

Table 6.3 Allogeneic blood tranfusion outcomes in patients undergoing total joint replacement in the USA 1996–1997: percentages of patients receiving allogeneic blood[a]

Procedure	No (n = 3741)	Yes (n = 5741) Non-anemic	Yes (n = 5741) Anemic (hematocrit < 0.39)
Knee:			
Unilateral	18	6	11
Revision	30	11	18
Bilateral	57	16	21
Hip:			
Unilateral	32	9	14
Revision	59	21	33

[a]Modified by permission from Bierbaum BE et al. *J Bone Joint Surg* 1999; 81A: 2–10. © 1999 *J Bone Joint Surg.*

Safety considerations

Autologous blood donation and the transfusion of autologous blood are each associated with risks. One in 16 783 autologous donations is associated with an adverse reaction severe enough to require hospitalization, which is 12 times the risk associated with community donations by healthy individuals.[63] Ischemic events have also been reported to occur in association with autologous blood donation.[61] The transfusion of autologous blood has many of the same complications as transfusion of allogeneic units, including bacterial contamination, hemolysis due to errors in the administration of units, and volume overload. Advantages and disadvantages of PAD are summarized in Table 6.4. Since mortality from allogeneic blood transfusion is now more likely to be due to administrative error[65] than to blood-transmitted infection,[39] the risks of banked autologous blood units are similar to banked allogeneic blood units.

Acute normovolemic hemodilution

ANH is a technique that involves the removal of whole blood from a patient while restoring the circulating blood volume with a cellular fluid shortly before an anticipated significant surgical blood loss. Blood is collected in standard blood bags containing anticoagulant on a tilt-rocker with automatic cut-off via volume sensors. The blood is then stored at room temperature, and reinfused in the operating room after major blood loss has ceased, or sooner if indicated. Simultaneous infusions of crystalloid (3 ml crystalloids to 1 ml blood withdrawn) and colloid (dextrans, starches, gelatin, albumin, 1 ml : 1 ml) have been recommended. Subsequent intraoperative fluid management is based on the usual surgical requirements. Blood units are reinfused in the

Table 6.4 Advantages and disadvantages of autologous blood donation	
Advantages	Disadvantages
• Prevents transfusion-transmitted disease	• Risk of bacterial contamination or volume overload remains
• Prevents red cell alloimmunization	• Does not eliminate risk of administrative error with ABO incompatibility
• Supplements the blood supply	• More costly than allogeneic blood
• Provides compatible blood for patients with alloantibodies	• Wastage of blood not transfused
• Prevents some adverse transfusion reactions	• Causes perioperative anemia and increased likelihood of transfusion

reverse order of collection. The first unit collected – and therefore the last unit transfused – has the highest hematocrit and concentration of coagulation factors and platelets.

Withdrawal of whole blood and replacement with crystalloid or colloid solution decreases arterial oxygen content, but compensatory hemodynamic mechanisms and the existence of surplus oxygen-delivery capacity make ANH safe. A sudden drop in red cell mass increases cardiac output and lowers blood viscosity, thereby decreasing peripheral resistance. If cardiac output can effectively compensate, oxygen delivery to the tissues at a hematocrit of 0.25–0.30 is as good as, but no better than, delivery at a hematocrit of 0.35–0.45.

Because blood collected by ANH is stored at room temperature and is usually returned to the patient within eight hours of collection, there is little deterioration of platelets or coagulation factors. The hemostatic value of blood collected by ANH is of questionable benefit for orthopedic or urologic surgery because plasma and platelets are rarely indicated in this setting. Its value in protecting plasma and platelets from the acquired coagulopathy of extracorporeal circulation in cardiac surgery (known as 'blood pooling') is better established.[66]

Efficacy

The chief benefit of ANH has been recognized to be the reduction of red cell losses when whole blood is shed perioperatively at lower hematocrit levels after ANH is complete. Mathematical modeling has suggested that severe hemodilution to preoperative hematocrit levels of less than 0.20, accompanied by substantial blood losses, would be required before the red cell volume 'saved' by hemodilution became clinically important.[67] An analysis of patients who had undergone 'minimal' ANH (representing 15% of patients' blood volume) estimates that only 100 ml red cells (the equivalent of half a unit of blood) is 'saved' under these conditions.[68] With moderate hemodilution (target hematocrit levels of 0.28), the 'saving' becomes more substantial, as illustrated in Figure 6.3. The removal of three blood units in a patient who subsequently undergoes a blood loss of 2600 ml results in an estimated 732 ml of red cells lost, compared with 947 ml of red cells that would have been lost if hemodilution had not been performed. The surgical red cell losses 'saved' in this instance by hemodilution are 215 ml, or the equivalent of one allogeneic blood unit. The safety and efficacy of more extensive hemodilution is controversial, and may provide little additional blood conservation.

Clinical studies

It had been recommended previously that patients scheduled for radical prostatectomy predonate three units of autologous blood; this reduced the prevalence of allogeneic exposure from 66–70% in patients without autologous blood to 14–16% in patients who have pre-donated three units of autologous blood.[69] A study of 250 patients in this setting reported that 21% of patients undergoing ANH alone received allogeneic blood.[70] Two prospective randomized trials[71,72] and a case-controlled retrospective comparison[73] of ANH and PAD in patients undergoing radical prostatectomy demonstrated that subsequent allogeneic blood exposure (10–20%) was not different for patients undergoing either method of autologous blood procurement.

The benefit of ANH as determined in a mathematical model[74] is illustrated in Figure 6.4. For an adult with an estimated 5000 ml blood volume and an initial hematocrit of

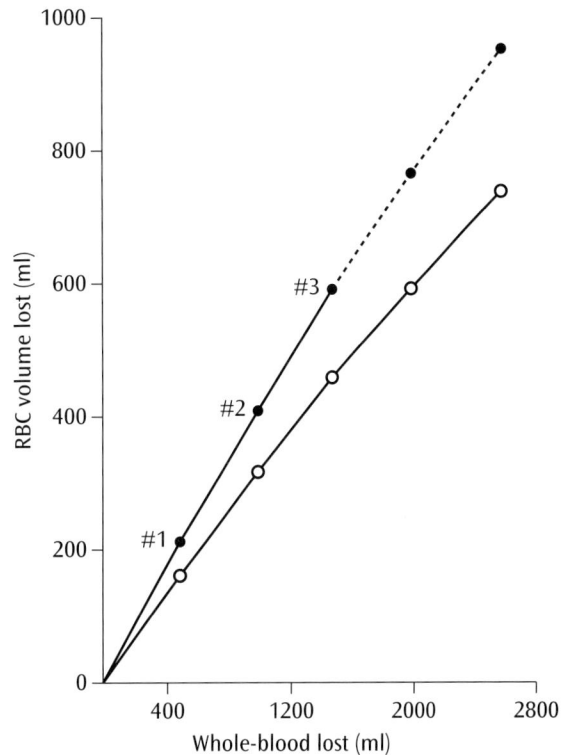

Figure 6.3
The relationship between whole-blood volume lost and red blood cell (RBC) volume lost in a 100 kg patient undergoing hemodilution: o—o, RBC volume lost with 2800 ml whole blood lost intraoperatively after hemodilution of 1500 ml whole blood. •—•, RBC volume lost with 2800 ml whole blood lost during hemodilution at each of three 500 ml volumes; •----•. Cumulative RBC volume lost intraoperatively, derived for 2800 ml whole blood lost if hemodilution had not been performed. A net 215 ml reduction in RBC volume lost with hemodilution is illustrated by the divergence of the two curves. Reprinted by permission from Goodnough LT et al. *Anesth Analg* 1994; 78: 932–7.

0.40, surgical blood losses of up to 3000 ml would result in a hematocrit that would remain at 0.25 postoperatively without autologous blood intervention. This level of hematocrit is generally considered safe for patients

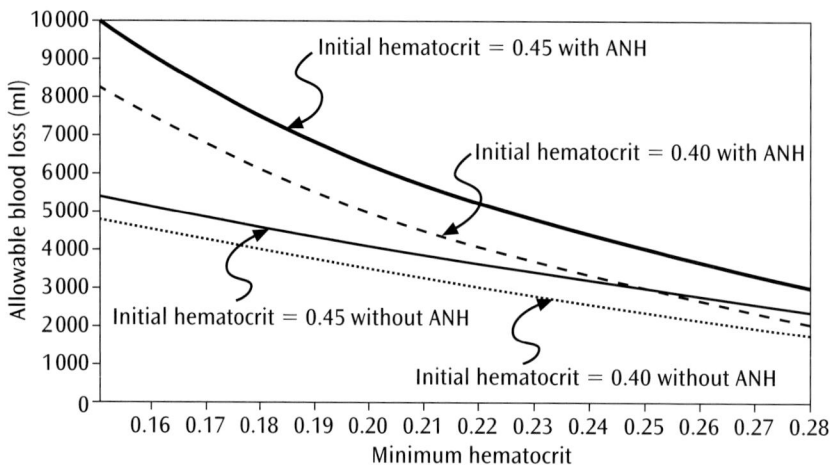

Figure 6.4
The maximum allowable blood loss in a patient with a blood volume of 5000 ml and an initial hematocrit of 0.45 (solid lines) or 0.40 (dotted lines), with and without acute normovolemic hemodilution (ANH). Reprinted by permission from Goodnough LT et al. *Hematology* 1997; **2**: 413–20.

with known risk factors.[16] Note that in this model, the performance of ANH with initial hematocrits of 0.40–0.45 would allow up to 2500–3500 ml surgical blood losses – yet the nadir hematocrit could be maintained at 0.28. The benefit of ANH in this model is to protect patients who have substantial blood losses that cannot be predicted, and maintain perioperative levels of hematocrit that minimize risks related to ischemia.

A more recent mathematical model[38] concluded that for a usual (5000 ml blood volume) surgical patient, 70–120% of the blood volume (representing 3500–6000 ml blood loss) must be lost before ANH can save 180 ml of RBC, or approximately the equivalent of one blood unit (Figure 6.5). However, this model assumed a transfusion trigger hematocrit of 0.18–0.21, a recommended level that has not been established as safe,[40,41] particularly in critically ill patients[9] or in elective surgical patients with or without identified risk factors for ischemic cardiac or cerebral vascular disease.[17,75] The guidelines that have recommended blood conservation

strategies such as ANH for patients who are anticipated to have surgical blood losses greater than 20% of their baseline blood volume, reflect the value of ANH as an 'insurance policy'[74] that serves not only to maintain higher levels of hematocrit for any given surgical blood losses, but also to reduce RBC losses in those patients who have greater than expected blood losses, as illustrated in Figure 6.4. Blood conservation strategies need to address both of these issues.[76]

In a randomized trial in patients undergoing total hip arthroplasty, 23 patients were randomized to ANH and 25 to PAD.[77] No differences were noted between the two groups, including estimated interoperative blood losses and calculated RBC losses for the surgical hospitalization. Four (17%) of 23 ANH patients received allogeneic blood – not significantly different from the figure of none in the PAD group ($p = 0.30$).

Since ANH represents 'point of care' autologous blood procurement, it is less costly than PAD. First, autologous blood units procured by ANH are re-transfused before leaving

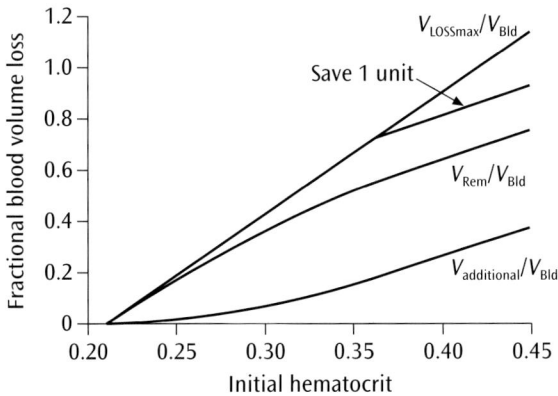

Figure 6.5

Fractional blood volume loss required before any erythrocyte-saving strategy is required (V_{Rem}/V_{Bld}), fractional blood volume loss permitted with the use of ANH ($V_{LOSSmax}/V_{Bld}$), and fractional blood volume loss required to save 1 unit of erythrocytes ('Save 1 unit'), for an initial hematocrit of 0.21. All but the third of these are independent of blood volume; the fractional blood volume loss indicated as required to save 1 unit of erythrocytes is shown for a blood volume of 5000 ml. Reprinted by permission from Weiskopf RB. *Anesthesia* 2001; **94**: 439–46.

the operating room and require no inventory or testing costs. ANH therefore eliminates the possibility of an administrative error that could lead to an ABO-incompatible blood transfusion and death, while PAD does not eliminate this risk; the estimated risk of death from a hemolytic transfusion reaction[65] now approximates the risk of mortality from HIV or hepatitis infection from blood transfusion.[39] Since ANH and reinfusion is accomplished in the operating room by on-site personnel, procurement and administration costs are minimized. In addition, blood obtained during ANH does not require the commitment of patient time, transportation, and loss of work associated with PAD. Finally,

the wastage[56] of autologous blood units (approximately 50% of units collected) is eliminated with ANH. Hemodynamic monitoring and absence of adverse events in 250 consecutive patients undergoing ANH[70] indicate that moderate hemodilution can be performed safely. A pro and con debate on the merits of ANH has been published.[78,79]

Intraoperative autologous blood recovery and reinfusion

Intraoperative recovery of blood involves the collection and reinfusion of autologous red cells lost by a patient during surgery. Cell-washing devices can provide the equivalent of up to 10 units of banked blood per hour to a patient with massive bleeding. The survival of the red cells that are recovered appears to be similar to that of transfused allogeneic red cells.[80] Relative contraindications include the potential for the aspiration of malignant cells, the presence of infection, and the presence of other contaminants such as amniotic or ascitic fluid in the operative field. Because washing does not completely remove bacteria from the recovered blood, intraoperative recovery should not be used if the operative field has gross bacterial contamination.[81]

As with other strategies of autologous blood procurement, the relative benefits, safety, and costs of intraoperative recovery of autologous blood should be carefully scrutinized. A prospective randomized trial of patients who were undergoing repair of abdominal aortic aneurysms or aorta–femoral artery bypass procedures found that intraoperative recovery and reinfusion of blood did not result in a need for fewer blood transfusions.[82] Four deaths related to intraoperative blood recovery were reported to the New York Department of Health from 1990 through 1995, for an estimated rate of one per 35 000 procedures.[83] With the use of automated cell-washing devices, the equivalent of at least two units of washed blood needs to be recovered in order for this method to be cost-effective.[84,85] Intraoperative recovery of blood may be of most value not because it reduces the requirements for blood transfusion, but because it provides blood that is less costly to obtain and is more immediately available in the event of rapid blood loss.

Postoperative autologous blood recovery and reinfusion

Postoperative recovery of blood involves the collection of blood from surgical drains, followed by reinfusion, with or without processing. The blood recovered is dilute, is partially hemolyzed and defibrinated, and may contain high concentrations of cytokines. For these reasons, programs set an upper limit on the volume of unprocessed blood (1400 ml at one of the hospitals in which we work) that can be reinfused.

The safety and the benefit of the use of unwashed blood obtained from surgical drains after orthopedic surgery remains in question.[86] One center that initially found this approach to be beneficial subsequently reported that this costly practice is of no clinical benefit.[87] Because the blood cell volume of the fluid collected is low (with a hematocrit of 0.20), the volume of red cells reinfused is often small. Selective use of the method in situations in which large postoperative blood losses are anticipated, such as in bilateral joint-replacement surgery, would improve the efficacy of the procedure – but such blood losses are difficult to predict.

CONCLUSIONS

The use of blood transfusion has declined, probably as a result of more conservative transfusion practices during an era of concerns about the safety of the blood supply. It is unlikely that any level of hemoglobin can be used as a universal threshold for transfusion. Increased attention to the costs and safety of healthcare delivery has caused the relative benefits and costs of both blood transfusion and conservation to be scrutinized. The prospective identification of surgical candidates who will need transfusion and will therefore truly benefit from blood conservation must be based on patient-specific factors, such as the baseline hematocrit and the anticipated blood loss during surgery. The decision to conserve blood needs may no longer be based on the safety of the blood supply, but on evidence that blood conservation is safe and of value for individual patients.

REFERENCES

1. Finch CA, Lenfant C. Oxygen transport in man. *N Engl J Med* 1972; **286**: 407–15.
2. Levy PS, Chavez RP, Crystal GJ et al. Oxygen extraction ratio: a valid indicator of transfusion need in limited coronary reserve? *J Trauma* 1992; **32**: 769–74.
3. Levy PS, Kim SJ, Eckel PK et al. Limit to cardiac compensation during acute isovolemic hemodilution: influence of coronary stenosis. *Am J Physiol* 1993; **265**: H340–9.
4. Goodnough LT, Despotis GJ, Hogue CW. On the need for improved transfusion indicators in cardiac surgery. *Ann Thorac Surg* 1995; **60**: 473–80.
5. Kitchens CS. Are transfusions overrated? Surgical outcome of Jehovah's Witnesses. *Am J Med* 1993; **94**: 117–19.
6. Carson JL, Duff A, Poses RM et al. Effect of

anaemia and cardiovascular disease on surgical mortality and morbidity. *Lancet* 1996; **348**: 1055–60.

7. Carson JL, Terrin ML, Barton FB et al. A pilot randomized trial comparing symptomatic vs hemoglobin-level driven red blood cell transfusions following hip fractures. *Transfusion* 1998; **38**: 522–9.

8. Carson JL, Duff A, Berlin JA et al. Perioperative blood transfusion and postoperative mortality. *JAMA* 1998; **279**: 199–205.

9. Hebert PC, Wells G, Blajchman MA et al. A multicenter, randomized, controlled clinical trial of transfusion requirements in critical care. *N Engl J Med* 1999; **340**: 409–17.

10. Hebert PC, Yetisir E, Martin C et al. Is a low transfusion threshold safe in critically ill patients with cardiovascular diseases? *Crit Care Med* 2001; **29**: 227–34.

11. Gore DC, DeMaria EJ, Reines HD. Elevations in red blood cell mass reduce cardiac index without altering the oxygen consumption in severely burned patients. *Surg Forum* 1992; **43**: 721–3.

12. Babineau TJ, Dzik WH, Borlase BC et al. Reevaluation of current transfusion practices in patients in surgical intensive care units. *Am J Surg* 1992; **164**: 22–5.

13. Mangano DT, Browner WS, Hollenberg M et al. Association of perioperative myocardial ischemia with cardiac morbidity and mortality in men undergoing noncardiac surgery. *N Engl J Med* 1990; **323**: 1781–8.

14. Rao TLK, Montoya A. Cardiovascular, electrocardiographic and respiratory changes following acute anemia with volume replacement in patients with coronary artery disease. *Anesth Dev* 1985; **12**: 49–54.

15. Practice guidelines for blood component therapy: a report by the American Society of Anesthesiologists Task Force on Blood Component Therapy. *Anesthesiology* 1996; **84**: 732–47.

16. Hogue CW Jr, Goodnough LT, Monk TG. Perioperative myocardial ischemic episodes are related to hematocrit level in patients undergoing radical prostatectomy. *Transfusion* 1998; **38**: 924–31.

17. Welch HG, Mehan KR, Goodnough LT. Prudent strategies for elective red blood cell transfusion. *Ann Intern Med* 1992; **116**: 393–402.

18. Kim DM, Brecher ME, Estes TJ, Morrey BF. Relationship of hemoglobin level and duration of hospitalization after total hip arthroplasty: implications for the transfusion target. *Mayo Clin Proc* 1993; **68**: 37–41.

19. Johnson RG, Thurer RL, Kruskall MS et al. Comparison of two transfusion strategies after elective operations for myocardial revascularization. *J Thorac Cardiovasc Surg* 1992; **104**: 307–14.

20. Wu W-C, Rathore SS, Wang Y, Radford MJ, Krumholtz KM. Blood transfusion in elderly patients with acute myocardial infarction. *N Engl J Med* 2001; **345**: 1230–6.

21. Blajchman MA. Transfusion-associated immunomodulation and universal white cell reduction. Are we putting the cart before the horse? *Transfusion* 1999; **39**: 667–70.

22. Goodnough LT. The case against universal leukoreduction (and for the practice of evidence-based medicine. *Transfusion* 2000; **40**: 1522–7.

23. Toy PTCY. Effectivenss of transfusion audits and practice guidelines. *Arch Pathol Lab Med* 1994; **118**: 435–7.

24. Barnette RD, Fish DJ, Eisenstaedt RS. Modification of fresh-frozen transfusion practices through educational intervention. *Transfusion* 1990; **30**: 253–7.

25. Lam HTC, Schweitzer SO, Petz L et al. Are retrospective peer-review transfusion monitoring systems effective in reducing red blood cell utilization? *Arch Pathol Lab Med* 1996; **120**: 810–16.

26. Goodnough LT, Audet AM. Retrospective utilization review for blood transfusions. Are we just going through the motions? *Arch Pathol Lab Med* 1996; **120**: 802.

27. Audet AM, Goodnough LT, Parvin CA. Evaluating the appropriateness of red blood cell transfusions: The limitations of retrospective medical record reviews. *Int J Qual Health Care* 1996; **8**: 41–9.

28. Despotis GJ, Grishaber J, Goodnough LT. The effect of an intraoperative transfusion algorithm on physician transfusion behavior in cardiac surgery. *Transfusion* 1994; **34**: 290–6.

29. Toy PTCY, Kaplan EB, McVay PA et al. Blood loss and replacement in total hip arthroplasty: a multicenter study. *Transfusion* 1992; **32**: 63–7.

30. Churchhill WH, McGurk S, Chapman RH et al. The Collaborative Hospital Transfusion Study: variations in use of autologous blood account for differences in red cell use during primary hip and knee surgery. *Transfusion* 1998; **38**: 530–9.

31. Goodnough LT, Verbrugge D, Vizmeg K, Riddell J IV. Identification of elective orthopedic surgical patients transfused with blood volumes in excess of blood needs: the 'transfusion trigger' revisited. *Transfusion* 1992; **32**: 648–53.

32. Goodnough LT, Johnston MFM, Toy PTCY, Transfusion Medicine Academic Award Group. The variability of transfusion practice in coronary artery bypass graft surgery. *JAMA* 1991; **265**: 86–90.

33. Stover EP, Siegel LC, Parks R et al. Variability in transfusion practice for coronary artery bypass surgery persists despite national consensus guidelines. *Anethesiology* 1998; **88**: 327–33.

34. Surgenor DN, Churchill WH, Wallace EL et al. The specific hospital significantly affects red cell and component transfusion practice in coronary artery bypass graft surgery: a study of five hospitals. *Transfusion* 1998; **37**: 122–34.

35. Consensus Conference: Perioperative red cell transfusion. *JAMA* 1988; **260**: 2700–3.

36. American College of Physicians. Practice strategies for elective red blood cell transfusion. *Ann Intern Med* 1992; **116**: 403–6.

37. Expert Working Group. Guidelines for red blood cell and plasma transfusions for adults and children. *Can Med Assoc J* 1997; **156**: (Suppl 11): S1–24.

38. Weiskopf RB. Efficacy of acute normovolemic hemodilution assessed as a function of fraction of blood volume lost. *Anesthesia* 2001; **94**: 439–46.

39. Goodnough LT, Brecher ME, Kanter MH, Aubuchon JP. Medical Progress: Transfusion medicine, Part I. Blood transfusion. *N Engl J Med* 1999; **340**: 439–47.

40. Valeri CR, Crowley JP, Loscalzo J. The red cell transfusion trigger: Has a sin of commission now become a sin of omission? *Transfusion* 1998; **38**: 602–10.

41. Lenfant C. Transfusion practices should be audited for both undertransfusion and overtransfusion. *Transfusion* 1992; **32**: 873–4.

42. Goodnough LT, Bach RG. Anemia, transfusion and mortality. *N Engl J Med* 2001: **345**: 1272–4.

43. NHLBI Expert Panel. Transfusion alert: use of autologous blood. *Transfusion* 1995; **35**: 703–11.

44. Goodnough LT, Brecher ME, Kanter MH, Aubuchon JP. Medical Progress: Transfusion medicine, Part II. Blood conservation. *N Engl J Med* 1999; **340**: 525–33.

45. Brecher ME, Goodnough LT. The rise and fall of preoperative autologous blood donation. *Transfusion* 2001; **41**: 1459–62.

46. National Blood Data Resource Centre. *Comprehensive report on blood collection and transfusion in the USA, 1999.* American Association of Blood Banks: Bethesda MD, 2001: 9.

47. Hutchinson AB, Fergusson D, Graham ID, Laupacis A, Herrin J, Hillyer CD. Utilization of technologies to reduce allogenic blood transfusion in the US. *Transfusion Med* 2001; **11**: 79–85.

48. Goodnough LT, Skikne B, Brugnara C. Erythropoietin, iron, and erythropoiesis. *Blood* 2000; **96**: 823–33.

49. Kasper SM, Gerlich W, Buzello W. Preopera-

tive red cell production in patients undergoing weekly autologous blood donation. *Transfusion* 1997; **37**: 1058–62.

50. Kasper SM, Lazansky H, Stark C et al. Efficacy of oral iron supplementation is not enhanced by additional intravenous iron during autologous blood donation. *Transfusion* 1998; **38**: 764–70.

51. Weisbach V, Skoda P, Rippel R et al. Oral or intravenous iron as an adjunct to autologous blood donation in elective surgery: a randomized, controlled study. *Transfusion* 1999; **39**: 465–72.

52. Goodnough LT, Rudnick S, Price TH et al. Increased preoperative collection of autologous blood with recombinant human erythropoietin therapy. *N Engl J Med* 1989; **321**: 1163–7.

53. Goodnough LT, Price TH, Rudnick S, Soegiarso RW. Preoperative red blood cell production in patients undergoing aggressive autologous blood phlebotomy with and without erythropoietin therapy. *Transfusion* 1992; **32**: 441–5.

54. Goodnough LT, Price TH, Friedman KD et al. A phase III trial of recombinant human erythropoietin therapy in non-anemic orthopedic patients subjected to aggressive autologous blood phlebotomy: dose, response, toxicity, efficacy. *Transfusion* 1994; **34**: 66–71.

55. Goodnough LT, Price TH, Parvin CA et al. Erythropoietin response to anaemia is not altered by surgery or recombinant human erythropoietin therapy. *Br J Haematol* 1994; **87**: 695–9.

56. Renner SW, Howanitz PJ, Bachner P. Preoperative autologous blood donation in 612 hospitals. *Arch Pathol Lab Med* 1992; **116**: 613–19.

57. Mintz PD, Nordine RB, Henry JB, Weble, R. Expected hemotherapy in elective surgery. *NY State J Med* 1976; **76**: 532.

58. Weisbach V, Corbiere C, Strasser E et al. The variability of compensatory erythropoiesis in repeated autologous blood donation. *Transfusion* 2001; **41**: 179–83.

59. Kanter MH, Van Maanen D, Anders KH et al. Preoperative autologous blood donation before elective hysterectomy. *JAMA* 1996; **276**: 798–801.

60. Bierbaum BE, Callaghan JJ, Galante Jo et al. An analysis of blood management in patients having total hip or knee arthroplasty. *J Bone Joint Surg* 1999; **81A**: 2–10.

61. Etchason J, Petz L, Keeler E et al. The cost-effectiveness of preoperative autologous blood donations. *N Engl Joint Med* 1995; **332**: 7.

62. Larocque BJ, Gilbert K, Brien WF. Prospective validation of a point score system for predicting blood transfusion following hip or knee replacement. *Transfusion* 1998; **38**: 932–7.

63. Popovsky MA, Whitaker B, Asrnold NL. Severe outcomes of allogeneic and autologous blood donations: frequency and characterization. *Transfusion* 1995; **35**: 734–7.

64. Goodnough LT, Monk TG. Evolving concepts in autologous blood procurement. Case reports of perisurgical anemia complicated by myocardial infarction. *Am J Med* 1996; **101**: 33S–37S.

65. Linden JV, Wagner, K, Voytovich AE, Sheehan J. Transfusion errors in New York State: an analysis of 10 years' experience. *Transfusion* 2000; **40**: 1207–13.

66. Petry AF, Jost T, Sievers H. Reduction of homologous blood requirements by blood pooling at the onset of cardiopulmonary bypass. *J Thorac Cardiovasc Surg* 1994; **109**: 1210.

67. Brecher ME, Rosenfeld M. Mathematical and computer modeling of acute normovolemic hemodilution. *Transfusion* 1994; **34**: 176–9.

68. Goodnough LT, Grishaber JE, Monk TG, Catalona WJ. Acute preoperative hemodilution in patients undergoing radical prostatectomy: a case study analysis of efficacy. *Anesth Analg* 1994; **78**: 932–7.

69. Goodnough LT, Grishaber JE, Birkmeyer JD et al. Efficacy and cost-effectiveness of autologous blood predeposit in patients undergoing radical prostatectomy procedures. *Urology* 1994; **44**: 226–31.

70. Monk TG, Goodnough LT, Brecher ME. Acute normovolemic hemodilution can replace preoperative autologous donation as a method of autologous blood procurement in radical prostatectomy. *Anesth Analg* 1997; **85**: 953–8.

71. Monk TG, Goodnough LT, Brecher ME et al. A prospective randomized trial of three blood conservation strategies for radical prostatectomy. *Anesthesia* 1999; **91**: 24–33.

72. Ness PM, Bourke DL, Walsh PC. A randomized trial of perioperative hemodilution versus transfusion of preoperatively deposited autologous blood in elective surgery. *Transfusion* 1991; **31**: 226–30.

73. Monk TG, Goodnough LT, Birkmeyer JD et al. Acute normovolemic hemodilution is a cost-effective alternative to preoperative autologous blood donation by patients undergoing radical retropubic prostatectomy. *Transfusion* 1995; **35**: 559–65.

74. Goodnough LT, Monk TG, Brecher ME. Acute normovolemic hemodilution in surgery. *Hematology* 1997; **2**: 413–20.

75. Andriole GL, Smith DS, Rao G et al. Early complications of contemporary anatomic radical retropubic prostatectomy. *J Urol* 1994; **152**: 1858–60.

76. Goodnough LT, Monk TG, Brecher, ME. A review of autologous blood procurement in the surgical setting: lessons learned in the last 10 years. *Vox Sang* 1996; **71**: 13–21.

77. Goodnough LT, Despotis GJ, Merkel K, Monk TG. A randomized trial of acute normovolemic hemodilution compared to preoperative autologous blood donation in total hip arthroplasty. *Transfusion* 2000; **40**: 1054–7.

78. Goodnough LT, Monk TG, Brecher ME. Acute normovolemic hemodilution should replace preoperative autologous blood donation before elective surgery. *Transfusion* 1998; **38**: 473–6.

79. Rottman G, Ness PM. Is acute normovolemic hemodilution a legitimate alternative to allogeneic blood transfusions? *Transfusion* 1998; **38**: 477–80.

80. Williamson KR, Taswell HF. Intraoperative blood salvage: a review. *Transfusion* 1991; **31**: 662–75.

81. Napier JA, Bruce M, Chapman J et al. Guidelines for autologous transfusion II. Perioperative haemodilution and cell salvage. *Br J Anaesth* 1997; **78**: 768–71.

82. Clagett GP, Valentine RJ, Jackson MR et al. A randomized trial of intraoperative transfusion during aortic surgery. *J Vasc Surg* 1999; **29**: 22–31.

83. Linden JV, Tourault MA, Scribner CL. Decrease in frequency of transfusion fatalities. *Transfusion* 1997; **37**: 243–4.

84. Bovill DF, Moulton CW, Jackson WS et al. The efficacy of introperative autologous transfusion in major orthopaedic surgery: a regression analysis. *Orthopedics* 1986; **9**: 1403–7.

85. Goodnough LT, Monk TG, Sicard G et al. Intraoperative salvage in patients undergoing elective abdominal aortic aneurism repair. An analysis of costs and benefits. *J Vasc Surg* 1996; **24**: 213–18.

86. Clements DH, Sculco TP, Burke SW et al. Salvage and reinfusion of postoperative sanguineous wound drainage. *J Bone Joint Surg* 1993; **74A**: 646–51.

87. Ritter MA, Keating EM, Faris PM. Closed wound drainage in total hip or total knee replacement. *J Bone Joint Surg* 1994; **76A**: 35–8.

7 Major obstetric haemorrhage

Simon Bricker

INTRODUCTION

Successive reports into maternal mortality have testified to the frightening speed with which obstetric haemorrhage can become life-threatening. This should come as no surprise: blood flow to the uterus at term may approach 600–800 ml/min, and irreversible circulatory shock can occur within minutes of the onset of uncontrolled blood loss. Imagine, therefore, a young primigravida who attends the labour ward. She weighs 75 kg and so has a blood volume of about 8 litres. Imagine further that her pregnancy is complicated by uncontrollable uterine haemorrhage. Much of her circulating blood volume will be lost in minutes, and within a few hours a young woman who was previously fit and healthy, expectant and excited, might well have become a maternal death. If this scenario seems melodramatic then go to the most recent maternal mortality reports. These confirm that in the years 1991–1999, no fewer than 34 mothers died in the UK as a direct result of major obstetric haemorrhage.[1,2,3] For every one of these deaths, it is probable that there are many more near-misses – an assertion that is supported by the statistics produced by one typical district general hospital with 3000 annual deliveries. In the latest 12-month period, no fewer than 18.5% of mothers satisfied the criterion for postpartum haemorrhage, namely blood loss exceeding 500 ml, while 3.7% of mothers lost in excess of a litre. Three women required

urgent replacement of more than their entire blood volumes (Countess of Chester Hospital, local audit data). Given that visual estimations of blood loss are notoriously unreliable,[4-6] and that these figures are probably an underestimate, it is likely that the actual situation may be even worse.

DEFINITIONS

By convention, postpartum haemorrhage (PPH) is defined as blood loss greater than 500 ml within 24 hours after birth. At least one study, however, has used accurate methods of measurement to confirm that 500 ml is in fact the average volume that routinely is lost by women undergoing normal vaginal delivery,[7] and so the value of this definition is questionable. It may even have inherent dangers. Most women who lose 500 ml of blood in the first 24 hours after delivery will compensate effortlessly. They may be classified for local statistical purposes as having 'significant PPH', but they will show no signs of circulatory compromise. It will not be long, therefore, before clinicians and midwives understandably become complacent and so may be slower to react when the haemorrhage clinically is important. It has been argued that it would be more logical to define significant PPH as any blood loss after delivery that threatens the haemodynamic stability of the mother,[8] although there are few signs that this more rational approach is being adopted. The term 'massive haemorrhage' is also one that requires clarification. Commonly used definitions include the loss of one blood volume within 24 hours,[9] 50% loss of blood volume within 3 hours, or a rate of loss of 150 ml/min.[10] With the exception of the last, all of these definitions are retrospective, and so while statistically they may have some relevance, clinically they are much less useful. One crucial factor in successful management is early recognition of the potential problem, the first step towards which is an understanding of the causes of obstetric haemorrhage, together with any predisposing factors that make it more likely.

CAUSES

Of the 34 deaths reported in the last three confidential enquiries, 14 were associated with uterine atony, 10 with placenta praevia, and 10 with placental abruption, and it is these three conditions that are numerically the most important. Other causes of major blood loss include uterine and genital tract trauma, retained products of conception, and coagulation failure.

Uterine atony

The uterus that fails to contract following delivery is the primary cause of all PPH, and may account for as many as 90% of cases.[11] Inasmuch as there are parturients in whom this complication is much more likely, at least some of these cases are predictable. The capacity of the uterus to contract is compromised by overdistension, and so PPH is more common in those with multiple pregnancy, in those who have polyhydramnios, and in those

with large babies (>4 kg). It is also more common in the multiparous, in women in whom labour has been prolonged, and in those in whom labour has been augmented with oxytocics. It may also occur in mothers who have been hypotensive: poor perfusion of the uterus is associated with relative ischaemia, and this diminishes the capacity of the myometrium to contract effectively. Other risk factors include a previous PPH due to uterine atony and the use of some drugs. These include not only β_2-agonists and magnesium sulfate, but also the volatile anaesthetic agents that may be used as part of a general anaesthetic technique for operative or instrumental delivery, and which have been shown to cause a dose-dependent reduction in uterine contractility.[12]

Placenta praevia

Some degree of placenta praevia, in which the placenta is sited abnormally near to or actually covering the internal os, is common, and complicates approximately 0.5% of pregnancies. Accurate prenatal ultrasound scanning allows precise localization in the majority of cases, and planned management by elective caesarean section is usually uneventful. The mothers who run into problems are those who have the unfortunate combination of an anterior placenta praevia in the presence of a previous caesarean section scar. Almost a quarter of such women will have placenta accreta,[13] and this risk increases with the number of previous caesarean deliveries that a mother has undergone. The placenta may be abnormally adherent (accreta), may infiltrate the myometrium (increta), or may invade through the myometrium (percreta) to attach to bladder or bowel. Paradoxically, it may even be the most severe of these variations, placenta percreta, that is associated with lower overall blood loss. This is because it is usually immediately obvious that part of the myometrium is effectively destroyed and that the only way to secure swift haemostasis is to proceed to emergency caesarean hysterectomy. Once surgical clamps have been applied to the uterine pedicles, massive further blood loss is less likely. If the mother has placenta accreta, however, the obstetrician may be more reluctant to proceed early to hysterectomy, particularly if preservation of fertility is important. Under these circumstances, the patient may continue to bleed massively. In one recent large study, blood loss exceeded 10 litres in 6.5% of patients and 20 litres in 3% of patients, and over 70 units of blood products were required by 5% of the cases.[14]

Placental abruption

Placental abruption, in which the implanted placenta separates prematurely from the endometrial wall, gives no warning and, unlike placenta praevia, cannot be predicted. It has a quoted incidence of 1 in 150 deliveries.[15] There are, however, some predisposing conditions, which include maternal hypertension, previous abruptio placentae, and premature rupture of the membranes. The separation may be complete or only partial, and in the latter case it may be concealed. Retroplacental bleeding occurs at the separation site, and may continue uncontrolled because of the inability of the gravid uterus to contract and compress the disrupted vessels. These large open venous sinuses may then act as portals to the systemic circulation through

which amniotic debris and coagulation activators such as tissue thromboplastin may be forced by the high intrauterine pressure. Disseminated intravascular coagulation (DIC) is therefore a well-recognized complication of placental abruption and occurs in some 10% of cases. It is the commonest precipitant of a consumption coagulopathy in pregnancy. Abruption may also be associated with uterine atony, particularly if the myometrium becomes suffused with blood (the so-called Couvelaire uterus).

Other causes

Trauma to the lower genital tract
Minor lacerations are common as a result of vaginal birth, but excessive maternal haemorrhage may be associated with delivery of a large infant relative to the mother's size or a difficult instrumental delivery. Bleeding can occur from vaginal or cervical lacerations or tears, and can be insidious. It may also be confused with normal post-delivery vaginal loss.

Retained products of conception
Retained placenta complicates 1–2% of all deliveries, and is sometimes (but not invariably) associated with blood loss. Retained products of conception almost always prevent the uterus from contracting down effectively, and will cause some bleeding.

Uterine rupture and uterine inversion
A previous caesarean section scar may dehisce during labour without causing significant bleeding. If, however, there is extension into previously unscarred uterus, or if there is uterine rupture elsewhere, bleeding may be substantial. Uterine rupture complicates about one-third of cases who have had a previous

classical (vertical) incision and about 0.7% of those who have had previous transverse caesarean section.[16] Other less common causes of rupture include traumatic forceps delivery, uterine abnormalities, and uterine overstimulation.

Uterine inversion is a rare cause of obstetric shock in which the haemodynamic collapse caused when the fundus of the uterus inverts through the cervix (which is vagally mediated) may be compounded by blood loss, which may not always be evident vaginally and so may be masked. It is associated both with precipitate delivery and with prolonged labour, and may also follow excessive traction during attempted delivery of the placenta.

Combination factors

Classification of major obstetric haemorrhage into discrete conditions should not obscure the fact that not infrequently there is more than one cause. Traumatic delivery of a large baby after prolonged labour, for example, may be complicated both by uterine atony and by lower genital tract trauma. Placental abruption may cause massive uterine blood loss as well as triggering DIC, and is frequently associated with uterine atony. All contributory causes should be excluded before it can safely be assumed that a mother's condition has stabilized.

Coagulation failure

Massive obstetric haemorrhage can be fatal before coagulation failure supervenes, but DIC may complicate some 10% of cases of placental abruption and 40% of cases of the much rarer condition of amniotic fluid embolism syndrome (AFE). DIC may also complicate intrauterine fetal death, pre-eclampsia and Gram-negative septicaemia.

The condition is believed to develop when a thrombogenic trigger, probably tissue thromboplastin, gains access to the circulation and activates one or both coagulation pathways. DIC is life-threatening, and its management requires immediate and expert haematological help.

THE PHYSIOLOGICAL RESPONSE TO ACUTE BLOOD LOSS

Recognition of the clinical signs of blood loss is helped by an understanding of the normal compensatory mechanisms. The circulation functions to distribute the cardiac output to all tissues in amounts sufficient to meet their metabolic demands. Any progressive loss of circulating volume is accompanied by a redistribution of flow to ensure that the brain and myocardium continue to receive oxygenated blood. As blood loss continues, the decreases in venous return, right atrial pressure, and cardiac output immediately activate baroreceptor reflexes. The decreased afferent input to the medullary cardiovascular centres inhibits parasympathetic and enhances sympathetic activity. This results both in an improvement in cardiac output and in the maintenance of tissue perfusion by alterations in the resistance of various vascular beds. Cardiac output is thereby redistributed from skin, muscle, and viscera to the heart and to the brain. These alterations are mediated not only via direct sympathetic innervation but also by circulating humoral vasopressors such as adrenaline, angiotensin, noradrenaline, and vasopressin, and by a large number of local tissue mediators, which include hydrogen ions, potassium, adenosine, and nitric oxide. The renal vasculature is especially sensitive.

At local tissue level, hypovolaemia encourages movement of fluid into capillaries: the decreased capillary hydrostatic pressure favours absorption of interstitial fluid, with a resultant increase in plasma volume and restoration of arterial pressure towards normal. These mechanisms are particularly efficient in situations in which blood loss is slow, such as occurs with insidious postpartum haemorrhage.

The hypothalamo-pituitary adrenal response is also important, although it is slower. Reduced renal blood flow stimulates intrarenal baroreceptors, which mediate renin release from the juxta-glomerular apparatus. This in turn leads to the conversion of circulating angiotensinogen to angiotensin I and then angiotensin II (in the lung). Angiotensin II is a powerful arteriolar vasoconstrictor that also stimulates aldosterone release from the adrenal cortex, and arginine vasopressin (AVP – also known as antidiuretic hormone, ADH) release from the posterior pituitary. AVP release is also stimulated by atrial receptors, which respond to the decrease in extracellular volume. These changes enhance sodium-ion and water reabsorption at the distal renal tubule as the body attempts to conserve fluid.

Shock is a potent stimulus to respiration, and so respiratory rate and minute ventilation increase, mediated partly by metabolic changes as carotid chemoreceptors respond to alterations in arterial partial pressures of oxygen and carbon dioxide (PaO_2 and $PaCO_2$) and hydrogen ion. Haemorrhage may cause substantial metabolic derangements: with decreased tissue perfusion, there is a progressive decline in aerobic metabolism, which is accompanied by a compensatory increase in anaerobic metabolism as tissue ischaemia progresses. The shift to anaerobic metabolism results in a decrease in energy production and the development of a metabolic acidosis. In the aerobic (tricarboxylic acid, TCA) cycle, the hydrogen ions produced are carried by NADH and $NADH_2$ to the electron transport chain, in which the final acceptor is molecular oxygen, which is then converted to water. In the absence of molecular oxygen, the final acceptor (oxygen) is lacking, and so NADH accumulates. The lack of NAD^+ effectively blocks the TCA cycle, and so pyruvate accumulates (at the 'entrance' to the cycle). NADH and pyruvate react to form lactate and NAD^+. The lactate then diffuses out of the cell and accumulates as lactic acid; NAD^+ meanwhile allows anaerobic glycolysis to proceed. This process is important because severe metabolic acidosis is deleterious to tissue and organ function, particularly that of the myocardium.

RECOGNITION

The physiological compensatory responses described above help to explain the clinical features that accompany major haemorrhage. Redistribution of blood flow is responsible for the typical pallor, cold peripheries, peripheral cyanosis, and oliguria. Sympathetic stimulation explains the tachycardia, which is an important early sign, even in low-volume loss, as well as the increase in respiratory rate. An outline of the response to varying degrees of blood loss is seen in Table 7.1, although this should be viewed only as a guide because not all patients will behave so predictably. Most healthy mothers can lose up to 15% of their circulating blood volume without developing marked clinical symptoms, but in the short term the rate of bleeding is as important as the

Table 7.1 Response to varying degrees of blood loss				
	Blood loss[a]			
	<15% (<1200 ml)	15–30% (1200–2400 ml)	30–40% (2400–3200 ml)	>40% (>3200 ml)
Heart rate	<100	>100	>120	>140
Systolic blood pressure	↔	↔	↓	↓
Pulse pressure	↔	↓	↓	↓
Capillary refill (normal <2 s)	↔	↓	Absent	Absent
Central venous pressure	↔	↓	↓	↓
Respiratory rate	14–20	20–30	30–40	>40
Mental state	Anxious	Anxious++	Confused	Obtunded

[a]The volumes shown assume a body weight of 80 kg.

total loss. Sudden brisk bleeding may well be accompanied by transient cardiovascular collapse, even if the total loss does not approach the 15% above which symptoms are said usually to appear. Equally, a mother may compensate for a much greater postpartum loss, provided that it takes place over a number of hours. Tachycardia is an important early sign of bleeding, but it has to be remembered that this has many other causes, including pain, anxiety, and drug treatment. It is also important to note that the systolic blood pressure – which is the measurement that seems to dominate all others in this context – is a relatively crude index that may show little change until 30–40% of the blood volume (2 litres or more in a pregnant woman) has been lost. This masking of massive blood loss will be less in situations when the bleeding is acute. The pulse pressure, however, which is the difference between the systolic and diastolic pressures, may give earlier warning of a

problem, particularly if other indices are considered at the same time. As blood loss continues, the pulse pressure narrows and the mean arterial pressure, rather than falling, may actually increase. This occurs because diastolic blood pressure is under the influence of catecholamines, which rise in response to haemorrhage. Close monitoring of trends is vital during this time. Capillary refill time, which is measured by blanching an extremity by continuous pressure for 5 seconds before releasing the pressure and timing reperfusion of the skin, is a simple and effective measure. A delay of more than 2 seconds is abnormal, and trends can be used to gauge the effectiveness of fluid resuscitation: as the intravascular compartment is stabilized, the refill time will decrease towards normal. Shock is a potent stimulus to respiration, but tachypnoea, like tachycardia, may also be associated with pain and anxiety. Urine output starts to fall early following intravascular depletion, but this too may have other causes, particularly if the mother has impaired renal function associated with pre-eclampsia. Changes in cerebration, manifested by confusion or obtunded mental state, are indicative of cerebral hypoxaemia and hypoperfusion, and indicate that the clinical situation is perilous. Confusional states, however, may also be associated with other conditions, such as sepsis or amniotic fluid embolism. It is essential, therefore, when obstetric haemorrhage is being gauged, to use a thorough approach that looks at each system separately before assessing the whole.

CONFOUNDING FACTORS

The assessment of major obstetric haemorrhage can be made even more difficult by the presence of the numerous confounding factors that may have to be considered. Tachycardia may be due to other factors, such as pain, infection, or the use of drugs (e.g. oxytocin). Tachypnoea equally may be due to pain, sepsis, or anxiety. In any mother who is bleeding antepartum, it is important to remain alert to the likelihood of supine hypotension due to aorto-caval compression, and so a wedge or tilt must be used throughout the resuscitation. A woman who has undergone operative delivery may also be hypotensive because of the residual effects of spinal (subarachnoid) anaesthesia. In such cases, low blood pressure may not only result from sympathetic blockade due to local anaesthesia but may also be an effect of one of the intrathecal adjuncts such as diamorphine or clonidine that are finding increasing use. The hypotensive effects of general anaesthesia may also persist into the immediate postoperative period to confuse the clinical picture. Most

difficult of all may be a mother who is bleeding but whose pregnancy has been complicated by severe pre-eclampsia. Such patients typically exhibit labile changes in blood pressure that may be clinically deceptive, and they are often managed according to protocols that restrict fluids, typically to 85 ml/h. It is essential to appreciate that this is the maintenance regimen, and should be given in addition to any fluids that are administered to replace blood loss. Mothers with hypertension may also have been treated with a β-adrenoceptor blocker, typically labetalol, which will limit the capacity of the sympathetic nervous system to compensate for fluid loss. The same will be true of women who have undergone operative delivery under epidural anaesthesia. Any such block that is adequate for surgery will always be accompanied by effective sympathetic blockade in the region that is anaesthetized.

SPECIFIC MONITORING

No single monitor can provide all the crucial information that is necessary for the optimal management of major obstetric haemorrhage. It is important to be able to interpret the available information as a whole, to be aware of the value of monitoring trends, and to recognize some of the potential pitfalls that are associated with particular devices.

Arterial blood pressure

Hypotension is a late sign of hypovolaemia in an otherwise-fit patient who is able to compensate. The accepted gold standard of measurement is direct intra-arterial blood pressure monitoring, which is the only method that gives beat-to-beat information.

This is particularly useful when blood loss is rapid, substantial, and unpredictable. The absolute numbers recorded are not the only information that is provided: a systolic pressure variation (the difference between the maximum and minimum pressures recorded during the respiratory cycle) of more than 10 mmHg during positive-pressure ventilation indicates a 10% reduction in circulating blood volume. This may be a more sensitive indicator than central venous pressure.[17] Direct intra-arterial monitoring, however, is not readily available on most labour wards, where non-invasive methods are much more familiar. While the automated oscillometric devices are useful, it is worth noting some of their inherent problems: they tend to under-read at high pressures and over-read at low pressures. At systolic pressures below 100 mmHg, they may overestimate by 20–25 mmHg. They have difficulty in producing readings if heart rates are slow (around 40 beats per minute) or if the pulse is irregular in conditions such as ventricular bigeminy or atrial fibrillation. If the blood pressure is very low, many automated machines may continue to cycle until a value falls within the manufacturer's algorithm.[18] Under these circumstances, traditional non-automated methods of blood pressure measurement can still be useful.

Central venous pressure

Very early data suggested that central venous pressure (CVP) rapidly reflects changes in circulating blood volume such that pressure in the right atrium decreases by some 0.7 cmH$_2$O for each 100 ml of blood removed from a healthy 70 kg adult. Blood loss of 500–800 ml in healthy volunteers leads to a decrease in CVP of up to 7 cmH$_2$O, even though the arterial pressure shows no fall.[19] Modern practice is to measure the CVP at the reference level of the right atrium, where the mean venous pressure is about 4 cmH$_2$O, and since an intravascular pressure cannot become persistently negative, the absolute numerical falls cannot be great. Clinical experience suggests, moreover, that – in some patients at least – compensatory venoconstriction may maintain the CVP during the early stages of major haemorrhage. It will also remain high if fluid is being infused rapidly. The best way of determining whether or not a patient has adequate intravascular volume by using CVP measurements is to use a fluid challenge. If, after a bolus of 250 ml of an appropriate fluid, the CVP rises but then falls back over 10–15 minutes to its previous level then it is probable that the central circulation can accept more fluid. It will be obvious, however, that in acute massive obstetric haemorrhage, this relatively leisurely approach is of modest value – although in the case of insidious postpartum loss, it can provide useful information.

It should be remembered that the anaesthetic and other literature contains abundant evidence of the many complications with which central venous cannulation has been associated, from nerve and vessel injury to pneumothorax and cardiac tamponade. Ultrasound-guided techniques increase the safety of the procedure, but if such a device is not available then a long line that is inserted, for example, via the antecubital fossa may be a satisfactory alternative.

CVP monitoring is likely to be the most invasive and technical of the devices used on the labour ward in the management of major blood loss, and its importance should not, because of this, be overestimated. It can be helpful in guiding resuscitation, but only when taken in conjunction with the overall clinical picture.

Oximetry

Arterial hypoxaemia is a very late sign of hypovolaemia, but nobody would dispute that pulse oximetry should be used continuously. Tachycardia, in contrast, is a useful early sign of blood loss, and so a pulse oximeter will provide timely evidence of possible bleeding. It may also give more subtle information: as the central venous pressure falls, there may be a variation in the plethysmographic waveform of the oximeter that is analogous to the changes that may be seen in a directly measured arterial trace. During the respiratory cycle in a ventilated patient, therefore, the peak of the waveform may fall during the phase of positive pressure. The usefulness of this sign may be limited by the fact that, with poor peripheral perfusion, the waveform, although it is usually corrected and amplified by the device, may almost disappear. This in itself is an important clinical sign that indicates failure of the peripheral circulation and possible compromise of organ perfusion.

Urine output

Urine output is another useful indicator of organ perfusion, because it decreases early in hypovolaemia and will cease completely once the percentage blood loss approaches 20–25%. Awake normotensive healthy humans produce urine at about 1 ml/kg/h; volumes of less than 0.5 ml/kg/h indicate poor renal perfusion.

Arterial blood gases

Major haemorrhage is associated usually with a normal PaO_2 and a low $PaCO_2$. As shock worsens, there is an increase in anaerobic metabolism and the development of a metabolic acidosis with decreased pH and increased base deficit despite the low $PaCO_2$. At tissue level, there is hypoxia and hypercapnia. Arterial acidosis indicates prolonged inadequacy of tissue perfusion suggestive of severe hypovolaemia. This will be reflected in mixed venous blood gases: the normal value for O_2 is 43 mmHg and for CO_2 46 mmHg, whereas in shock these values change to about 20 and 55–60 mmHg respectively. In major obstetric haemorrhage, however, it is improbable that these will be recorded early, since mixed venous blood gases require a pulmonary arterial catheter to allow sampling.

Haemoglobin estimation

Haemoglobin values are of limited value in the acute stages of major blood loss and can be difficult to interpret. Transient haemoconcentration may be superseded by marked haemodilution if large volumes of non-blood colloid or crystalloid solution are used for initial resuscitation. It is only when the fluid shifts have stabilized that a haemoglobin determination will provide reliable information.

MANAGEMENT

The priorities for management should be the restitution of blood volume; the correction of coagulopathy by judicious use of blood component therapy, and the restoration of haemostasis by treatment of any surgical source of blood loss. As soon as bleeding is suspected, high-flow oxygen should be administered via a fixed-performance face-mask. If the mother has not yet delivered, left uterine displacement must be maintained using a right pelvic wedge. Occlusion of the vena cava has been demonstrated by invasive methods to occur in almost all parturients at term, with venous drainage dependent on tortuous collateral diversion through the paravertebral and azygos veins. Venous return is delayed, and cardiac output may decrease by as much as 50%.[20,21] If the supine hypotensive syndrome is not recognized, it may compromise fatally any attempt at resuscitation. In some cases, aorto-caval compression is relieved completely only by turning the patient into the full decubitus position.

Aggressive fluid resuscitation should begin while the cause of the blood loss is being investigated. Rapid diagnosis is essential. Although the overriding priority of management is maintenance of tissue perfusion and oxygen delivery by the rapid restoration of circulating blood volume, given the hyperdynamic nature of the uteroplacental circulation, even the most vigorous fluid resuscitation will eventually fail unless the primary cause is addressed and the source of the bleeding is stopped. In every case, the importance of early recognition cannot be overemphasized, nor can effective communication between the clinical specialties. Senior anaesthetists, obstetricians, and haematologists should be involved early, as must transfusion laboratory staff.

Fluid resuscitation

Intravascular volume must be restored as quickly as possible so as to maintain tissue perfusion, oxygen delivery, and, in the mother who has not yet delivered, fetal viability. Resuscitation should begin using short, wide-bore peripheral intravenous cannulae. This advice follows from the frequently quoted Poiseuille–Hagen equation, which states that flow through a tube is inversely proportional to its length and directly proportional to the fourth power of its radius. This relationship is not academic: double the length of a cannula and fluid flow through it is halved, double its diameter and flow increases by 16 times. This does not necessarily mean, however, that anything smaller than a 14G cannula is useless: an 18G cannula and a pressure infuser are enough to initiate effective fluid resuscitation pending the establishment of more definitive intravenous access. It should also be remembered that cannulae are not standardized and that flow characteristics may differ between cannulae of the same gauge. Flow through a 16G Venflon, for example, is quoted by the manufacturer as 180 ml/min, which is greater than the 150 ml/min claimed for a 16G Wallace but less than the 210 ml/min quoted for a 16G Optiva. Fluid can be given through central venous catheters, although these tend to be much longer than peripheral cannulae. Cold blood should not be administered via this route: extracellular potassium in a unit of blood that has not been warmed to body temperature can have a concentration some ten times greater than normal, and if delivered directly into the right heart may act as a cardioplegic solution and cause cardiac standstill.

In respect of the optimal fluid for volume replacement, clinicians are unable to agree whether crystalloid solutions or non-blood colloids are better for initial resuscitation – and there is no sign, certainly in obstetric practice, of the studies that will provide a definite answer. A pragmatic view is that the type of fluid that is given is less important than that adequate volume is given, and that crystalloid solutions, colloids, or a mixture of both probably can be used in the healthy obstetric patient without clinical detriment. Rational management does demand, however, an understanding of the fluid compartments of the body and how the various infused solutions distribute within those compartments. The three fluid spaces are the intravascular space (comprising about 10% of the whole), the interstitial space (comprising some 30% of the whole), and the largest space, the intracellular space (containing the remaining 60% of the body's fluid). The extracellular fluid (ECF) space consists, therefore, of the interstitial and intravascular spaces. These compartments have different compositions and different functions. Intracellular sodium is kept low by active extrusion, while the sodium concentration in the ECF remains high. The intravascular compartment is maintained by the presence of oncotically active plasma proteins, which exert a colloid oncotic pressure (COP) across the capillary endothelium. An infusion of glucose 5%, therefore, will distribute evenly across all fluid spaces, and so – at the very most – only 10% can remain within the circulation. An infusion of isotonic saline, however, will distribute evenly only between the intravascular and interstitial spaces, so that 1.5 hours after infusion of a litre of sodium chloride 0.9%, the plasma volume, predictably, will have increased by only about 250–275 ml.[22] An oncotically active colloid, by contrast, is more likely to be retained within the intravascular compartment. But not all non-blood colloidal solu-

tions are the same, and the effectiveness of a particular substance in maintaining intravascular volume depends on the molecular weight, the renal and capillary thresholds for the solution, and its specific water-binding capacity. If the plasma volume restitution at 1.5 hours after administration is expressed as a percentage of the original volume infused then the most effective colloid is the glucose polymer dextran-70 at 79%, followed by hydroxyethylstarch (HES) at 72%, human albumin at 48%, and the gelatine solution Haemaccel at 24%. The figure for sodium chloride 0.9% is about 18%.[23] In many hospitals, the colloid that is immediately available is one of the gelatins, either Haemaccel or Gelofusine, and these data suggest that, in terms of volume expansion, their advantages over crystalloid may be limited. Albumin solutions, meanwhile are viewed with undeserved suspicion following a controversial meta-analysis that ensured that many clinicians ceased using them.[24] Dextrans have also suffered from adverse publicity that is probably unwarranted. Renal failure has been associated with high-volume infusion of dextran 40, which may accumulate in the renal tubules of dehydrated patients, but the actual number of cases is very low.[25] The allergic reactions that once were common have been all but eliminated by the use of hapten inhibition, but the charge that dextrans interfere with blood crossmatching by coating red blood cell surfaces continues to be influential, and they are not used widely in the UK. The manufacturers recommend that the total infused should not exceed 20 ml/kg because of concerns about the effect on haemostasis. The same restriction is applied to HES by the manufacturer, because above this level it too may depress factor VIII and platelet activity, and a number of significant haemorrhagic complications have been described in the literature. It appears, however, that the guideline of 20 ml/kg is not supported by the evidence, which suggests on the contrary that adverse effects on haemostasis can appear independently of the dose given.[26] HES also has the disadvantage of being a synthetic colloid that is not fully metabolized. Non-degraded high-molecular-weight residues are sequestered indefinitely within the reticuloendothelial system with long-term effects that are as yet unknown. In obstetric practice in the UK, therefore, the main fluids that are used are crystalloid solutions and gelatins.

Haematological assistance

Expert haematological help is essential, and should be sought early. A senior haematologist will expedite the provision of blood and blood products, advise on investigations, particularly those relating to coagulation status, and guide component therapy.

Blood replacement

A recent study into transfusion requirements in critical care suggested that in patients who were randomized to a restrictive transfusion policy, in which blood transfusion was triggered by a haemoglobin concentration of 7.0 g/dl, outcome was improved.[27] Such data should be extrapolated to obstetric patients with caution, if at all. While it is true that the primary problem is loss or intravascular volume, loss of red cell mass inevitably compromises oxygen delivery to the tissues, whose metabolic demands in the peripartum period are increased by up to 35%.[28] Oxygen consumption in the third trimester rises to 60% above baseline levels. There are isolated reports of Jehovah's Witnesses who have survived falls in haemoglobin to below 3.0 g/dl,[29] but it takes an iron nerve to withhold blood transfusion from a young mother who is exsanguinating, on the basis of a case report or a contentious meta-analysis. One problem with obstetric haemorrhage is that it is rarely clear what is the likely endpoint. It is never certain at the outset whether a mother is going to lose 25% or 250% of her blood volume. Nor is it common for fluid replacement to match precisely at any given time during a very labile situation the exact intravascular losses. At any one point during resuscitation, therefore, a mother is likely either to be under- or over-transfused. It is not until the situation has stabilized that volaemic status can be assessed accurately. In the meantime a bleeding obstetric patient should receive red cells, because crystalloid and the immediately available non-blood colloids do not carry oxygen. In extreme emergency, up to two units of non crossmatched group O Rhesus-negative blood can be given. As soon as the blood group has been identified by the laboratory, group-specific red cells should be given. This simplified crossmatching procedure is swift and can be performed in under 5 minutes, although published figures suggest that it more typically takes between 10 and 30 minutes. Standard full crossmatching and antibody screening are likely to take an hour or longer.[30] Further crossmatching is not necessary after one blood volume has been replaced.[31] A blood warmer should be used from the outset, and a rapid infusion device should be available. One disadvantage of these devices is their potential to overload the circulation, but, alarming though it may be both for patient and clinician, it is much easier to treat acute pulmonary oedema than acute renal failure secondary to hypovolaemic hypoperfusion. Over-transfusion with packed cells should, however, be avoided, because of the microcirculatory compromise consequent upon a high haematocrit.

Fresh-frozen plasma

Before it became routine practice to provide red cell replacement in the form of plasma-poor blood suspended in optimal additive solution, both whole-blood and plasma-reduced blood were available. This explained the US National Institutes of Health consensus view in 1985 that residual and adequate coagulation factor activity meant that there was no evidence to support the routine administration of fresh-frozen plasma (FFP) as part of therapy for transfusion-associated coagulopathy.[32] This advice is no longer appropriate. After 1.5 blood volumes have been lost, the level of fibrinogen will fall to the critical level of 0.1 g/dl, and after 2 volumes have been replaced, the coagulation activity reduces to about 25% of normal.[33] 'Formula replacement' in which, for example, one unit of FFP is given for every 4 units of blood is no longer advocated, and administration should be guided both by the laboratory results and by the advice of a senior haematologist. As a general rule, however, once it has been decided, either empirically or in response to laboratory results, to give FFP to a mother who is bleeding, it should be administered in a volume of 15 ml/kg.[31] Coagulation factors ideally should be given according to laboratory results such that the activated partial thromboplastin time (APTT) and prothrom-

bin time (PT) are prolonged by less than 1.5 times control.

Cryoprecipitate

If investigations confirm that a woman is defibrinating then cryoprecipitate should be given to restore fibrinogen levels to at least 0.1 g/dl, for which 1–1.5 packs per 10 kg body weight may be necessary.[31]

It should be remembered that these blood products may need to be transported to the hospital from a distant site and will also require thawing after arrival – a process that takes about 30 minutes. If a woman is bleeding sufficiently to warrant blood transfusion with plasma-poor red cells then the requirement for FFP and cryoprecipitate should be anticipated and the products ordered early.

Platelets

The current consensus is that platelets should not be allowed to fall below $50 \times 10^9/l$ in any patient who is bleeding acutely, because a level of 50 (assuming that plasma-poor blood has been used for replacement) suggests that up to two blood volumes have been lost.[33] Platelet numbers, however, may not reflect the adequacy of platelet function, and haematological guidance must be sought early. Massive obstetric haemorrhage is almost certain to require platelet transfusion, and so this should be requested as soon as it becomes clear that major blood loss is a possibility. Platelets frequently need to be ordered from a blood centre that may be some miles distant, and so it is important to anticipate any requirement.

Obstetric, surgical, or radiological intervention: stopping the bleeding at source

Uterine atony

A uterus may fail to contract effectively after delivery because its cavity contains residual products of conception. It will continue to bleed until these are removed. At the same time, any drugs that relax the uterus should, if possible, be discontinued. This may be more difficult in the case of a bleeding parturient in whom magnesium sulfate is being used as part of the treatment of pre-eclampsia, but it should be possible to avoid volatile anaesthetic agents, which relax the uterus except when given in very low concentrations. Any general anaesthetic technique that is used should be based ideally upon total intravenous anaesthesia.

Primary uterine atony should be treated pharmacologically with appropriate stimulants. First-line management is usually the administration of oxytocin (Syntocinon) in a bolus dose of 5 units. This drug has a short half-life of 12–17 minutes,[34] and so the bolus should be followed by an infusion of 5–10 units an hour. If this is ineffective then ergometrine can be given as a bolus of 500 µg. As this drug has potent haemodynamic effects and is associated with nausea and vomiting in 50% of patients, a better option may be to use prostaglandin. Prostaglandin $F_{2\alpha}$ (carboprost, Hemabate) is effective in the management of refractory uterine atony. It can be given in a dose of 250 µg by the intramuscular route, although many obstetricians find it most effective when it is injected directly into the myometrium. Its datasheet emphasizes that it should not be given intravenously. It should

be remembered that none of these drugs is free from cardiovascular effects: oxytocin can cause tachycardia and hypotension, both ergometrine and prostaglandin $F_{2\alpha}$ may provoke hypertension and tachycardia. If bleeding is not controlled by these measures then surgical or radiological intervention may be required.

Non-conservative measures

If all else fails, it may prove necessary to proceed to peripartum hysterectomy. Abnormal placental implantation is the most common precipitant, accounting for 64% of cases in one series, while uterine atony was responsible for 21%.[35] This can be a difficult procedure and the operative course may be stormy. If preservation of fertility is important, but torrential haemorrhage is complicating surgery, then packing the abdomen may be a lifesaving temporizing manoeuvre. A pack within the uterine cavity, however, will prevent its effective contraction and should not be used. Obstetricians are not used to crossclamping the aorta, but this too may be lifesaving and without adverse sequelae. A healthy woman will stand this potential insult much better than a patient with an abdominal aortic aneurysm in whom crossclamping is employed as a routine. If the appropriate surgical instruments are not immediately available then manual compression may achieve the same effect. (This can also be used externally – a fist pressed dorsally in the midline and just above the umbilicus will compress the aorta against the vertebral column and abolish (55%) or reduce (10%) lower limb perfusion.[36]) Ligation of the internal iliac arteries can be used, as can direct ligation of the uterine arteries themselves. This is not as effective as might be expected – the collateral blood supply to the uterus is impressive and internal iliac artery ligation reduces blood flow by less than 50%. The procedure is successful in only half of those treated. Surgical ligation does, however, approach 100% success if as sequential approach is taken, with successive ligation of the internal iliac, the uterine, and then the ovarian arteries.[37] The technical difficulties of accurate identification in a surgical field that is awash with blood should not, however, be underestimated. An alternative may be the use of interventional radiology in which the bleeding vessels can be identified accurately via percutaneous transfemoral angiography prior to being embolized. It may not even be necessary to embolize the vessels if bleeding can be controlled by the intravascular inflation of a balloon-tipped catheter. Experience of interventional radiology to date suggests that the success rate of embolization approaches 90%, although it should be noted that the reported numbers remain small. A recent review concluded that the technique is underused,[38] but the logistical difficulties of transferring a bleeding parturient to an area with imaging facilities will be evident to all those who work in maternity units that are not immediately adjacent to a radiology department.

Intraoperative blood salvage

The use of cell-savers to salvage intraoperative blood has been avoided in obstetric practice because of concerns about the presence of fetal squames or amniotic fluid components that, were they to gain access to the maternal circulation, would cause amniotic fluid embolism. It appears, however, that modern cell-saver devices can separate out these potentially undesirable components, which suggests that they may in due course prove as useful in massive haemorrhage in obstetrics as they are everywhere else.[39]

CONCLUSIONS

Obstetric haemorrhage can be torrential and catastrophic, and the stakes are very high. Successful management demands that the potential for major haemorrhage be recognized early, that it should be treated aggressively by vigorous fluid resuscitation, and that the bleeding should be stopped at source. Senior anaesthetists, obstetricians, and haematologists must be mobilized as early as possible, because it may be their combined efforts only that can help ensure survival with minimal morbidity.

REFERENCES

1. *Report of Confidential Enquiries into Maternal Deaths in the United Kingdom 1991–1993.* London: HMSO, 1996.
2. *Why Mothers Die. Report on Confidential Enquiries into Maternal Deaths in the United Kingdom 1994–1996.* London: HMSO, 1998.
3. *Why Mothers Die. The confidential enquires in maternal deaths in the United Kingdom, 1997–1999.* London: RCOG Press, 2001.
4. Gilbert L, Porter W, Brown VA. Postpartum haemorrhage – a continuing problem. *Br J Obstet Gynaecol* 1987; **94**: 67–71.
5. Duthie SJ, Yung LK, Guang DZ et al. Discrepancy between laboratory determination and visual estimation of blood loss during normal delivery. *Eur J Obstet Gynecol Reprod Biol* 1990; **38**: 119–24.
6. Duthie SJ, Ghosh A, Ng A, Ho PC. Intraoperative blood loss during elective lower segment caesarean section. *Br J Obstet Gynaecol* 1992; **99**: 364–7.

7. Combs CA, Murphy EL, Laros RK. Factors associated with postpartum hemorrhage with vaginal birth. *Obstet Gynecol* 1991; **70**: 69–76.

8. Hurley R, Ostheimer GW. Postpartum hemorrhage and uterine atony. In: *Complications in Anesthesiology*, 2nd edn (Gravenstein N, Kirby RR, eds). Philadelphia: Lippincott-Raven, 1996.

9. Hewitt PE, Machin SJ. Massive blood transfusion. In: *ABC of Transfusion* (Contreras M, ed). London: BMJ Publishing, 1992.

10. Fakhry SM, Sheldon GF. Massive transfusion in the surgical patient. In: *Massive Transfusion* (Jeffries LC, Brecher ME, eds). Bethesda, MD: American Association of Blood Banks, 1994.

11. Phillips OC. Uterine atony. In: *Complications in Anesthesiology* (Orkin FK, Cooperman, LH, eds). Philadelphia: Lippincott, 1983.

12. Munson ES, Embro WJ. Enflurane, isoflurane, and halothane on isolated human uterine muscle. *Anesthesiology* 1977; **46**: 11–14.

13. Clark SL, Koonings P, Phelan JP et al. Placenta praevia/accreta and prior cesarean section. *Obstet Gynecol* 1985; **66**: 89–92.

14. Miller DA, Chollet JA, Goodwin TM. Clinical risk factors for placenta praevia–placenta accreta. *Am J Obstet Gynecol* 1997; **177**: 210–14.

15. Rasmussen S, Irgens LM, Bergsjo PB et al. The occurrence of placental abruption in Norway 1967–1991. *Acta Obstet Gynecol Scand* 1996; **75**: 222–8.

16. Farmer RM, Kirschbaum T, Potter D et al. Uterine rupture during trial of labor after previous caesarean section. *Am J Obstet Gynecol* 1991; **165**: 996–1001.

17. Perel A, Pizov R, Cotev S. Systolic blood pressure variation is a sensitive indicator of hypovolaemia in ventilated dogs subject to graded haemorrhage. *Anesthesiology* 1987; **67**: 498–502.

18. Lawes EG. In praise of mercury sphygmomanometers. *BMJ* 2000; **321**: 1534.

19. Gauer OH, Henry JP, Sieker HO. Changes in central venous pressure after moderate haemorrhage and transfusion in man. *Circul Res* 1956; **4**: 79–83.

20. Lees MM, Scott DB, Kerr MG et al. A study of cardiac output at rest throughout pregnancy. *J Obstet Gynaecol Br Commonwealth* 1967; **74**: 319–28.

21. Weaver JB, Pearson JF, Rosen M. Posture and epidural block in pregnant women at term. *Anaesthesia* 1975; **30**: 752–6.

22. Imm A, Carlson RW. Fluid resuscitation in circulatory shock. *Crit Care Clin* 1993; **9**: 313–33.

23. Lamke L-O, Liljedahl S-O. Plasma volume changes after infusion of various plasma expanders. *Resuscitation* 1976; **5**: 93–102.

24. Cochrane Injuries Group Albumin Reviewers. Human albumin administration in critically ill patients: systematic review of randomized controlled trials. *BMJ* 1998; **317**: 235–40.

25. Ljungström K-G. Safety of dextran in relation to other colloids – ten years experience with hapten inhibition. *Infusionsther Transfusionsmed* 1993; **20**: 206–10.

26. Warren BB, Durieux ME. Hydroxyethyl starch: safe or not? *Anesth Analg* 1997; **84**: 206–12.

27. Hebert PC, Wells G, Blajchman MA et al. A multicenter, randomized controlled clinical trial of transfusion requirements in critical care. *N Engl J Med* 1999; **340**: 409–17.

28. Prentice AM, Goldberg GR, Davies HL et al. Energy-sparing adaptations in human pregnancy assessed by whole-body calorimetry. *Br J Nutr* 1989; **62**: 5–22.

29. Rasanayagam SR, Cooper GM. Two cases of severe postpartum anaemia in Jehovah's Witnesses. *Int J Obstet Anaesth* 1996; **5**: 202–5.

30. Kretschmer V, Karger R, Weippert-Kretschmer M. Emergency and massive transfusion. *Baillière's Clin Anaesthesiol* 1997; **11**: 261–76.

31. Stainsby D, MacLennan S, Hamilton PJ. Man-

agement of massive blood loss: a template guideline. *Br J Anaesth* 2000; **85**: 487–91.

32. NIH Consensus Conference. Fresh frozen plasma: indications and risks. *JAMA* 1985; **253**: 551–3.

33. Hiippala ST, Myllyla GJ, Vahtera EM. Hemostatic factors and replacement of major blood loss with plasma-poor red cell concentrates. *Anesth Analg* 1995; **81**: 360–5.

34. Amico JA, Seitchik J, Robinson AG. Studies of oxytocin in plasma of women during hypocontractile labour. *J Clin Endocrinol Metab* 1984; **58**: 274–9.

35. Zelop CM, Harlow BL, Frigoletto FD Jr et al. Emergency peripartum hysterectomy. *Am J Obstet Gynecol* 1993; **168**: 1443–8.

36. Riley DP, Burgess RW. External abdominal aortic compression: a study of a resuscitation manoeuvre for postpartum haemorrhage. *Anaesth Intensive Care* 1994; **22**: 571–6.

37. Abd Rabbo SA. Sequential uterine devascularisation: a novel technique for management of uncontrollable postpartum hemorrhage with preservation of the uterus. *Am J Obstet Gynecol* 1994; **171**: 694–700.

38. Vedantham S, Goodwin SC, McLucas B et al. Uterine artery embolization: an underused method of controlling pelvic haemorrhage. *Am J Obstet Gynecol* 1997; **176**: 938–48.

39. Bernstein HH, Rosenblatt MA, Gette S, Lockwood C. The ability of the haemanetics and cell saver system to remove tissue factor from blood contaminated with amniotic fluid. *Anesth Analges* 1997; **85**: 81–3.

8 Paediatric and neonatal transfusions

Paula HB Bolton-Maggs

INTRODUCTION

Transfusion of blood or blood products to children and infants requires special consideration for a number of reasons. Careful thought needs to be given both to the clinical indication for blood and blood products and to any special requirements of the products resulting from the age of the recipient. Children receiving transfusions are largely expected to have a normal life expectancy and therefore to have longer in which to manifest any long term ill-effects of the transfusion process. Transfusion of any blood component is a potentially hazardous procedure; the parents of a child requiring blood products often worry about possible transmission of infection, but do not realize that the greatest risk is that a child will get a product intended for someone else as a result of one or more human errors at some stage of the process.[1,2] It is important to be clear that any transfusion of blood product is clearly needed and that the indication is recorded in the case record. Unfortunately, there are many areas of paediatric transfusion practice where evidence for efficacy is lacking. Despite this, guidelines based upon opinion and standard of practice can be very useful – at least as a base against which to audit practice and outcomes.

Long-term sequelae of blood transfusion have been tragic where human immunodeficiency virus (HIV) or hepatitis C virus (HCV) was inadvertently transmitted,[3–8] donor screening has reduced but not completely eliminated these risks in developed countries,[9] but these risks vary and may be higher in other parts of the world.[10–15] In all cases, clinicians should think carefully whether there are alternatives to transfusion. It is clear that in high-risk areas, strict attention to defining criteria for transfusion can reduce the risks of transfusion-transmitted infections.[16–20] These are important lessons from which we can learn.

For practical purposes, the transfusion of children can be divided into transfusion of neonates and infants up to four months of age, who have special requirements in terms of products, and transfusion of older children, whose requirements are more akin to those of adults.

PHYSIOLOGY

When are transfusions of red cells required? Red cell transfusion will be of benefit when tissue oxygenation is compromised. Unfortunately this is very difficult to measure, so that surrogate indicators have to be used, which may be misleading (such as the haemoglobin level). Oxygen delivery to the tissues is normally two- or fourfold more than is required, and is influenced by the haemoglobin concentration, the percentage haemoglobin oxygen saturation, and the cardiac output. Each of these has a large reserve, so that several compensating mechanisms come into play. Tissues may extract more oxygen from the blood, and blood with reduced red cell concentration has a lower viscosity and so flows better. In some tissues, normal oxygen extraction is only 25%; but in the brain and heart, the normal extraction is 55–70%, so that for these tissues an increase in flow is required to counteract the effect of anaemia. In animals, coronary lactate production starts at a haemoglobin level of less than 3.5 g/dl, and in the presence of coronary stenosis this anaerobic state occurs at a haemoglobin level of 6–7 g/dl.[21,22] Children have higher 2,3-diphosphoglycerate (2,3-DPG) levels in red cells compared with adults, which may be one mechanism for tolerating a lower haemoglobin level. This shifts the oxygen dissociation curve to the right, i.e. oxygen is more easily released to the tissues. There is no easy way to measure precisely when oxygen consumption exceeds oxygen delivery, and this will vary in different clinical situations. The haemoglobin level is a very poor surrogate marker for this. There are very few adequate clinical trials in the literature addressing these issues. Those available address clinical situations that are specialized (e.g. transfusion for malaria and anaemia in Africa) or that have changed since the publication of the reports (e.g. the use of hypertransfusion in children treated for malignant disease). The data from Africa – based on risk of death – suggested that children should receive red cells when the haemoglobin level is below 5 g/dl and there are signs of respiratory or cardiac decompensation, and at a haemoglobin level below 3 g/dl irrespective of symptoms.[23] Certainly children tolerate lower haemoglobin levels without symptoms than do adults, so that in general the threshold for

transfusion in anaemia can be lower (see below).

INDICATIONS FOR BLOOD TRANSFUSION IN CHILDREN

The following are the clinical situations in which blood transfusion may be indicated in children:

- blood loss;
- haemolysis;
- chronic anaemia caused by a variety of different aetiologies.

Blood loss

Acute haemorrhage in children occurs as a result of trauma, or, more rarely, from the gastrointestinal tract (e.g. varices from portal hypertension, ulceration). The principles of management are essentially as for adults – but the compensatory mechanisms differ in the very young, so that hypotension, for example, is a very late and serious sign. In any serious injury, vascular access should be urgently established, preferably by more than one large-bore cannula; an intraosseous infusion (using the tibia or lower end of the femur) can be lifesaving, and is the recommended route of access in cardiac arrest – these and other techniques are well described in the recent third edition of *Advanced Paediatric Life Support*.[24] In a shocked child, initial boluses of fluid can either be crystalloid or colloid at a dose of 20 ml/kg, repeated if the response is inadequate. In an emergency, the weight of the child may not be known, but if the age is known then the weight (for children between 1 and 10 years) can be estimated according to the following formula: weight (kg) = 2 (age + 4). Only after this should blood be given; this should give sufficient time to obtain group-specific blood rather than using group O Rhesus (Rh) D-negative blood.

Chronic blood loss is rare in children, and likely to manifest as iron-deficiency anaemia, but by far the commonest cause of iron deficiency in childhood is diet. Transfusion for iron deficiency is almost never required; children can tolerate low haemoglobin levels down to 3 g/dl or less without significant symptoms, and respond very quickly to oral iron providing there is good compliance with treatment (the haemoglobin concentration rises at a rate of 1 g/dl per week, sometimes faster). Chronic blood loss should be considered and appropriately investigated in the presence of gastrointestinal symptoms and in the older child where dietary deficiency is relatively less common.

Haemolysis

Transfusion strategies in haemoglobinopathies

Thalassaemia

Children with β-thalassaemia major will manifest anaemia within 6–12 months of birth and will become transfusion-dependent. It should be noted, however, that some children have a milder phenotype (thalassaemia intermedia), and can be variably maintained without transfusion. The management of this group can be particularly difficult; they may not have severe anaemia, but can develop skeletal deformities due to marrow hyperplasia, which may benefit from a period of transfusion. A specialist with an interest should manage such children. The molecular diagnosis may be helpful in predicting the clinical course. Current transfusion

practice in thalassaemia major aims at maintaining an average haemoglobin level of 12 g/dl, with a pretransfusion level of 9–10 g/dl.[25] This regimen produces less iron overload and better growth of the children than the 'hypertransfusion' policy used in the past. Hypersplenism must be considered if the transfusion requirements are unexpectedly high. Iron-chelation therapy (normally with parenteral desferrioxamine) is usually started after the ferritin reaches more than 1000 ng/ml (often after 10 transfusions) and preferably over 2 years of age.[26] Attention to detail with desferrioxamine chelation is often the key to success – finding the most acceptable type of subcutaneous needle and delivery systems. The use of young red cells extracted by cell processing methods has been tried, with the idea that these 'neocytes' would last longer and reduce the transfusion requirements. However, the gains have only been modest and at the price of increased donor exposure, so that this is not generally practised.[27]

Sickle cell disease

Transfusions in sickle cell disease are not routine but only given for certain indications – for example exchange transfusion for acute emergencies such as acute chest syndrome, and simple transfusion for splenic sequestration or parvovirus-related aplastic crisis. Following a stroke, there is evidence that regular transfusion to keep the haemoglobin S (HbS) level below 30% in the first two years and thereafter below 50% reduces the risk of recurrence.[28] There is also clear clinical trial evidence that transcranial Doppler ultrasonography can identify high-risk children, and that in these children transfusion to reduce the

HbS to less than 30% is associated with a 90% reduction in the risk of stroke.[29]

Other causes of haemolysis

Inherited enzyme disorders

Although glucose-6-phosphate dehydrogenase (G6PD) deficiency is the commonest congenital red cell enzyme deficiency worldwide, it rarely causes chronic haemolysis. Children may have acute haemolytic crises that require transfusion, usually before the diagnosis is made. Once advised about diet and drugs, such crises are rare, but may be triggered by infection.

Many other red cell enzyme deficiencies (of which pyruvate kinase deficiency is the commonest) may lead to a chronic haemolytic state, but these are rarely transfusion-dependent. Individuals may need top-up transfusions occasionally when viral infections lead to temporary decompensation. Individuals with more severe haemolysis may benefit from splenectomy.

Hereditary spherocytosis

This is common in northern Europe, but is rarely transfusion-dependent. Clinical manifestations are considerably improved by splenectomy, which should be undertaken in transfusion-dependent cases, preferably after the age of 6 years.[30] Because of the risk (lifelong) of post-splenectomy sepsis, splenectomy is only indicated for symptomatic individuals, and the risks and benefits should be carefully weighed up.

Autoimmune haemolysis

This is rare in children. It is usually an acute self-limiting illness related to an acute viral infection. Most commonly, the antibodies are IgM and 'cold' reacting. It is important to obtain as much information as possible about the antibody. Such children need close monitoring (e.g. measurement of the haemoglobin twice daily), since the haemoglobin may drop very quickly; then transfusion may be required, using red cells that are 'least incompatible'. Chronic IgG immune haemolysis is less common, but can occur particularly as part of a more generalized autoimmune disorder. Transfusion may be avoided in such individuals by the use of immunosuppressive therapy, particularly corticosteroids.

Other chronic anaemias

There are a variety of rare constitutional bone marrow failure syndromes that may present in children with anaemia or pancytopenia. The treatment of choice for idiopathic aplastic anaemia is bone marrow transplantation. As soon as this diagnosis has been made, a search should begin for an HLA-compatible donor, preferably a sibling. Transfusion of red cells and other products should be minimized to prevent HLA sensitization, although this is much less likely if all the cellular products are leukodepleted. Donors should be cytomegalovirus (CMV)-negative. Children for whom a marrow donor cannot be found will be transfusion-dependent.

Children with pure red cell aplasia (Diamond–Blackfan anaemia) may be maintained for a period (sometimes years) on steroids, but frequently come to transfusion dependence (50–60% of patients[31]) because the dose of steroids required to maintain a response is unacceptably high. These individuals should have an extended red cell phenotype prior to starting regular transfusion, so that the risk of alloimmunization can be reduced.

Children starting chronic transfusion regimens should also be vaccinated against hepatitis B virus (HBV).

INDICATIONS FOR TRANSFUSIONS OF PLATELETS AND OTHER BLOOD PRODUCTS

Platelet transfusions

The main uses of platelet concentrates in paediatric practice are as follows:

- marrow failure – support for children undergoing chemotherapy for malignant disease;
- cardiac surgery;
- the sick neonate or child with evidence of disseminated intravascular coagulation (DIC), usually in an intensive care setting.

Marrow failure

The platelet 'triggers' are controversial. In marrow aplasia, the threshold for transfusing the non-bleeding patient has come down in adults from 20 to $10 \times 10^9/l$,[32] or lower.[33] Recent evidence has shown that it is safe to use $5 \times 10^9/l$ as a threshold in aplastic anaemia patients.[34] Paediatric units vary, but in the light of this evidence in adults, a count of $5–10 \times 10^9/l$ is probably an acceptable cut-off in the non-bleeding child, but each case should be considered individually.[35]

Cardiac surgery

In cardiac surgery, the requirement for platelets is related to a variety of contributing factors, including the functional defect induced by bypass surgery, effects of anticoagulation with heparin, and possibly the induction of DIC. Platelet transfusions may be required to arrest bleeding, even in the face of a normal platelet count.

The sick child with sepsis

In the sick child in intensive care with sepsis, thrombocytopenia is multifactorial. It is important to consider the cause of the low count, since there are some important conditions where platelet transfusions are contraindicated in the acutely sick child – these are haemolytic uraemic syndrome and heparin-induced thrombocytopenia – because they may make the condition worse. In the septic child, thrombocytopenia is often related to a combination of relative marrow dysfunction and DIC. Platelet transfusions are often required, but it is important to monitor the post-transfusion increment, since this may be less than expected. Children with DIC will require other blood product support, depending upon the severity of the accompanying coagulation defect. Platelet transfusions are also not indicated for the treatment of immune thrombocytopenia.[36] Neonatal thrombocytopenia is considered below.

Fresh-frozen plasma and cryoprecipitate transfusions

Fresh-frozen plasma (FFP) and cryoprecipitate are only indicated for the management of documented coagulation derangements, either with bleeding or prior to interventions that might induce bleeding. The indications have been reviewed by Hume.[27] The level of coagulation derangement at which blood products should be given prophylactically is not clear. Children should not be given plasma products without a clear clinical indication.

Granulocyte transfusions

Transfusion of neutrophils is rarely required, but may be lifesaving in the child with a severe bacterial or fungal infection, unresponsive to antibiotics, in the presence of prolonged neutropenia. This topic has been reviewed by Strauss.[37,38] It is important to use ABO and Rh-compatible HLA-matched donors and to obtain an adequate dose of neutrophils ($1-2 \times 10^9$ neutrophils/kg), which must also be irradiated and transfused within 12 hours of preparation.

CHOICE AND VOLUME OF PRODUCT FOR OLDER CHILDREN

All blood and blood products should as a minimum be infused through a 170 μm mesh filter (part of a standard blood-giving set).

Red cells

It should be noted that whole blood with a haematocrit of 0.30–0.40 is almost never required. The possible exception to this is for cardiac surgery, where in some centres whole blood is used for priming the bypass circuit.

Red cell products must be compatible, i.e. those to which the recipient does not possess antibodies in the plasma – naturally occurring (anti-A, anti-B, or anti-A/B), or (in infants) acquired across the placenta (maternal IgG antibodies, e.g. anti-D), or provoked by previous exposure to the antigen. Minor ABO incompatibility (where the donor plasma contains antibodies to the recipient's own red cells) is generally less important both because the amount of plasma transfused with red cells is minimized and because many tissues contain the A and B antigens, which can also absorb the antibodies. These factors are not sufficient to prevent potentially important reactions in infants,[39] where the volume of plasma transfused may be relatively large in relation to the plasma volume. Transfusion services normally screen group O donors to exclude or at least label those with strongly active (high-titre) or IgG anti-A and anti-B.

Any child who is about to embark on a long-term transfusion regimen (e.g. β-thalassaemia major, Diamond–Blackfan anaemia, and other bone marrow failure syndromes, including aplastic anaemia) should have a more extended red cell phenotype performed. This is particularly important where the child is of a different ethnic origin from the local blood donor population, since the frequency of some common and immunogenic antigens is different. Such patients should then receive red cells that are matched for at least the extended Rh groups and for Kell, which are the most common causes of irregular antibody development. This is also important in sickle cell disease, where transfusions may be less frequent, but where red cell transfusion may be required in an emergency.

How much blood is required for transfusion in a child? In adults, the rule of thumb of one unit of blood raising the haemoglobin by 1 g/dl is convenient, but this cannot apply to children, whose body weight and blood volume is age-dependent. A number of formulae are in general use, and are given below for guidance:

- red cells with haematocrit 0.70–0.75 (concentrated red cells): 10 ml/kg will raise the haemoglobin by about 2.5 g/dl;
- red cells with haematocrit 0.50–0.60 (plasma-reduced or cells in optimal additive solutions): 14 ml/kg will raise the haemoglobin by about 2.5 g/dl;
- a whole-blood transfusion of 8 ml/kg will raise haemoglobin by 1 g/dl.

These calculations (from Hume[27]) are not suitable where a child has a very low haemoglobin level (e.g. <5 g/dl) that has developed slowly. An alternative strategy in this situation is to perform an exchange transfusion or to give packed red cells at a rate of 2 ml/kg/h until the desired haemoglobin level is reached.[40] An alternative formula used for infants and children is:

volume of blood (ml) = [desired haemoglobin − actual haemoglobin] (g/dl) × weight (kg) × k

where $k = 3$ for packed cells, $k = 4$ for plasma-reduced blood, and $k = 6$ for whole blood.[41] Note that in severe chronic anaemia, the haemoglobin should not be increased too rapidly, for example not by more than 6 g/dl/day.

Plasma

FFP must be group-compatible as shown in Table 8.1. It is important to alert medical practitioners to the differences between compatibility of red cells and plasma because of the widespread and mistaken notion that group O is the 'universal donor' for all products – not only red cells. FFP is indicated for correction of coagulopathies. The choice of product then lies between standard single-donor FFP and a pathogen-inactivated equivalent. These are available either as a commercial pooled solvent–detergent (SD) virally inactivated FFP or as single-donor units treated with methylene blue. Many clinicians continue to have reservations concerning pooled plasma products because of the potential risk for transmission of new unknown viruses. The SD method protects against lipid-enveloped viruses such as HIV, HBV, and HCV.[42] Methylene blue is activated by light treatment and inactivates viruses by intercalation into their DNA. The quantity of methylene blue in the final product is very small, and has been shown not to be toxic to neonates. Virally inactivated single-donor units are probably preferable to a pooled product, if locally available. The argument for using such products is less convincing for children exposed to numerous other non-pathogen-inactivated products such as red cells and platelets.

For correction of coagulation derangements, a dose of 10–20 ml/kg is estimated to

Table 8.1 Choice of ABO groups for red cell, plasma, and platelet transfusions for children

Recipient blood group	Compatible red cells	Compatible plasma	Compatible platelets
O	O	O, A, B, or AB	O, A, B, or AB
A	A or O	A or AB	A or AB
B	B or O	B or AB	B or AB
AB	AB, A, B, or O	AB	AB

produce a 20% rise in coagulation factors. The main indication in children is in relation to DIC occurring in the context of sepsis, where other products such as cryoprecipitate and platelets are likely to be required, or for severe coagulopathies produced by liver failure. FFP should not be used to correct severe congenital coagulation factor deficiencies such as factor VIII or IX deficiency, since there are highly effective genetically engineered concentrates available. Children with congenital coagulation factor deficiencies should be referred to a specialist haemophilia centre.

Platelets

These should be group-compatible. In an attempt to reduce wastage, some transfusion services have issued platelets to patients irrespective of ABO group, usually without any adverse clinical consequences in adults. This may be hazardous in infants (see below). ABO-incompatible platelets have been shown to have a reduced survival compared with the patient's own group, suggesting they may not be as effective clinically, and may result in an increased risk of the development of platelet refractoriness in the multitransfused patient.[43] A suitable platelet dose calculated to raise the count by $50 \times 10^9/l$ is one single-donor unit per 10 kg body weight, or 5 ml/kg from apheresis donations. Another dose calculation is to give an apheresis donation if the child's body weight is more than 25 kg, 100 ml if it is 10–25 kg, 50 ml if it is 5–10 kg, and 5 ml/kg for infants less than 5 kg. Platelet concentrates are usually contaminated with red cells. As Rh D-positive cells can induce an immune response in D-negative recipients even when immunosuppressed by chemotherapy, platelet

transfusions must be Rh D-compatible. In an emergency, platelets containing A/B antibodies in the plasma may be transfused to recipients with those antigens on their red blood cells. This is safe in adults and older children, but in small children and infants such antibodies may give rise to demonstrable haemolysis.[39] A single-donor platelet concentrate contains about 40 ml of plasma, which is a significant quantity when infused into a baby of weight 3 kg, whose total plasma volume is only 150 ml, compared with 2000–3000 ml in an adult.[44] Infants under 4 months of age may have maternal antibodies, which must be taken into account.

Cryoprecipitate

This is only indicated for correction of fibrinogen deficiency (<0.8–1.0 g/l). This is usually in the context of DIC, when other products, particularly platelets, may also be required. The suggested dose is one unit per 5–10 kg recipient weight, but since the content of each bag can vary between 100 and 250 mg of fibrinogen, it is important to confirm that the anticipated correction has occurred. Although cryoprecipitate is a rich source of factor VIII and von Willebrand factor, there are better products for treatment of these deficiencies. Units must be ABO-compatible, but the Rh type does not matter.

TRANSFUSION IN NEONATES

Physiology of neonatal haematopoiesis and indications for transfusion

At birth, the oxygenation of a baby improves as oxygen is much more easily extracted from the lungs than from maternal blood (HbA) via the placenta. The haemoglobin switching that usually begins at about 32 weeks gestation continues to replace the high-oxygen-affinity HbF with the lower-affinity HbA. With this, the drive to red cell production is much reduced, leading to a reduction in haemoglobin over the first 4–8 weeks of life (physiological anaemia). This trough occurs earlier and is more profound in premature infants. There are many reasons for transfusion in the neonatal period, but preterm neonates receiving supportive intensive care from early gestation (e.g. 24 weeks) are an intensively transfused group. This is related to repeated blood sampling required for monitoring these sick infants – removal of 1 ml of blood from a 600 g baby represents about 1.5% of the infant's blood volume.[45] These infants are unlikely to survive a sojourn in intensive care without transfusion; infants with birth weight less than 1.5 kg had an 80% likelihood of transfusion in 1991,[46] and almost all infants of less than 1.0 kg require transfusion at some stage.[47] The mean number of donor exposures was reported as 8 in 1989.[48] A number of strategies can reduce this, and are discussed below. Apart from the blood loss, needlesticks are painful and can cause sudden rises in blood pressure, which may result in periventricular haemorrhage.[49] Unfortunately, despite the need for transfusion, the evidence upon which to base criteria for transfusion is conflicting, resulting in differences in practice between centres[50] and significant differences in national guidelines,[41,51,52] which have been well reviewed.[53] One guideline sets the haemoglobin trigger for the stable newborn with clinical manifestations of anaemia at 8 g/dl and another at 10.5 g/dl. All agree that a higher haemoglobin trigger of 13 g/dl is suitable for infants with severe pulmonary or cyanotic heart disease, or heart failure. The need for blood transfusion arises from a number of factors: these infants require intensive monitoring and therefore blood sampling; their haemoglobin is usually lower than term neonates, and falls to a lower nadir in the first 8 weeks (e.g. as low as 7 g/dl in infants whose birth weight was less than 1 kg); many require ventilatory support where it is thought that a higher haematocrit optimizes oxygen delivery to the tissues. Transfusions may be given to enhance weight gain (four studies, two showing an increase[54,55] and two no change,[56,57]) and to reduce respiratory irregularities such as periodic breathing and apnoea (7 studies reviewed by Ramasethu and Luban[53]) or tachycardia (8 studies of cardiac function).[53] However, the outcomes may be similar if simple volume expansion is given, suggesting that simple dehydration may be more important.[53] Perhaps the most relevant criterion is an elevated serum lactic acid, which reflects anaerobic metabolism secondary to inadequate oxygenation of tissues.[58,59] More restrictive guidelines (including a cut-off haematocrit of 0.20) were used in one erythropoietin trial without adverse events,[60] and more recently the College of American Pathologists have published new criteria shown in Table 8.2.[61] Similar criteria have been suggested by neonatologists.[62] These are largely empirical, and their use needs to be carefully audited, since the limits are lower than any previously published guidelines. Over the past few years, there has already been a trend in some units towards a more restricted transfusion policy, although less stringent than these, which has not resulted in any adverse outcomes.[63]

> **Table 8.2 Neonatal red blood cell transfusion guidelines – College of American Pathologists 1998[61]**
>
> 1. Hct ⩽ 0.20 or Hb < 7 g/dl and reticulocyte count <4% (or absolute reticulocyte count <100 000/ml)
>
> 2. Hct ⩽ 0.25 or Hb ⩽ 8 g/dl and any of the following conditions:
>   (a) Apnoea/bradycardia ⩾10 episodes/24 h or ⩾2 episodes requiring bag-mask ventilation
>   (b) Sustained tachycardia >180 bpm or sustained tachypnoea >80 breaths/min over 24 h by averaging 3-hourly measurements
>   (c) Cessation of adequate weight gain over 4 days (⩾10 g/day despite 420 kJ/kg/day)
>   (d) Mild RDS with FiO_2 = 0.25–0.35 or nasal cannula 1/8–1/4 or IMV or NCPAP with Paw < 6 cmH$_2$O
>
> 3. Hct ⩽ 0.30 or Hb ⩽ 10 g/dl with moderate RDS + FiO_2 > 0.35 or nasal cannula O_2 or intermittent mandatory ventilation with Paw = 6–8 cmH$_2$O
>
> 4. Hct ⩽ 0.35 or Hb ⩽ 12 g/dl with severe RDS requiring mechanical ventilation and Paw ⩾ 8 cmH$_2$O and FiO_2 > 0.50 or severe congenital heart disease associated with cyanosis or heart failure.
>
> 5. Acute blood loss with shock: blood replacement to re-establish adequate blood volume and Hct = 0.4.
>
> 6. Do not transfuse to replace blood removed for laboratory tests or low Hct alone unless the above criteria are met.
>
> ---
>
> FiO_2, fraction of inspired oxygen; Hb, haemoglobin; Hct, haematocrit; IMV, intermittent mandatory ventilation; NCPAP, nasal continuous positive airway pressure; Paw, mean airway pressure; RDS, respiratory distress syndrome.
> Reproduced from reference 61, by permission of the College of American Pathologists.

Special requirements and choice of products for transfusion in neonates

A number of features of the fetus and neonate lead to special requirements for transfusion products:

- The infant has an immature immune system and cannot easily eliminate transfused lymphocytes (which have been reported to persist for up to 25 years after intrauterine transfusion).[64] Under some circumstances, these may cause graft-versus-host disease (GvHD). The infant is also more susceptible to viral infections transmissible by blood that are not usually a problem to the (often immune) adult, such as cytomegalovirus (CMV) and Epstein–Barr virus (EBV).

- The infant has a small blood volume relative to priming equipment that may be required for manipulations such as exchange transfusion and cardiac bypass.
- The infant's plasma may contain irregular red cell (and anti-HLA or antiplatelet) antibodies from the maternal plasma.
- The sick premature neonate is metabolically unstable, with many immature organ systems, and so unable to adapt easily to biochemical insults that may be associated with blood transfusion, especially when of large volume.
- Under some circumstances (sepsis), there may be exposure of T antigens, resulting in a tendency to haemolysis with standard blood products (see below).

Blood suitable for neonatal use therefore has the following requirements:

Donors and screening of donations
Donors of blood and blood products for neonates and infants up to a year of age should be as safe as possible; blood should only be accepted from those who have given at least one donation in the previous 2 years that is negative for all mandatory microbiological markers. The red cells are plasma-reduced (and may be suspended in optimal additive solution, but this is not suitable for exchange or massive transfusion). The pretransfusion testing of such units will include a more extended screening for irregular antibodies. Red cells should be screened to exclude sickle cell trait.

Leukocyte depletion
Cellular components should be leukocyte-depleted ($<5 \times 10^6$/unit), which has been standard practice in the UK since November 1999.

CMV status
In the UK, it is recommended that for infants under 1 year of age the blood should be CMV-seronegative. It is likely that leukocyte reduction will reduce considerably the risk of CMV transmission, and it is known that infants or fetuses weighing less than 1.5 kg are at highest risk. In an emergency, therefore, non-CMV-screened blood is probably safe, and in recent US guidelines leukocyte depletion is considered equivalent to CMV seronegativity for practical purposes.[61]

Irradiation
Leukocyte reduction by filtration is not sufficient on its own to eliminate the risk of transfusion-associated GvHD; the most vulnerable children must therefore receive irradiated cellular products (i.e. red cells and platelets). These groups are:

- infants undergoing intrauterine transfusion; any postnatal transfusions (whether for top-up or exchange) in these infants should continue to be irradiated in the neonatal period;
- when the infant has suspected or confirmed immune deficiency, for example children undergoing cardiac surgery who have (or are suspected to have) DiGeorge syndrome, children suspected to have HIV infection, and children with any other of the rarer congenital cellular or combined immune deficiency disorders;
- when the donation comes from a first-degree relative or has been HLA-matched.

Irradiation should be to a minimum of 25 Gy. If the blood is for top-up only, it may be irradiated up to 14 days from collection and stored for a further 14 days. Blood for exchange transfusion should be irradiated within 5 days of collection and transfused within 24 hours to ensure optimal red cell function and low plasma potassium levels.[65] It has been demonstrated that the transfusion of large volumes of irradiated blood 14 days post irradiation contributed to hyperkalaemic cardiac arrest in a child during craniofacial surgery.[66] The irradiated units were shown to have a markedly increased potassium concentration of 30 to >40 mmol/l compared with a 3-day-old non-irradiated bag (8.2 mmol/l).

Pretransfusion testing

The blood group of the neonate is determined usually only by the red cell group, since the 'naturally occurring' antibodies that determine the reverse group are absent or present only in small amounts. It is recommended that the ABO group be repeated with a second set of reagents. The infant in addition may possess irregular IgG antibodies from the mother that have crossed the placenta, and which can persist for 12–16 weeks after birth. It is easiest to test for these in a sample of maternal blood, but careful attention must be paid to the identification and labelling of such samples so that it is completely clear which mother and infant are a pair. The mother's sample should include the information 'mother of baby x', with the baby's unique hospital number and date of birth. If maternal serum is not available, the infant serum must be screened by an indirect antiglobulin test. A direct antiglobulin test (DAT) must be done to detect antibodies on the red cells of the neonate, which, if present, indicate haemolytic disease of the newborn. This must be fully and appropri-

ately investigated. This can be clinically particularly important in infants of mothers with anti-D. An infant may erroneously group as Rh D-negative when all the Rh D-antigen sites are occupied by antibody, but the presence of a positive DAT will indicate the correct interpretation. Such infants may be asymptomatic, but must be very closely followed-up to detect the development of significant anaemia within the first few weeks of life.

If there are no irregular antibodies, and the DAT is negative, then repeated small volume transfusions can be given over the first 4 months of life without further serological testing, since neonates and infants are unlikely to make irregular red cell antibodies in response to transfusion of red cells.

The blood group transfused may either be the infant's own ABO group or an alternative ABO-compatible group; it must also be compatible with any maternally derived irregular antibodies.

T-antigen activation

The T antigen is present on all red cells, but is only exposed when sialic acid residues are stripped from the cells by an enzyme, neuraminidase, that is produced by some bacteria causing necrotizing enterocolitis (NEC) in neonates. The incriminated organisms are *Clostridium* spp., *Bacteroides fragilis*, and *Streptococcus pneumoniae*. Anti-T antibodies (IgM) are 'naturally occurring' in all normal sera. Transfusion of any blood product in affected infants may therefore produce haemolysis due to agglutination, which, at worst, can be fatal. The diagnosis of milder degrees of haemolysis in premature infants is not straightforward, and laboratory screening for T activation, although relatively easy with a lectin panel, is not currently widely available in most hospitals. Any infant with NEC who has a less-than-expected rise in haemoglobin or evidence of haemolysis (with haemoglobinuria) should be screened. Management may be difficult in the severely ill infant. Antibiotic therapy to eradicate the offending organisms is essential; the infant may need exchange transfusion with plasma-reduced blood, preferably red cells in optimal additive solution, but these septic infants may also have deranged coagulation and bleeding, requiring correction with potentially hazardous plasma products.[67] Platelets should be washed before transfusion, and, if possible, FFP and cryoprecipitate should be transfused from adults with low anti-T levels. This may not be practical in an urgent situation. NEC is a well-recognized risk in premature infants and may develop in up to 10% of babies in neonatal intensive care units. The incidence of T activation has been reported at 11% of all infants with NEC, but is most likely to occur in those requiring surgical intervention, where the incidence has been reported to be as high as 28%.[68] Other variants of T antigen are reported; one of these (Tx) has been reported transiently in association with *Streptococcus pneumoniae* infection in children. Another variant (Tn) arises as an abnormal structure on a clone of cells in some haematological malignancies. These have been reviewed by Horn.[69]

Platelet transfusions in neonates

Thrombocytopenia is common in the neonatal intensive care unit population for a variety of reasons. Often these infants have increased platelet destruction together with reduced megakaryocyte reserve and a relatively low thrombopoietin level.[70] These infants may also have defective function, although the evidence is conflicting. Platelet transfusions in neonates are thought to be required at relatively higher platelet counts than in older children, although there is little published evidence for this.[27,71,72] Recent guidelines suggest a threshold of $20 \times 10^9/l$ for the stable non-bleeding infant, $50 \times 10^9/l$ if an invasive procedure is required, and $100 \times 10^9/l$ for a bleeding or unstable infant.[70] Some neonatologists would transfuse platelets in the very preterm infant at a threshold of $100 \times 10^9/l$ because of the higher risk of intracranial haemorrhage in this population, but there is no evidence that this therapy reduces the incidence. It is important to exclude maternal antibodies (due either to maternal autoimmune thrombocytopenia or to alloimmunization), since the treatment of these conditions is not with platelet transfusions but with immune modulation.[73]

Granulocyte transfusions in neonates

The neonate is particularly susceptible to severe sepsis. Several studies have been published using neutrophil transfusions in this setting; these are reviewed by Strauss.[70] The studies are heterogeneous, and the dose of neutrophils was inadequate in some. There may be circumstances under which neutrophil transfusions are justified (suggested guidelines are infants in the first week of life with neutropenia $<3 \times 10^9/l$ and fulminant sepsis, or after the first week of life with a count $<1 \times 10^9/l$ and fulminant sepsis.[70] Donors should be ABO- and Rh-compatible, CMV-seronegative, with other criteria as indicated above.

EXCHANGE OR MASSIVE TRANSFUSION IN INFANTS

Exchange transfusion is most commonly indicated for:

- severe hyperbilirubinaemia at birth, most often due to Rh haemolytic disease (but also other antibodies, G6PD deficiency, or metabolic causes);
- severe anaemia, especially in the presence of heart failure.

Although these are general groups, there is a lack of standard indications or guidelines.[74] Massive transfusion in the neonate has been well reviewed by Luban.[75]

Exchange transfusion

The introduction of anti-D treatment for Rh D-negative women has reduced the mortality and incidence of haemolytic disease due to anti-D, but this antibody remains the commonest indication for exchange transfusion. Other antibodies (anti-c and ABO incompatibility) account for about half the cases.[76] Many of these instances of sensitization could be avoided by transfusing women of childbearing age with fully Rh-genotyped and Kell-typed blood. One audit of neonatal units requesting blood for exchange transfusion showed that in about half the cases, the ordered blood tends not to be used.[74] Often two units were requested where one was sufficient. This is a waste of blood with high specification and cost, and demonstrates the need for close collaboration between paediatrician, haematologist, and the transfusion service.

Before the discovery of anti-D prophylaxis for Rh D-negative women, Rh haemolytic disease was not uncommon, and most neonatal units had ample opportunity to gain experience of exchange transfusion. This is now an uncommon and highly specialized procedure that should be carried out only by staff with adequate training and experience. Blood should be less than 5 days old, because with storage the potassium leaks out of the red cells and has been associated with fatal hyperkalaemia in infants. In addition, stored red cells become depleted of 2,3-DPG, which affects oxygen transport. Ideal donors will be at low risk of having developed irregular antibodies (untransfused and women with no children). The units will be either group O Rh D-negative or group O Rh D-positive (R1R1), Kell-negative and screened for irregular antibodies, low titre for anti-A and anti-B, CMV-negative, and negative for HbS by a screening test. Debate continues about whether whole blood or plasma-reduced blood should be used for exchange. An audit of 20 neonatal units in 1998 showed that 73% of respondents would prefer plasma-reduced blood, and only 2 of 19 would choose whole blood.[74] A more recent survey of UK neonatologists showed that the preferred product would be plasma-reduced blood with a haematocrit of 0.45–0.55. Whole blood with a haematocrit of 0.35–0.45 can result in unacceptably low haemoglobins (<12 g/dl) post exchange for anaemia, and packed cells with a haematocrit of 0.75 can result in an unacceptably high post-transfusion haematocrit. The volume exchanged may be a 'single' or 'double' volume, based upon theoretical models that calculate how much is required to remove most of the infant's own red cells. A single-volume exchange (80–90 ml/kg) will remove 75%, and a double-volume exchange

(160–180 ml/kg) 90%. The only published randomized controlled trial has shown that a single volume exchange is as effective.[77] If the exchange is being performed primarily for hyperbilirubinaemia, a slower procedure will remove more, and a double-volume exchange can remove 50% of circulating bilirubin. However, it should be noted that the bilirubin is in equilibrium with tissue stores that will continue to move into the plasma compartment, and the vilirubin should continue to be monitored 4-hourly. It is not usually necessary to give any additional plasma or saline when using plasma-reduced blood. The blood must be given through a blood warmer, and the preferred method is to use two lines (in addition to a line for continued maintenance fluids), either via the umbilical vessels or through peripheral lines, with blood being given at a constant rate (e.g. from 60 ml/h in an infant less than 1 kg weight up to 180 ml/h for those over 3 kg) through one while aliquots are removed at timed intervals (5 minutes) through the other. The use of a two-line technique probably causes less haemodynamic instability. The procedure takes 2–3 hours to perform, and needs very close monitoring with electrocardiogram and pulse oximetry, temperature recordings, and a naso- or oro-gastric tube in place on free drainage.

Massive transfusion

Massive transfusion occurs where infants require a large part of their circulating volume replaced, either because of acute blood loss (twin-to-twin transfusion or fetomaternal haemorrhage) or in cardiopulmonary bypass surgery or equivalent (such as extracorporeal membrane oxygenation, ECMO). In these cases, similar criteria to those for exchange blood are required.

Cardiac surgery

This is an important use of blood in the neonatal period: in the UK, about 3500 children undergo cardiac surgery per annum, of whom more than 70% are on bypass. Protocols and requirements for bypass surgery are not well standardized – there are variations between units and between surgeons and anaesthetists within the same centres, demonstrating a clear need to set some standards against which practice may be audited. General principles are that blood should be fresh – usually within 5 days of donation for infants less than 1 year of age, and not collected into additive solutions (because of theoretical hazards of a large mannitol load). Some sources have reported better results with blood anticoagulated with heparin and used within 48 hours,[78] but this is not practical for most units. Experience with Jehovah's Witnesses has demonstrated that the amount of homologous blood transfused in relation to surgery could almost certainly be considerably reduced. Fifteen children aged 1–16 years underwent cardiac bypass surgery without transfusion using isovolaemic haemodilution and bloodless priming of the bypass circuit.[79] Other blood products are not required as a routine for cardiac surgery, but children undergoing complex or re-do operations are more likely to bleed when platelet transfusions and possibly plasma may be required. The haemostatic derangements produced by cardiac bypass surgery are complex.[80] Numerous strategies have been tried both in adults and children; strategies successful for adults (use of desmopressin and tranexamic acid and aprotinin) have in general not been as useful in children.

Extracorporeal membrane oxygenation

ECMO is a very specialized variant of cardiac bypass where a child with life-threatening respiratory failure undergoes prolonged support until the lung disease recovers. This procedure is only carried out in a small number of approved centres in the UK, and the reader is referred to an excellent review by Luban[75] for further information.

Acute blood loss

Massive transfusion can also occur in the setting of acute blood loss, from trauma or surgery or other causes. It is defined as the loss of one blood volume within a 24-hour period, or 50% blood volume loss within 3 hours, or a rate of loss of 150 ml/min in an adult. A template for the management of massive transfusion has been published[81] that is helpful in indicating the order in which blood products are likely to be required and the likely time taken to obtain these. It is important to note that good communication between the clinicians at the emergency and transfusion staff is essential so that blood products can be provided most efficiently – particularly platelet concentrates, which may not be available on site.

STRATEGIES TO AVOID ALLOGENEIC TRANSFUSION EXPOSURE IN CHILDREN AND NEONATES

As there are anxieties about the long-term effects of transfusion of red cells and other blood products, it is important to consider ways in which transfusion of allogeneic products in children might be reduced. The following can be contributory.

Limiting of transfusions

Transfusion should be limited to clear clinical indicators that are regularly audited against outcome measures. Phlebotomy losses in neonates should be reduced to a minimum.

Minimizing donor exposure

Donor exposure in neonates should be minimized by using several aliquots from the same donation up to its expiry date. While it used to be considered safe only to give blood within 5–7 days of collection to neonates, it is now clear that blood can be used for small 'top-up' transfusions until its expiry date.[41,82] Single units divided into multiple (4–8) small satellite packs can therefore be allocated to a specific child and used sequentially.

Use of directed donations

Parents not infrequently ask if they can give blood for their own child. This is usually due to their unrealistic fears of the infection risks (especially HIV) associated with blood transfusion. When informed of the very low risk of viral transmission (e.g. <1 in 2 million for HIV in the UK) and the safety of transfusion, generally parents are able to accept standard allogeneic blood for their child. In addition, there are particular hazards that may be associated with transfusion from the mother or father. Maternal plasma may contain HLA antibodies against the child's platelets or white cells. The baby has an underdeveloped immune system and is at risk for the development of GvHD from transfused parental lymphocytes. Blood from first-degree relatives must therefore be irradiated as well as leukocyte-depleted. In children who require regular transfusions for chronic anaemia (such as β-thalassaemia), it has proved possible to restrict the number of donors[83] by using a limited panel of donors. Directed donations from relatives may have a higher incidence of infectious disease markers and be less safe than volunteer allogeneic transfusion.[84]

Use of erythropoietin in neonates

Several trials of the use of erythropoietin (EPO) have been reported (and summarized by Ohls[85]). The entry criteria (birth weight and gestational age) were variable, and the doses of EPO used ranged from 500 units/kg/week to 1250 units/kg/week, administered subcutaneously in some trials, and intravenously in others. The use of EPO is still a matter of controversy in the sense that the criteria for selection of suitable infants for therapy are not clear. Normal neonates have a decline in haemoglobin over the first 8 weeks of life, which relates to many factors, including the switch from HbF (high oxygen affinity) to HbA (lower oxygen affinity); the red cell mass is relatively less as the body weight doubles. The premature infant starts with a lower haemoglobin and has a lower nadir, together with a relatively reduced EPO response. Early trials showed little benefit in terms of reducing blood transfusions, particularly in the first 2 weeks of life, but this may have been due to inadequate dosing (750 units/kg/week[86]), since infants were shown to require relatively larger doses (e.g. 1250 units/kg/week[87]) than adults. The volume of distribution in infants is much larger than in adults (approximately 300 ml/kg in infants, compared with approximately 70 ml/kg in

adults[85]). One useful influence of the trials has been to define red cell transfusion policies more clearly, leading to a lower incidence of transfusion in placebo groups (by 50%, with no adverse consequences[85]) compared with similar infants not in trials. The anaemia does respond to exogenous EPO with adequate supplemental iron therapy (at least 6 mg/kg/day orally, but recent evidence suggests that intravenous iron may be more effective[88]). In several studies, the outcome measures were not significantly improved and EPO did not alter transfusion requirements in the very low-birth-weight group (<800 g) in the first 2 weeks. EPO may have a place in an intermediate group (birth weight 800–1300 g) where the transfusion exposure can thereby be decreased. However, EPO is an expensive drug, and careful attention to other factors, such as multisatellite packs dedicated to single infants used up to their expiry date, careful attention to reduction of phlebotomy losses, and in particular, setting clear transfusion guidelines, may well be as effective in reducing donor exposure.[27] A structured approach to the use of EPO has been suggested, and the algorithm is reproduced in Figure 8.1.[62] It is also important to note that EPO has effects on many tissues in addition to its role in red blood cell production – there are EPO receptors on bowel cells – perhaps treatment with EPO offers some protection against necrotizing enterocolitis.[89] Conversely, it will be very important to be sure that EPO, through its stimulatory effect on angiogenesis, has no adverse effect on retinopathy of prematurity (which is caused by neovascularization). Thus far, no long-term sequelae of EPO use have been identified.[90] The non-erythropoietic actions of EPO have been

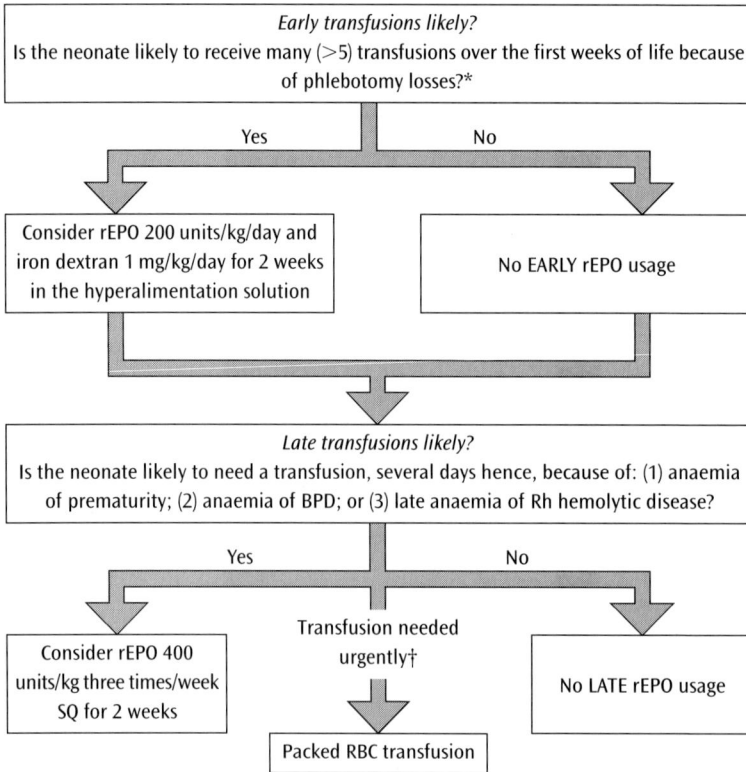

Figure 8.1
Algorithm for a consistent approach to using rEpo in the neonatal intensive care unit. BPD, bronchopulmonary displasia; RBC, red blood cell; SQ, subcutaneous. Reproduced by permission from reference 62.

reviewed.[91] EPO has been shown to be beneficial in the treatment of anaemia associated with bronchopulmonary dysplasia.[92] Infants with haemolytic disease due to Rh disease are likely to develop late anaemia at 4–12 weeks, particularly after intrauterine transfusion. EPO has been shown to be beneficial in this setting also,[93] and a collaborative trial is underway to confirm this.

Use of autologous transfusion

Autologous transfusion has become widely used in adult transfusion practice for elective procedures where 1–4 units can be collected in advance. Cell-saver techniques have also reduced the requirements for allogeneic blood transfusion. For a number of reasons, these are more difficult to translate into paediatric practice. Despite the constraints, autologous blood collections for paediatric orthopaedic surgery were reported as early as 1974 in 193 children aged from 7 years up (mean age 14 years). Several other studies have been reported, and are reviewed together by Thompson and Luban.[94] These studies suggest that children as young as 6–10 years of age may understand and be able to give consent.

The needle size (16G) attached to standard blood bags is uncomfortably large, and consideration should be given to using a smaller gauge, consistent with obtaining satisfactory flow. Careful attention must be paid to the volumes withdrawn in relation to the weight of the child (formulae and suggested schedules have been published[94]). The suggested volumes to withdraw range from 180 ml in a 20 kg child to 405 ml in a 45 kg child. Using a weekly collection schedule and appropriate anticoagulant, it is possible to collect up to 5 appropriate 'units'. Cord blood has been suggested as a source of autologous transfusion to preterm infants, but in practice it has been difficult to collect and separate sufficient quantities, particularly in the smallest babies, even with an experienced team. In addition, there are anxieties about the increased infection risk, so that this is unlikely to be of practical value in most units.[95]

CONCLUSIONS

Blood transfusion in children and neonates is sometimes necessary, and can usually be achieved safely. This requires close attention to donor screening, good blood-banking practice, and careful consideration of the reasons for blood or blood product transfusion. Clinicians have a clear responsibility to ensure that each blood product transfused is indicated, properly given, and recorded, and that the child and its parents understand the reasons for the procedure and the possible complications. More information is needed concerning indicators for blood transfusion, which will result from good audit and sharing of information between clinicians as well as from carefully constructed controlled trials.

REFERENCES

1. Williamson L, Cohen H, Love E et al. The Serious Hazards of Transfusion (SHOT) initiative: the UK approach to haemovigilance. *Vox Sang* 2000; **78**: 291–5.
2. Williamson LM, Lowe S, Love EM, Cohen H et al. Serious Hazards of Transfusion (SHOT) initiative: analysis of the first two annual reports. *BMJ* 1999; **319**: 16–19.
3. Vogt M, Lang T, Frosner G, Klingler C et al. Prevalence and clinical outcome of hepatitis C infection in children who underwent cardiac surgery before the implementation of blood-donor screening. *N Engl J Med* 1999; **341**: 866–70.
4. Paul IM, Sanders J, Ruggiero F et al. Chronic hepatitis C virus infections in leukemia survivors: prevalence, viral load, and severity of liver disease. *Blood* 1999; **93**: 3672–7.
5. Bhushan V, Chandy M, Babu PG et al. Transfusion associated HIV infection in patients with haematologic disorders in southern India. *Indian J Med Res* 1994; **99**: 57–60.
6. Hersh BS, Popovici F, Jezek Z et al. Risk factors for HIV infection among abandoned Romanian children. *AIDS* 1993; **7**: 1617–24.
7. DePalma L, Luban NL. Transmission of human T-lymphotrophic virus type I infection to a neonatal infant by transfusion of washed and irradiated red cells. *Transfusion* 1993; **33**: 582–4.
8. van den Berg H, Gerritsen EJ, van Tol MJ et al. Ten years after acquiring an HIV-1 infection: a study in a cohort of eleven neonates infected by aliquots from a single plasma donation. *Acata Paediatr* 1994; **83**: 173–8.
9. Regan FA, Hewitt P, Barbara JA, Contreras M Prospective investigation of transfusion transmitted infection in recipients of over 20 000 units of blood. TTI Study Group. *BMJ* 2000; **320**: 403–6.
10. Maeda M, Hamada H, Tsuda A et al. High rate of TTV infection in multitransfused patients with pediatric malignancy and hema-

tological disorders. *Am J Hematol* 2000; **65**: 41–4.

11. Patil RS, Wadgaonkar P, Joshi SH et al. Viral infections in newborns through exchange transfusion. *Indian J Pediatr* 1998; **65**: 723–8.

12. Aach RD, Yomtovian RA, Hack M. Neonatal and pediatric posttransfusion hepatitis C: a look back and a look forward. *Pediatrics* 2000; **105**: 836–42.

13. Jamal R, Fadzillah G, Zulkifli SZ, Yasmin M. Seroprevalence of hepatitis B, hepatitis C, CMV and HIV in multiple transfused thalassemia patients: results from a thalassemia day care center in Malaysia. *Southeast Asian J Trop Med Public Health* 1998; **29**: 792–4.

14. Jonas MM. Hepatitis C infection in children. *N Engl J Med* 1999; **341**: 912–13.

15. Kebudi R, Ayan I, Yilmaz G et al. Seroprevalence of hepatitis B, hepatitis C, and human immunodeficiency virus infections in children with cancer at diagnosis and following therapy in Turkey. *Med Pediatr Oncol* 2000; **324**: 102–5.

16. Lackritz EM, Ruebush TKd, Zucker JR et al. Blood transfusion practices and blood-banking services in a Kenyan hospital. *AIDS* 1993; **7**: 995–9.

17. Holzer BR, Egger M, Teuscher T et al. Childhood anemia in Africa: to transfuse or not transfuse? *Acta Trop* 1993; **55**: 47–51.

18. Jager H, N'Galy B, Perriens J et al. Prevention of transfusion-associated HIV transmission in Kinshasa, Zaire: HIV screening is not enough. *AIDS* 1990; **4**: 571–4.

19. Vos J, Gumodoka B, Ng'weshemi JZ et al. Are some blood transfusions avoidable? A hospital record analysis in Mwanza Region, Tanzania. *Trop Geogr Med* 1993; **45**: 301–3.

20. Craighead IB, Knowles JK. Prevention of transfusion-associated HIV transmission with the use of a transfusion protocol for under 5s. *Trop Doct* 1993; **23**: 59–61.

21. Wilkerson DK, Rosen AL, Sehgal LR et al. Limits of cardiac compensation in anemic baboons. *Surgery* 1988; **103**: 665–70.

22. Spahn DR, Smith LR, Veronee CD et al. Acute isovolemic hemodilution and blood transfusion. Effects on regional function and metabolism in myocardium with compromised coronary blood flow. *J Thorac Cardiovasc Surg* 1993; **105**: 694–704.

23. Lackritz EM, Campbell CC, Ruebush TKd et al. Effect of blood transfusion on survival among children in a Kenyan hospital. *Lancet* 1992; **340**: 524–8.

24. Group ALS. *Advanced Paediatric Life Support – The Practical Approach*, 3rd edn. London: BMJ Books, 2001.

25. Cazzola M, Borgna-Pignatti C, Locatelli F et al. A moderate transfusion regimen may reduce iron loading in beta-thalassemia major without producing excessive expansion of erythropoiesis. *Transfusion* 1997; **37**: 135–40.

26. Olivieri NF. The beta-thalassemias. *N Engl J Med* 1999; **341**: 99–109 [Erratum 1407].

27. Hume H. Blood components: preparation, indications and administration. In:*Pediatric Hematology*, 2nd edn (Lilleyman J, Hann I, Blanchette V, eds). London: Churchill Livingstone, 1999: 709–39.

28. Cohen AR, Martin MB, Silver JH et al. A modified transfusion program for prevention of stroke in sickle cell disease. *Blood* 1992; **79**: 1657–61.

29. Adams RJ. Stroke prevention in sickle cell disease. *Curr Opin Hematol* 2000; **7**: 101–5.

30. Bolton-Maggs PH. The diagnosis and management of hereditary spherocytosis. *Baillière's Best Pract Res Clin Haematol* 2000; **13**: 327–42.

31. Willig TN, Gazda H, Sieff CA. Diamond–Blackfan anemia. *Curr Opin Hematol* 2000; **7**: 85–94.

32. Slichter SJ. Platelet transfusions – a constantly evolving therapy. *Thromb Haemost* 1991; **66**: 178–88.

33. Gmur J, Burger J, Schanz U et al. Safety of stringent prophylactic platelet transfusion policy for patients with acute leukaemia. *Lancet* 1991; **338**: 1223–6.

34. Sagmeister M, Oec L, Gmur J. A restrictive platelet transfusion policy allowing long-term support of outpatients with severe aplastic anemia. *Blood* 1999; **93**: 3124–6.

35. Cahill MR, Lilleyman JS. The rational use of platelet transfusions in children. *Semin Thromb Hemost* 1998; **24**: 567–75.

36. Eden OB, Lilleyman JS. Guidelines for management of idiopathic thrombocytopenic purpura. The British Paediatric Haematology Group. *Arch Dis Child* 1992; **67**: 1056–8.

37. Strauss RG. Rebirth of granulocyte transfusions: Should it involve pediatric oncology and transplant patients? *J Pediatr Hematol Oncol* 1999; **21**: 475–8.

38. Strauss R. Granulocyte transfusion therapy. In: *Transfusion Therapy: Clinical Principles and Practice* (Mintz P, ed). Bethesda, MD: American Association of Blood Banks Press, 1999: 81–96.

39. Duguid JK, Minards J, Bolton-Maggs PH. Lesson of the week: incompatible plasma transfusions and haemolysis in children. *BMJ* 1999; **318**: 176–7.

40. Jayabose S, Tugal O, Ruddy R et al. Transfusion therapy for severe anemia. *Am J Pediatr Hematol Oncol* 1993; **15**: 324–7.

41. Voak D, Cann R, Finney RD et al. Guidelines for administration of blood products: transfusion of infants and neonates. British Committee for Standards in Haematology Blood Transfusion Task Force. *Transfus Med* 1994; **4**: 63–9 [Erratum 306].

42. Solheim BG, Rollag H, Svennevig JL et al. Viral safety of solvent/detergent-treated plasma. *Transfusion* 2000; **40**: 84–90.

43. Carr R, Hutton JL, Jenkins JA et al. Transfusion of ABO-mismatched platelets leads to early platelet refractoriness. *Br J Haematol* 1990; **75**: 408–13.

44. Chambers L, Luban N. Neonatal and intra-uterine transfusion. In: *Transfusion Therapy: Clinical Principles and Practice* (Mintz P, ed). Bethesda, MD: American Association of Blood Banks Press, 1999: 299–312.

45. Madsen LP, Rasmussen MK, Bjerregaard LL, Nohr SB, Ebbesen F. Impact of blood sampling in very preterm infants. *Scand J Clin Lab Invest* 2000; **60**: 125–32.

46. Strauss R. Neonatal anemia: pathophysiolopgy and treatment. In: *Improving Transfusion Practice for Pediatric Patients* (Wilson S, Levitt J, Strauss R, eds). Arlington, VA: American Association of Blood Banks Press, 1991: 1–17.

47. Widness JA, Seward VJ, Kromer IJ et al. Changing patterns of red blood cell transfusion in very low birth weight infants. *J Pediatr* 1996; **129**: 680–7.

48. Sacher RA, Luban NL, Strauss RG. Current practice and guidelines for the transfusion of cellular blood components in the newborn. *Transfus Med Rev* 1989; **3**: 39–54.

49. Wimberley PD, Lou HC, Pedersen H et al. Hypertensive peaks in the pathogenesis of intraventricular hemorrhage in the newborn. Abolition by phenobarbitone sedation. *Acta Paediatr Scand* 1982; **71**: 537–42.

50. Ringer SA, Richardson DK, Sacher RA et al. Variations in transfusion practice in neonatal intensive care. *Pediatrics* 1998; **101**: 194–200.

51. Fetus and Newborn Committee CPS. Guidelines for transfusion of erythrocytes to neonates and premature infants; position statement. *Can Med Assoc J* 1992; **147**: 1781–6.

52. Blanchette VS, Hume HA, Levy GJ et al. Guidelines for auditing pediatric blood transfusion practices. *Am J Dis Child* 1991; **145**: 787–96.

53. Ramasethu J, Luban N. Red blood cell transfusions in the newborn. *Semin Neonatal* 1999; **4**: 5–16.

54. Stockman JAd, Clark DA. Weight gain: a response to transfusion in selected preterm infants. *Am J Dis Child* 1984; **138**: 828–30.

55. Meyer J, Sive A, Jacobs P. Empiric red cell transfusion in asymptomatic preterm infants. *Acta Paediatr* 1993; **82**: 30–4.

56. Blank JP, Sheagren TG, Vajaria et al. The role of RBC transfusion in the premature infant. *Am J Dis Child* 1984; **138**: 831–3.

57. Lachance C, Chessex P, Fouron JC et al. Myocardial, erythropoietic, and metabolic adaptations to anemia of prematurity. *J Pediatr* 1994; **125**: 278–82.

58. Moller JC, Schwarz U, Schaible TF et al. Do cardiac output and serum lactate levels indicate blood transfusion requirements in anemia of prematurity? *Intensive Care Med* 1996; **22**: 472–6.

59. Izraeli S, Ben-Sira L, Harell D et al. Lactic acid as a predictor for erythrocyte transfusion in healthy preterm infants with anemia of prematurity. *J Pediatr* 1993; **122**: 629–31.

60. Shannon KM, Keith JF 3rd, Mentzer WC et al. Recombinant human erythropoietin stimulates erythropoiesis and reduces erythrocyte transfusions in very low birth weight preterm infants. *Pediatrics* 1995; **95**: 1–8.

61. Simon TL, Alverson DC, AuBuchon J et al. Practice parameter for the use of red blood cell transfusions: developed by the Red Blood Cell Administration Practice Guideline Development Task Force of the College of American Pathologists. *Arch Pathol Lab Med* 1998; **122**: 130–8.

62. Calhoun DA, Christensen RD, Edstrom CS et al. Consistent approaches to procedures and practices in neonatal hematology. *Clin Perinatol* 2000; **27**: 733–53.

63. Maier RF, Sonntag J, Walka MM et al. Changing practices of red blood cell transfusions in infants with birth weights less than 1000 g. *J Pediatr* 2000; **136**: 220–4.

64. Vietor HE, Hallensleben E, van Bree SP et al. Survival of donor cells 25 years after intrauterine transfusion. *Blood* 2000; **95**: 2709–14.

65. Guidelines on gamma irradiation of blood components for the prevention of transfusion-associated graft-versus-host disease. BCSH Blood Transfusion Task Force. *Transfus Med* 1996; **6**: 261–71.

66. Buntain SG, Pabari M. Massive transfusion and hyperkalaemic cardiac arrest in craniofacial surgery in a child. *Anaesth Intensive Care* 1999; **27**: 530–3.

67. Pisciotto P, Luban N. Complications of neonatal transfusions. In: *Transfusion Reactions* (Popovsky M, ed). Bethesda, MD: American Association of Blood Banks Press, 1996: 321–56.

68. Williams RA, Brown EF, Hurst D, Franklin LC. Transfusion of infants with activation of erythrocyte T antigen. *J Pediatr* 1989; **115**: 949–53.

69. Horn KD. The classification, recognition and significance of polyagglutination in transfusion medicine. *Blood Rev* 1999; **13**: 36–44.

70. Strauss R. Blood banking and transfusion issues in perinatal medicine. In: *Hematologic Problems of the Neonate* (Christensen R, ed). Philadelphia: WB Saunders, 2000: 405–26.

71. Blanchette VS, Kuhne T, Hume H, Hellmann J. Platelet transfusion therapy in newborn infants. *Transfus Med Rev* 1995; **9**: 215–30.

72. Hume H, Blanchette VS. Symposium on neonatal transfusion practices. *Transfus Med Rev* 1995; **9**: 185–6.

73. Blanchette VS, Johnson J, Rand M. The management of alloimmune neonatal thrombocytopenia. *Baillière's Best Pract Res Clin Haematol* 2000; **13**: 365–90.

74. Stern SC, Cockburn H, de Silva PM. Current practice in neonatal exchange transfusions: a retrospective audit based at one transfusion centre. *Transfus Med* 1998; **8**: 97–101.

75. Luban NL. Massive transfusion in the neonate. *Transfus Med Rev* 1995; **9**: 200–14.

76. Howard H, Martlew V, McFadyen I et al. Consequences for fetus and neonate of maternal red cell allo-immunisation. *Arch Dis Child Fetal Neonatal Ed* 1998; **78**: F62–6.

77. Amato M, Blumberg A, Hermann U Jr, Zurbrugg R. Effectiveness of single versus double volume exchange transfusion in newborn infants with ABO hemolytic disease. *Helv Paediatr Acta* 1988; **43**: 177–86.

78. Manno CS, Hedberg KW, Kim HC et al. Comparison of the hemostatic effects of fresh whole blood, stored whole blood, and components after open heart surgery in children. *Blood* 1991; **77**: 930–6.

79. Stein JI, Gombotz H, Rigler B et al. Open heart surgery in children of Jehovah's Witnesses: extreme hemodilution on cardiopulmonary bypass. *Pediatr Cardiol* 1991; **12**: 170–4.

80. Bevan DH. Cardiac bypass haemostasis: putting blood through the mill. *Br J Haematol* 1999; **104**: 208–19.

81. Stainsby D, MacLennan S, Hamilton PJ. Management of massive blood loss: a template guideline. *Br J Anaesth* 2000; **85**: 487–91.

82. Strauss RG, Burmeister LF, Johnson K et al. AS-1 red cells for neonatal transfusions: a randomized trial assessing donor exposure and safety. *Transfusion* 1996; **36**: 873–8.

83. Strauss RG, Barnes A Jr, Blanchette VS et al. Directed and limited-exposure blood donations for infants and children. *Transfusion* 1990; **30**: 68–72.

84. Pink J, Thomson A, Wylie B. Infectious disease markers in autologous and directed donations. *Transfus Med* 1994; **4**: 135–8.

85. Ohls RK. The use of erythropoietin in neonates. *Clin Perinatol* 2000; **27**: 681–96.

86. Maier RF, Obladen M, Scigalla P et al. The effect of epoetin beta (recombinant human erythropoietin) on the need for transfusion in very-low-birth-weight infants. European Multicentre Erythropoietin Study Group. *N Engl J Med* 1994; **330**: 1173–8.

87. Donato H, Vain N, Rendo P et al. Effect of early versus late administration of human recombinant erythropoietin on transfusion requirements in premature infants: results of a randomized, placebo-controlled, multicenter trial. *Pediatrics* 2000; **105**: 1066–72.

88. Meyer MP, Haworth C, Meyer JH, Commerford A. A comparison of oral and intravenous iron supplementation in preterm infants receiving recombinant erythropoietin. *J Pediatr* 1996; **129**: 258–63.

89. Ledbetter DJ, Juul SE, Erythropoietin and the incidence of necrotizing enterocolitis in infants with very low birth weight. *J Pediatr Surg* 2000; **35**: 178–81; discussion 182.

90. Soubasi V, Kremenopoulos G, Diamanti E et al. Follow-up of very low birth weight infants after erythropoietin treatment to prevent anemia of prematurity. *J Pediatr* 1995; **127**: 291–7.

91. Juul SE. Nonerythropoietic roles of erythropoietin in the fetus and neonate. *Clin Perinatal* 2000; **27**: 527–41.

92. Ohls RK, Hunter DD, Christensen RD. A randomized, double-blind, placebo-controlled trial of recombinant erythropoietin in treatment of the anemia of bronchopulmonary dysplasia. *J Pediatr* 1993; **123**: 996–1000.

93. Scaradavou A, Inglis S, Peterson P et al. Suppression of erythropoiesis by intrauterine transfusions in hemolytic disease of the newborn: use of erythropoietin to treat the late anemia. *J Pediatr* 1993; **123**: 279–84.

94. Thompson HW, Luban NL. Autologous blood transfusion in the pediatric patient. *J Pediatr Surg* 1995; **30**: 1406–11.

95. Eichler H, Schaible T, Richter E et al. Cord blood as a source of autologous RBCs for transfusion to preterm infants. *Transfusion* 2000; **40**: 1111–17.

9 Transfusion practice in resuscitation and critical illness

Gary Masterson

INTRODUCTION

There is great variation in attitudes towards the practice of administering blood products and other intravenous fluids to critically ill patients. Opinion is based largely on dogma supported by the results of experimental animal models rather than reliable clinical evidence. As a developing medical speciality, critical care medicine is now starting to address some of the unanswered questions in this field.

The decision to administer blood and other fluids to critically ill patients can be considered in two distinct phases. The first half of this chapter will concentrate on intravenous fluid resuscitation or the attempt to restore adequate circulatory volume in absolute or relative hypovolaemic states during the early stages of critical illness. Much of the discussion will centre on the choice of resuscitation fluids available. The colloid-versus-crystalloid argument will be revisited and reference will be made to the emerging role of hypertonic fluids in resuscitation.

The remainder of the chapter will focus on the decision-making process underlying whether blood transfusion is indicated or not in the later stages of critical illness as a treatment for normovoloemic anaemia. The reasons for the widespread adoption of a lower transfusion threshold trigger in haemodynamically stable critically ill patients will be discussed.

RESUSCITATION

Resuscitation strategies

The ultimate goal of resuscitation is to maintain oxygen delivery and therefore, hopefully, consumption to the vital organs and thereby sustain aerobic metabolism.[1] The determinants of oxygen consumption are identified in the following equation:

$$VO_2 = Q \times Hb \times 13 \times (SaO_2 - SvO_2) \quad (1)$$

where VO_2 is oxygen consumption, Q is cardiac output, Hb is haemoglobin concentration, SaO_2 is arterial oxygen saturation, and SvO_2 is mixed venous oxygen saturation.

The factors that pose a risk to VO_2 during haemorrhage are decreased cardiac output and decreased haemoglobin concentration. The consequences of a subnormal cardiac output are far more threatening than the consequences of anaemia. Therefore, the first priority in acute blood loss is to preserve cardiac output, while correcting the haemoglobin deficit is a secondary goal.

Flow-directed resuscitation

If restoration of cardiac output is the first priority in the management of acute haemorrhage, then blood cannot be considered an effective resuscitation fluid, because blood products do not promote blood flow as well as acellular resuscitation fluids (such as the colloid 'dextran'). The density of erythrocytes impedes the ability of blood products to promote blood flow. In fact, the administration of packed cell concentrates can actually reduce blood flow and aggravate tissue oxygen debts.[2,3]

As red cell blood products may be considered unacceptable fluids for, at least, early volume expansion in hypovolaemia, the choice of resuscitation fluid is restricted to two other classes of fluid: colloids and crystalloids. Colloids consist of large molecules that do not pass easily from one compartment to another, and so have a tendency to remain within the intravascular compartment. Crystalloids are isotonic sodium-rich fluids that are devoid of large molecules and tend to distribute between the intravascular and interstitial spaces. Although the choice of colloids over crystalloids for resuscitation of haemorrhage would at first hand appear obvious, this is not mirrored by clinical practice.[4-6] The reasons for this will be addressed in more detail later in this chapter.

Endpoints

Physiological endpoint measurements are used to guide both rate and extent of volume resuscitation. The endpoints commonly used in clinical practice include the following:

- central venous pressure[7] = 15 mmHg;
- pulmonary capillary wedge pressure[8] = 10–15 mmHg;
- cardiac index > 3 l/min/m^2;
- oxygen consumption > 100 ml/min/m^2;
- plasma lactate < 2 mmol/l;
- base deficit -3 to $+3$ mmol/l.

The base deficit has been shown to correlate with volume deficits and mortality in trauma patients.[9] As such, it is widely used as a guide to volume resuscitation in general. A persistently elevated base deficit during resuscitation usually indicates ongoing tissue hypoperfusion and ischaemia. Plasma lactate levels are now routinely used as a more precise index of tissue ischaemia.

Most critical care physicians would agree that these measurements are helpful in deciding whether a patient has been adequately resuscitated or not, but it is important to emphasize that reviewing the overall picture is a much more satisfactory approach than focusing on one or more physiological measurements as endpoints. Moreover, the quoted range of measurements above represent measurements from normal healthy adult patients and do not necessarily indicate the optimal pathophysiological status for a shocked patient.

Erythrocyte resuscitation

In the second stage of volume resuscitation, attention is directed away from volume status and the achievement of an adequate cardiac output towards correcting deficits in oxygen-carrying capacity. The current practice of transfusing red blood cells based on haemoglobin measurements has absolutely no scientific basis.[10,11] A serum haemoglobin concentration offers no information about tissue oxygenation, nor is it synonymous with oxygen-carrying capacity. A more rational approach would be to employ oxygen transport variables[12] and measurements of end-organ failure, such as plasma lactate levels, to make inferences about tissue oxygenation and the need for red blood cell transfusion. This approach, and transfusion triggers in normovoloemic, anaemic, critically ill patients, will be discussed in more detail later in this chapter.

Choice of resuscitation fluids

The large variety of resuscitation fluids available, both colloids and crystalloids, underlines our continued failure to identify the best choice of resuscitation fluid for the shocked patient.[13–15] The choice of fluids currently available will be described before discussing the potential roles for crystalloids and colloids in resuscitation.

Crystalloid fluids

The major constituent of all commonly available crystalloid fluids is the inorganic salt sodium chloride (NaCl), which is the most abundant solute in the extracellular space (Table 9.1). After administration, approximately 75–80% of sodium-based intravenous fluids are distributed in the interstitial space. Therefore the predominant effect of volume resuscitation with crystalloid fluids is to expand the interstitial space rather than the intravascular space.[15]

0.9% sodium chloride

Isotonic saline or normal saline (which is an inappropriate term, since a one-normal NaCl solution contains 58 g NaCl per litre rather than the 9 g NaCl in 0.9% NaCl) has higher sodium and chloride concentrations than plasma, is slightly hypertonic to plasma, and has a significantly lower pH than plasma. These rarely pose a problem in clinical practice, but hyperchloraemic metabolic acidosis has been reported following large-volume 0.9% NaCl resuscitation.[16]

Lactated Ringer's

Sidney Ringer, a British physician, who studied mechanisms of cardiac contraction, introduced Ringer's solution in 1880.[17] Fifty years later, Alexis Hartmann, an American paediatrician proposed the addition of sodium lactate buffer to treat metabolic acidosis. Lactated Ringer's solution, also known as Hartmann's solution, gained popularity and eventually replaced the standard Ringer's solution for routine intravenous therapy.

Lactated Ringer's solution contains potassium and calcium in concentrations that approximate those in plasma, and to maintain electrical neutrality the sodium content is less than that in isotonic saline. The addition of lactate similarly decreases the chloride concentration to more closely approximate plasma chloride concentrations than does isotonic saline. There is little current evidence that the lactate present provides any useful buffer effect. The calcium in lactated Ringer's

	Table 9.1 Composition of intravenous crystalloid fluids							
	Concentration (mmol/l)							Osmolality
Fluid	Na	Cl	K	Ca	Mg	Buffer	pH	(mOsm/l)
Plasma	141	103	4–5	5	2	Bicarbonate: 26	7.4	289
0.9% NaCl	154	154	—	—	—	—	5.7	308
Lactated Ringer's	131	111	5	2	—	Lactate: 29	6.4	273
Plasma-Lyte	140	98	5	—	1.5	Acetate: 27	7.4	295

can bind to certain drugs, resulting in decreased bioavailability and efficacy. Of particular note is calcium binding to the citrated anticoagulant in blood products, which promotes the formation of blood clots in donor blood if lactated Ringer's is used as a diluent.[18]

Plasma-Lyte

The most important feature of this crystalloid is the added buffer capacity that results in a pH equivalent to that of plasma. Magnesium is also a constituent, and may well be of benefit since hypomagnesaemia frequently accompanies critical illness. However, excessive administration of Plasma-Lyte to patients with renal insufficiency can cause hypermagnesaemia that may lead to vasodilatation and hypotension.

Dextrose solutions

5% dextrose was originally introduced to supply non-protein calories and thus provide a protein-sparing effect. However, enteral and parenteral nutrition is now the standard of care for providing daily calorie requirements, and the use of 5% dextrose as a source of energy is now obsolete. Dextrose solutions are ineffective plasma expanders as a result of their rapid intracellular distribution after administration. Other potentially detrimental effects of glucose infusions in critically ill patients include enhanced carbon dioxide production,[19] enhanced lactate production,[20,21] and aggravation of cerebral ischaemia.[22]

Colloid fluids

These fluids consist of large molecules that do not pass across diffusional barriers as readily as crystalloids, and therefore after infusion they have a greater tendency to enhance plasma volume than crystalloids. Colloids are generally more effective plasma expanders than crystalloids, and the potency of individual colloids as plasma expanders is related to the colloid oncotic pressure exerted by each fluid (Table 9.2).

Albumin

Albumin is predominantly a transport protein, and accounts for approximately 75% of the oncotic pressure of plasma.[23,24] Heat-treated

Fluid	Average molecular weight (kDa)	Oncotic pressure (mmHg)	Plasma volume expansion ratio	Serum half-life
5% albumin	69	20	0.7–1.3	16 hours
25% albumin	69	70	4.0–5.0	16 hours
6% hetastarch	69	30	1.0–1.3	17 days
10% pentastarch	120	40	1.5	10 hours
10% dextran 40	26	40	1.0–1.5	6 hours
6% dextran 70	41	40	0.8	12 hours

Table 9.2 Characteristics of intravenous colloid fluids

human serum albumin preparations are commercially available as 5% and 25% solutions in an isotonic saline diluent. As the sodium load in 25% albumin is comparatively low, 25% albumin is also termed salt-poor albumin. 5% albumin has a colloid oncotic pressure of 20 mmHg, which approximates that of plasma. Around half of the infused volume of albumin remains intravascular after infusion, and the oncotic effects last between 12 and 18 hours.

25% albumin has a greater oncotic pressure of 70 mmHg and expands the plasma volume by 4–5 times the volume infused. This plasma expansion occurs at the expense of the interstitial fluid volume, and so many do not consider 25% albumin to be an appropriate resuscitation fluid in hypovolaemic states. Salt-poor albumin is administered to attempt to shift fluid from the interstitial space to the intravascular space in hypoalbuminaemic states. However, there is little evidence to support this hypothesis.

Hetastarch

This is a synthetic colloid available as a 6% solution in isotonic saline. It consists of amylopectin molecules that vary in size between a few hundred to over one million daltons. The resulting oncotic pressure is similar to that of 5% albumin, and its major benefit over albumin is its lower cost. Although it has a very prolonged elimination half-life of 17 days, its oncotic effects disappear within 24 hours.

Hetastarch molecules are metabolized by serum amylase enzymes, and the breakdown products are cleared renally. This occasionally causes a mild elevation of serum amylase that usually returns to normal within 5–7 days. Serum lipase levels are not affected, and so a diagnosis of acute pancreatitis should not be considered. Anaphylactic reactions to hetastarch are very rare, with a reported incidence of 0.0004%.[25] In vitro coagulopathy, secondary to a prolonged partial thromboplastin time resulting from an interaction with factor VIII, has been described, but there is no evidence of increased risk of clinical bleeding following hetastarch administration.[26]

Pentastarch

This is a low-molecular-weight analogue of hetastarch that is available as a 10% solution in isotonic saline. Pentastarch contains smaller but greater numbers of starch molecules than hetastarch and thus has a higher colloid oncotic pressure. It is more effective as a volume expander than hetastarch, and increases the plasma volume, by 1.5 times the infused volume, and its plasma expansion effects last for approximately 12 hours.[27] Compared with hetastarch, pentastarch has fewer tendencies to interact with coagulation proteins, but the significance of this is unclear.[28]

Dextrans

Dextrans are glucose polymers produced by the bacterium *Leuconostoc* after incubation in a sucrose medium. Dextrans have fallen from clinical popularity because of a perceived risk of serious adverse reactions. Both of the commercially available preparations, 10% dextran 40 and 6% dextran 70, are hyperoncotic relative to plasma. Dextran 40 causes a greater increase in plasma volume than dextran 70, but its effects only last for a few hours and so dextran 70 is the preferred solution because of its longer duration of action.

Dextrans cause a dose-related bleeding tendency in vivo by inhibiting platelet aggregation, reducing activation of factor VIII, and promoting fibrinolysis.[25] To minimize the risk of bleeding, it is recommended to limit the daily dextran dose to 20 ml/kg. Anaphylaxis is now a rare complication of dextran administration with an incidence of 0.032%. Dextrans can also coat the surface of red blood cells, which may lead to difficulty in crossmatching blood and may increase the erythrocyte sedimentation rate. Dextrans have also been implicated as a cause of acute renal failure resulting from a reduced filtration pressure secondary to the hyperoncotic state following administration.[29] However, this mechanism is unproven, and renal failure occurs only exceptionally rarely with dextrans.

Gelatins

Haemaccel is a gelatin solution with an average molecular weight of 35 kDa and has the same oncotic pressure as plasma. Evidence suggests that it is safe to administer large volumes of gelatins, since they do not appear to cause coagulopathy or renal impairment. Gelatins are comparatively cheap, but the incidence of allergic reactions is believed to be greater than with dextrans and starch solutions. As the gelatin molecules cross the glomerular basement membrane without difficulty, gelatin solutions cause a diuresis and the oncotic effect lasts for only 2–3 hours.

The colloid-versus-crystalloid controversy

Little progress has been made in resolving the controversy over the choice of colloids versus crystalloids in resuscitation and critical illness. Any evidence in favour of either fluid has been overshadowed by personal opinion, anecdotal information, uncontrolled clinical trials, and animal models of doubtful relevance.

The crystalloid school of thought is based on the concept that reduced extracellular water is the primary defect in shock states. Before the Second World War, Collier et al[30] and Blalock[31] advocated the administration of large volumes of saline and glucose in the treatment of traumatic shock. In the 1950s and 1960s, Moyer[32] and Shires,[33–36] amongst others, used large volumes of sodium-rich solutions. Crystalloid supporters recommend the use of adequate volumes of isotonic fluids (Ringer's lactate or isotonic saline) to replace the deficit due to both intravascular and extracellular fluid losses in shock states. There are numerous experimental studies that support the presence of extracellular water losses in excess of the measured plasma volume losses and increased intracellular water resulting from leakage of fluid into the intracellular compartment during shock. However, other investigators have criticized the methods used to measure extracellular water in these studies, and have failed to reproduce the results of these studies.[37]

In contrast, the colloid school of thought believes that intravascular fluid depletion is the primary deficit in shock. They argue that none of the isotopes and tracers used to measure extracellular water in the above studies, such as ^{35}S-labelled sulfate, thiocyanate, inulin, ^{22}Na, ^{24}Na, ^{36}Cl, ^{38}Cl, and ^{82}Br, are either entirely confined to or evenly distributed within the extracellular compartment.[37] Moreover, it has not been convincingly demonstrated in either animals or patients that replenishing interstitial fluid deficits leads to any beneficial cardiorespiratory changes apart from those that may result from the associated slight increase in intravascular volume. In fact, there is much evidence that plasma volume expansion that decreases interstitial water resulting from the administration of concentrated colloids not only improves pressure and flow in shock states but also improves oxygen transport variables.[38,39] In fact, the colloid protagonists suggest that crystalloids merely expand the interstitial compartment, which has no established benefit and may be effective in replacing sublethal intravascular volume losses, but with limited efficacy. Moreover, the attempt to replenish intravascular volume with crystalloids causes indefinite expansion of the interstitial space and may lead to serious pulmonary sequelae. In summary, from the pathophysiological perspective, the logical conclusion is that circulatory volume losses are most effectively replenished using colloids, and interstitial losses with isotonic crystalloids.[40]

Despite the aforementioned discussion and resulting logical conclusions, there remains great uncertainty about whether to administer colloids or crystalloids in clinical practice. Clinical studies have suggested that resuscitation with crystalloids improves postoperative organ function with respect to cardiovascular,[41] respiratory,[42] renal,[43] coagulation,[44] and immunological systems.[45] In addition, crystalloids minimize the risk of anaphylactic reactions[46] and are considerably cheaper than colloids.[47] On the negative side, clinical studies suggest that crystalloids may predispose to pulmonary oedema,[48] and peripheral oedema (which itself may impair tissue oxygen delivery and wound healing).[49] In contrast, resuscitation with colloids requires less volume and time.[50,51] There is also clinical evidence that colloids enhance oxygen transport, myocardial contractility, and cardiac output.[52]

The most recent and, to date, highest quality systemic review addressing the colloid-versus-crystalloid question was published by Choi et al[53] from Ontario. They pooled the data for 814 patients from 17 primary, randomly controlled studies comparing crystalloid with colloid resuscitation. They concluded that there was no overall apparent difference in pulmonary oedema, mortality, or length of stay between isotonic crystalloid and colloid resuscitation. Subgroup analysis revealed that crystalloid resuscitation is associated with a lower mortality in trauma patients. However, methodological limitations, mainly from insufficient patient numbers, precluded the authors from making any evidence-based clinical recommendations. Until a large prospective randomized trial is conducted, the colloid-versus-crystalloid controversy will continue.

A role for albumin?

Many critical-care physicians consider human albumin solution to be the most effective, albeit costly,[54] intravascular replacement fluid for the resuscitation of critically ill patients. Moreover, serum hypoalbuminaemia in critical illness is associated with increased mortality and has led to the hypothesis that albumin replacement therapy in such patients may improve outcome.[55] However, systemic review of randomized, controlled trials by the Cochrane Injuries Group has shed a degree of doubt on this firmly held belief.[56] The aim of this review was to establish if albumin improved outcome sufficiently to justify the increased expense incurred.

The authors identified 30 randomized, controlled trials including a total of 1419 randomized patients who received albumin for hypovolaemia, burns, or hypoalbuminaemia. For each of the three patient groups, the risk of death was significantly higher for those patients who received albumin, with an excess mortality of 6%. The reasons offered to explain this detrimental effect of albumin included its anticoagulant properties, through the inhibition of platelet aggregation and the enhancement of the inhibition of factor Xa by antithrombin III,[57] and also the increased leakage of albumin across the capillary membrane into the extravascular space to reduce the oncotic pressure difference across the capillary wall, thus enhancing interstitial oedema formation.[58] The group concluded that the use of human albumin in critically ill patients should be urgently reviewed and that it should not be used outside the context of rigorously conducted randomized controlled trials. This review was widely publicized by the media and provoked the irrational withdrawal of human albumin from many institutions, enforcing changes in clinical practice.

The most important criticism of this review is that it was based on relatively small trials in which there were only a small number of deaths, and therefore it must be interpreted with caution. The populations of patients studied were extremely heterogeneous in that postoperative adult patients, preterm neonates, general intensive care patients, and patients with hypoalbuminaemia were all pooled together for the purpose of this review. The endpoint selected by the Cochrane Injuries Group, namely mortality, was not an endpoint in most of the comprising studies. The authors were statisticians, not critical-care physicians, and therefore may have inadvertently included inappropriate studies. These criticisms are ample enough to conclude that the question whether albumin is better or worse than other resuscitation fluids should remain unanswered until a large well-designed randomized trial is completed. At this time, a change in clinical practice as a result of this review is unwarranted.

Hypertonic fluids in resuscitation

In recent years, the use of small-volume hypertonic saline resuscitation for hypovolaemic shock has enjoyed intermittent popularity. An intravenous bolus of 250 ml of 7.5% saline to a 70 kg adult results in plasma expansion of approximately 500 ml, which is approximately the same intravascular volume achieved following 1000 ml of 5% albumin. In other words, hypertonic saline resuscitation can achieve equivalent volume expansion to colloids, but at one-quarter the infused volume. The excess volume results from the flux of fluid from the intracellular compartment down the resulting concentration gradient into the interstitial and intravascular spaces. This process results in cellular dehydration, but the significance of this in clinical practice remains uncertain.

Since the early 1980s, hypertonic saline has been demonstrated repeatedly, but not unanimously, to be safe and effective in the early resuscitation of hypovolaemia. The question that remains unanswered is whether hypertonic saline offers any benefit over conventional fluid choices. The most convincing evidence for using hypertonic saline comes from studies focusing on prehospital trauma resuscitation; however, a clear benefit with this approach has not been clearly demonstrated for all patients.[59] Select subgroups of patients, for example those with penetrating truncal injury who require surgery, may benefit from resuscitation with hypertonic saline, but these subgroups are small.[60] In summary, after 15 years of evaluation, hypertonic fluid resuscitation techniques have few advocates.

Minimal-volume resuscitation

The traditional management of haemorrhage favours aggressive volume resuscitation, but there is an emerging body of evidence from both animal studies and clinical trials that volume resuscitation to normotension in some clinical situations can actually promote continued blood loss. This concept is important for two reasons. First, it suggests that blood pressure is not an appropriate endpoint for the resuscitation of hypovolaemic shock (not, at least, until the source of ongoing blood loss is sealed). Second, it implies that the critical-care physician's attempt to achieve normal clinical parameters (which is the general approach in modern medicine) is inappropriate when the human body is subjected to abnormal conditions. Normal clinical parameters are a desirable goal only when abnormal conditions are corrected.

Currently there is substantial evidence to support the use of minimal-volume resuscitation in leaking/ruptured abdominal aortic aneurysms and penetrating truncal trauma, but many advocate that the application of these principles should be much more widespread.[61] Nevertheless, it would be inappropriate to replace the long-held dogma of aggressive fluid resuscitation in all situations with this potentially new practice of minimal-volume resuscitation in all situations. Instead, these different principles of resuscitation must be applied according to the individual patient's circumstances. The role of minimal-volume resuscitation in clinical practice awaits clarification.

Blood transfusion in early resuscitation

As already discussed, there is evidence that the administration of cellular blood products is an inefficient method of increasing cardiac output in hypovolaemic patients because of the comparatively high viscosity of transfused blood. It is also widely appreciated that correction of the low-cardiac-output state is more important than correction of anaemia during haemorrhage. The question arises as to when blood administration should be considered as part of the initial resuscitation fluid protocol. Whilst accepting that correction of intravascular volume, and hence cardiac output, in the haemorrhaging patient is vital, if the haemorrhage is excessive enough then a point must be reached when the decreasing haemoglobin concentration becomes a contributing factor to tissue hypoxia. To date, there is little evidence to help the clinician decide what should be considered an acceptable haemoglobin concentration in a patient undergoing resuscitation for ongoing haemorrhage. Attempting to disentangle the contributions of decreased cardiac output and anaemia to tissue hypoxia during haemorrhage is difficult – and ultimately may well prove impossible, particularly in the clinical arena. For now, the clinician must rely on experience and judgement to guide decisions about when to administer blood during volume resuscitation.

There is some evidence that blood administered during volume resuscitation can have detrimental sequelae, which emphasizes why it is important to consider whether blood is truly necessary during early resuscitation. Duke et al[62] studied 252 patients undergoing surgery for traumatic splenic injury and found that those patients who received early blood transfusions had a significantly increased risk of postoperative infections, respiratory complications, and admission to the intensive care unit. Therefore, apart from the issue of expense, there is well-established clinical evidence that blood should be transfused during early resuscitation only when absolutely necessary. The difficulty lies in deciding just what 'absolutely necessary' means in this context.

Resuscitation: conclusions

During haemorrhage, the replenishment of intravascular volume takes priority over red cell replacement; however, the huge choice of fluids available underlines the continued uncertainty about what the best resuscitation fluid is. Although there is a theoretical benefit in administering colloids compared with crystalloids, this benefit has not been supported by clinical studies. Until a large prospective trial comparing crystalloids with colloids in resuscitation is carried out, this question will remain unanswered.

The practice of administering human albumin solution – once considered the optimal, albeit expensive, volume expander in critically ill patients – has recently been questioned as a result of a single study. However, this study has been severely criticized, and it would be inappropriate to alter clinical prac-tice as a result. Despite well over a decade of research and evidence of improved outcome in some patient groups, the enthusiasm for using hypertonic fluids remains limited. Minimal-volume resuscitation has been demonstrated to reduce haemorrhage and improve outcome in patients with penetrating truncal injuries and leaking abdominal aortic aneurysms, but its use for other patients has not been substantiated. The decision to transfuse blood during the early phases of resuscitation should not be taken lightly, since there is evidence of an increased incidence of detrimental sequelae.

TRANSFUSION THRESHOLD

Aim of transfusion during critical illness

The ultimate goal of resuscitation and critical care is the establishment of an adequate oxygen delivery (DO_2) to bodily tissues in an attempt to prevent, or assist recovery from, organ dysfunction.[63] Equation (1), given earlier in this chapter demonstrates that DO_2 and therefore, hopefully, VO_2 can be maximized by manipulating either cardiac index or plasma haemoglobin concentrations. The first half of this chapter focused on the issue of intravenous fluid administration during resuscitation as a method of augmenting cardiac index and therefore global oxygen delivery. The remainder of this chapter will concentrate on the decision-making process surrounding the administration of blood to secure an adequate oxygen delivery after an adequate blood volume and therefore cardiac index have been achieved following initial resuscitation.

Does optimizing oxygen transport improve outcome in critical illness?

Although the concept of optimal oxygen transport improving outcome in critically ill patients is commonly used to justify the practice of transfusion and fluid administration, it remains a contentious issue. Under normal conditions, the average 70 kg body consumes 100–120 ml/min/m^2 of oxygen. If DO_2 decreases because of a decreased cardiac index or plasma haemoglobin concentration, VO_2 remains stable over a wide range of DO_2 as a result of increasing oxygen extraction. When DO_2 falls below a critical value, VO_2 will also decrease, because oxygen extraction eventually reaches its maximum capability. Under these circumstances, VO_2 is described as supply-dependent.[64]

The relationship between DO_2 and VO_2 has been studied in a variety of different disease states, including acute respiratory distress syndrome (ARDS),[65,66] chronic obstructive pulmonary disease (COPD),[67] pulmonary vascular disease,[68] and congestive cardiac failure.[69] Although these studies were all very different in design, an important recurring theme was the observation of a relationship between DO_2 and VO_2, or pathological supply-dependency, at values considerably greater than the DO_2 critical value of 300 ml/min/m^2 documented in healthy adults. These results suggest that the mechanisms controlling oxygen extraction may be impaired in disease states. The assumption that this pathological supply-dependency indicates a true oxygen debt gave rise to the popular practice of administering fluids, inotropes, and blood transfusions to promote supranormal DO_2 levels with the hope of improving outcome.

Nevertheless, in some patients, it remains difficult to explain how the apparent presence of supply-dependency can indicate an oxygen debt in the absence of a lactic acidosis. Furthermore, most of these studies measured DO_2 but calculated VO_2 using the reverse Fick method. As there are variables common to both dependent VO_2 and independent DO_2 values, there is a mathematical coupling of measurement errors shared in the common variables.[70,71] This adds further doubt to the concept of supply-dependency in critically ill patients.[72]

Some two decades ago, Shoemaker et al[73,74] demonstrated that surgical patients who achieved supranormal haemodynamic parameters had a greater chance of survival than patients who failed to do so (Table 9.3). The hypothesis was that the greater values observed in survivors indicated an ability to compensate physiologically for the increased metabolic demands caused by disease. These observations lead to the deduction that a therapeutically driven increase in DO_2, and hopefully VO_2, using fluids, transfusion, and inotropes would also result in an improved outcome. With time, this concept spread enthusiastically to different categories of critically ill patients

There have been a number of trials attempting to answer the question whether the therapeutic achievement of supranormal

---

Table 9.3 Shoemaker's supranormal haemodynamic goals

- Cardiac index > 4.5 l/min/m^2
- DO_2 > 600 ml/min/m^2
- VO_2 > 170 ml/min/m^2

haemodynamic goals improves outcome in different groups of critically ill patients. There is some evidence that such an approach improves outcome in high-risk surgical patients, particularly if the goals are achieved pre-emptively.[75,76] There is limited evidence that the achievement of supranormal haemodynamic parameters increases survival in trauma patients.[77,78] However, there is no substantial evidence that this goal-driven approach improves outcome in patients with sepsis[79] or ARDS[80] or in unselected critically ill patients.[81,82] Currently the consensus is that there is no place for setting supranormal haemodynamic goals in unselected groups of critically ill patients,[83] although there may be some justification for such an approach pre-emptively in high-risk surgical patients.

Effect of transfusion on oxygen transport

Although it remains controversial as to whether achieving increased oxygen transport actually benefits critically ill patients, it has always been assumed from a theoretical perspective that transfusion increases oxygen delivery, and therefore consumption, by increasing plasma haemoglobin concentration – see Equation (1). However, there is little evidence to support even this apparently logical deduction.

Dietrich et al[84] reported that augmenting red cell mass in non-surgical critically ill patients did not improve oxygen consumption, whereas Czer and Shoemaker[85] suggested that a haematocrit of 0.33 is associated with improved survival in surgical critically ill patients. Gramm et al[86] administered two units of packed red blood cells to a group of patients with sepsis syndrome and studied the observed changes in haemodynamic and oxygen transport measurements. Although plasma haemoglobin concentration and haematocrit increased significantly as a result, the anticipated increases in DO_2 and VO_2 were not documented. Babineau et al[87] also found that when a transfusion trigger of 10 g/dl was used in surgical critically ill patients, VO_2 did not increase appreciably following transfusion. These studies do not support the practice of improving oxygen transport by transfusion – at least when using currently popular transfusion triggers.

Although there is little evidence to support a survival advantage from delivering supranormal oxygen transport values, it remains intuitive that for each patient there must be a DO_2 value (contributed by plasma haemoglobin concentration and cardiac index) below which the patient is exposed to the risk of hypoxia and organ dysfunction. The remainder of this chapter will describe the current thinking on the lowest acceptably safe haemoglobin concentration (otherwise known as a transfusion trigger) in clinical practice.

Why change the transfusion threshold?

In addition to the current evidence that transfusion does not improve oxygen transport, it has been acknowledged in recent years that blood transfusion carries a number of risks. As a result, clinicians now question the inappropriately held belief that a plasma haemoglobin concentration of 10 g/dl or less should trigger a blood transfusion in critically ill patients. Blood is expensive and is becoming an increasingly limited resource. There is also a definite risk of transmission of infections, including hepatitis C and human immunodeficiency virus.[88] These well-recognized complications of transfusion are discussed in more detail elsewhere in this text.

Of conceivably more relevance to the critically ill patient is the less appreciated complication of blood transfusion-associated immunosuppression and subsequent infection. There is an extensive literature, both experimental and clinical, addressing the effects of blood transfusion on the immunological system.[89] Although the underlying mechanisms remain unclear, many immunological effector systems are affected by transfusion: increased prostaglandin E_2 production,[90] decreased interleukin-2 release,[91] decreased production of tumour necrosis factor, interferon-γ, and granulocyte–macrophage colony-stimulating factor,[92] decreased $CD4^+/CD8^+$ T-cell ratio,[93] diminished natural killer cell activity,[94] reduced antigen presentation by macrophages,[95] unspecified suppressor cells,[96] anti-idiotypic antibodies,[97] T-suppressor cells,[98] mixed lymphocyte culture (MLC) blocking factors,[99] and donor-specific chimerism.[100] This transfusion-associated immunosuppression can only exacerbate the already-established immunosuppression resulting from critical illness itself, and therefore further increases the risk of infection.

Most of the evidence for transfusion-associated immunosuppression has been documented in surgical rather than critically ill patients, and it remains uncertain whether the immunosuppression results from the transfusion itself or from other associated confounding factors. Heiss et al[101] addressed this question by comparing postoperative infection rates in matched colorectal cancer patients receiving either allogeneic blood or autologous transfusion (which is thought to cause less immunosuppression). There were significantly more infections in the allogeneic group compared with the autologous group, suggesting that allogeneic transfusion causes immunosuppression and increases the risk of infection. A number of other clinical studies support this conclusion, and other authors have concluded that no other variable was more consistently associated with postoperative infection than perioperative allogeneic blood transfusion.[89,102] Although transfusion-associated immunosuppression has been most clearly demonstrated in surgical patients, it nevertheless suggests that the decision to transfuse a critically ill patient should be considered with caution.

Variations in transfusion practice

A plasma haemoglobin threshold of 10 g/dl is commonly used as a trigger for transfusion of allogeneic blood in critically ill patients, but the reasoning for this approach is based on dogma rather than scientific or clinical evidence. Amongst others, Moss and co-workers[103–105] suggested that a more physiological trigger might be a pretransfusion extraction ratio VO_2/DO_2 greater than 50%. However, most of their work was performed with non-critically ill animal models undergoing controlled euvoloemic haemodilution to achieve an anaemic state. These results cannot be extrapolated directly to critically ill patients, and, in fact, the adoption of any physiological transfusion trigger is fraught with theoretical and practical difficulties. For the foreseeable future, numerical transfusion triggers will continue to dominate clinical practice.

In 1941, Adams and Lundy[106] recommended transfusion for haemoglobin concentrations between 8 and 10 g/dl in the perioperative period. It has even been suggested that the widespread adoption of 10 g/dl as a transfusion trigger (a term coined by Friedman et al[107]) may be because it is an easy figure to remember.[108,109] As a result of increasing appreciation of transfusion-associated complications, as discussed above, recent guidelines emphasize that the decision to transfuse should not be based on a single haemoglobin concentration measurement.[110-112] Nevertheless, surveys of transfusion practice have repeatedly documented the importance attributed to transfusion triggers.[113-115]

Hebert et al[117] surveyed transfusion practice in Canadian intensive care units and found significant variation in critical-care transfusion practice. Even in 1997, the majority of critical-care physicians were adhering to a 10 g/dl transfusion trigger, whereas others practised a more restrictive approach to blood transfusion. Clinical factors, such as age, admitting pathology, comorbidity, presence of chronic anaemia, and ongoing coronary ischaemia, all influenced transfusion triggers significantly. There was also a geographical influence on transfusion triggers. Guidelines[112] have also recommended that blood should be administered one unit at a time according to clinical judgement, but over 90% of clinicians in this survey elected to transfuse two or more units of blood at a time.

Current best practice

Much progress has been made in recent years in addressing what the new transfusion trigger should be in critically ill patients. This is largely due to the efforts of the Transfusion Requirements in Critical Care (TRICC) Investigators and the Canadian Critical Care Trials Group. This group has published a series of landmark papers that have helped to define the most evidence-based approach to transfusion triggers in critical illness.

Evidence for liberal and restrictive approaches to transfusion

As previously discussed, the liberal administration of red cells to critically ill patients (or the adoption of a high transfusion trigger) may be justified on the basis that oxygen transport should be maintained at levels sufficient to avoid tissue hypoxia. This concept has limited supporting evidence and remains controversial. The argument that pathological supply-dependency indicates ongoing tissue ischaemia and the development of multiple organ failure is supported by two prospective observational studies that suggested a significant association between mortality and the occurrence of pathological supply-dependency.[66,117] To date, all randomized clinical trials that have attempted to define optimal levels of oxygen transport in critically ill and high-risk surgical patients used therapeutic interventions other than red cell transfusion to enhance oxygen delivery.[76,79-82,118,119] All of these trials maintained haemoglobin levels greater than 10 g/dl, and it is therefore difficult to draw conclusions about optimal red cell transfusion strategies from these data. As discussed above, the majority of studies addressing the impact of red cell transfusion on oxygen transport failed to identify a presumed beneficial increase in VO_2 following transfusion. This may reflect methodological errors or the absence of pathological supply-dependency rather than the fact that red cells were actually unnecessary. In summary, it is difficult to justify a transfusion trigger of 10 g/dl resulting in a liberal transfusion practice when the evidence for the very existence of pathological supply-dependency, and its contribution towards poor outcome, in critically ill patients is so controversial.

Many critical-care physicians transfuse more liberally in patients at risk of coronary artery disease or with established cardiac pathology. One large cohort study suggested that critically ill patients with cardiac disease had a trend towards increased mortality when haemoglobin concentrations were less than 9.5 g/dl compared with anaemic critically ill patients with other diagnoses.[120] In Jehovah's Witness patients undergoing surgery, anaemia increased mortality significantly in patients with cardiac disease compared with those without cardiac pathology.[121] This constitutes indirect evidence that critically ill patients with cardiac disease may benefit from a higher transfusion threshold than critically ill patients with other diagnoses.

The aforementioned reasons for attempting to reduce transfusion triggers in critically ill patients are complemented by the emerging volume of literature that red cell transfusion may decrease microcirculatory DO_2 despite an increase in global DO_2.[122–125] Sepsis may decrease red cell deformability and the ability to off-load oxygen in the microcirculation.[126–128]

There have been a number of small randomized controlled trials, including a pilot study by the TRICC Investigators, specifically addressing the question of different transfusion triggers on mortality and morbidity in high-risk surgical and critically ill patients.[129–133] However, the small numbers of patients studied in all of these studies precludes any definitive conclusions about which transfusion strategy is the best in critical illness. Until recently, the published literature on this topic was not able to establish an optimal and safe lower limit of transfusion threshold in critically ill patients. The recognized need to answer this question resulted in the TRICC trial.[134]

TRICC trial

In 1999, the TRICC Investigators and the Canadian Critical Care Trials Group published a large multicentre randomized controlled clinical trial of transfusion requirements in critical care.[134] The aim of this study was to finally answer the question whether a restrictive strategy of red cell transfusion produces equivalent results to a liberal transfusion strategy in terms of mortality and organ dysfunction in critically ill patients.

The study recruited patients from 25 centres throughout Canada between 1994 and 1997 who were expected to require intensive care for more than 24 hours and whose plasma haemoglobin had decreased to less than 9 g/dl within 72 hours of admission and were considered to be euvoloemic. Consecutive patients were randomly allocated to one of two treatment groups, stratified according to disease severity and centre. The patients assigned to the restrictive transfusion strategy group had their plasma haemoglobins maintained between 7 and 9 g/dl, with the transfusion trigger set at 7 g/dl. The group of patients assigned to the liberal transfusion strategy group had their plasma haemoglobin concentrations maintained between 10 and 12 g/dl, with the transfusion trigger set at 10 g/dl. Transfusions were administered one unit at a time, and plasma haemoglobin was checked before considering further transfusion. These transfusion protocols were discontinued after discharge from the intensive care unit.

The primary outcome measure was death from all causes in the 30 days after randomization. Secondary outcome measures included 60-day rates of death from all causes, mortality rates during the stay in the intensive care unit and during hospitalization, and survival times in the first 30 days. Measures of organ failure and dysfunction were also documented.

Of the 838 patients enrolled, 418 were allocated to receive a restrictive transfusion strategy and the remaining 420 were assigned to a liberal strategy of transfusion. Only 1% of enrolled patients did not complete the study. It would appear that the transfusion protocols were followed successfully in that the average daily haemoglobin concentrations in the restrictive-strategy group were 8.5 g/dl, compared with 10.7 g/dl in the liberal-strategy group. An average of 2.6 units of blood was administered to the restrictive-strategy patients, compared with 5.6 units in the liberal-strategy group. This represents a relative decrease of 54% in the number of transfusions when the restrictive strategy was used. Interestingly, 33% of patients in the restrictive-strategy group did not require transfusion compared with zero in the liberal-strategy group.

The primary outcome measure, namely the mortality from all causes in the 30 days after randomization, was 18.7% in the restrictive-strategy group and 23.3% in the liberal-strategy group, but the difference did not reach statistical significance ($p = 0.11$). The mortality rates during hospitalization were statistically significantly lower for the restrictive-strategy group (22.2% versus 28.1%). Intensive care (13.9% versus 16.2%) and 60-day (22.7% versus 26.5%) mortality rates were also lower for the restrictive-strategy patients – but not significantly so.

The number of patients with multiple organ failure (defined as greater than three-organ failure) were similar between the two groups, and the mean multiple-organ-dysfunction score was slightly less in the restrictive-strategy group – but not significantly so. Cardiac events, including myocardial infarction and pulmonary oedema, were significantly more common in the liberal-strategy group.

Subgroup analysis revealed that the primary outcome measure was significantly better for patients receiving the restrictive-strategy who were less unwell with APACHE II scores of 20 or less or were younger than 55 years. There were no significant differences between the groups for patients with APACHE II scores greater than 20 or older than 55 years. There was no significant difference in primary outcome measurements for subgroups of patients with cardiac disease, severe infections and septic shock, and trauma. Interestingly, adjusted multiple-organ-dysfunction scores were significantly lower for patients with APACHE II scores of 20 or less and for patients younger than 55 years who were allocated to the restrictive-strategy compared with the liberal-strategy transfusion protocol.

The authors concluded that the use of a transfusion trigger as low as 7 g/dl, combined with the maintenance of haemoglobin concentrations in the range of 7–9 g/dl, was at least as effective as and conceivably better than a liberal transfusion strategy, with a trigger of 10 g/dL and a maintenance range of 10–12 g/dl, in critically ill patients with normovoloemia. Although not significant, there was a trend towards a decreased 30-day mortality rate in patients treated by a restrictive strategy. The restrictive strategy was also favoured by the significant differences in mortality rates during hospitalization, rates of cardiac complications, and rates of organ dysfunction.

Significantly, the restrictive strategy also resulted in a decrease in the average number of red cell unit transfusions by 54% and a decrease in exposure to any red cell unit transfusions by 33%. Limited availability and concerns about blood-transfusion-associated risks have encouraged the increased use of expensive drugs, such as erythropoietin and aprotinin, which have not been demonstrated to have any overall effectiveness. By comparison, the adoption of a simple restrictive transfusion policy in this study not only proved cost-effective in terms of reducing red cell unit transfusions but also produced clinical benefit.

Two previous cohort studies found that increasing severity of anaemia was associated with a disproportionate increase in mortality rates amongst patients with ischaemic heart disease. However, the TRICC study did not demonstrate an increase in adverse events in patients with cardiac disease when a transfusion trigger of 7 g/dl was used. This discrepancy between the TRICC study and previous observational studies may have arisen because of confounding factors or the inability of observational studies to document detrimental effects of transfusion. The authors of the

TRICC study concluded that a restrictive strategy could be used in patients with coronary artery disease, but that such a strategy should be considered with caution in patients with acute myocardial infarction or unstable angina.

Transfusion threshold: conclusions

The long-held dogma of a transfusion trigger of at least 10 g/dl for critically ill patients was fuelled by the belief that the plasma haemoglobin concentration contributes to the achievement of a supranormal DO_2, and subsequently VO_2, which helps resolve the suspected oxygen debt in apparent pathological supply-dependency. Further studies have cast doubt not only on whether transfusion improves oxygen transport significantly when such transfusion triggers are used, but also on the concept that achieving supranormal oxygen transport improves outcome and even on the very existence of pathological supply-dependency.

The limited availability, costs, and increasingly appreciated risks of blood transfusion in critically ill patients have resulted in an attempt to identify a lower and perhaps better transfusion trigger. The TRICC study offers reliable clinical evidence that a transfusion trigger of 7 g/dl, with a maintenance range of 7–9 g/dl, should be adopted for most critically ill patients. This strategy appears to be of most benefit to younger, less sick patients, and should probably only be considered with caution in patients with acute myocardial infarction and unstable angina.

REFERENCES

1. Shoemaker WC. Relationship of oxygen transport patterns to the pathophysiology

and therapy of shock states. *Intensive Care Med* 1987; **213**: 230–43.

2. Marik PE, Sibbald WJ. Effect of stored-blood transfusion on oxygen delivery in patients with sepsis. *JAMA* 1993; **269**: 3024–9.

3. Silverman HJ, Tuma P. Gastric tonometry in patients with sepsis. Effects of dobutamine infusions and packed red blood cell transfusions. *Chest* 1992; **102**: 184–8.

4. Falk JL, O'Brien JF, Kerr R. Fluid resuscitation in traumatic hemorrhagic shock. *Crit Care Clin* 1992; **8**: 323–40.

5. Imm A, Carlson RW. Fluid resuscitation in circulatory shock. *Crit Care Clin* 1993; **9**: 313–33.

6. Domsky MF, Wilson RF. Hemodynamic resuscitation. *Crit Care Clin* 1993; **9**: 715–26.

7. Shoemaker WC, Fleming AW. Resuscitation of the trauma patient. Restoration of hemodynamic functions using clinical algorithms. *Ann Emerg Med* 1986; **12**: 1437–44.

8. Packman MI, Rackow EC. Optimum left heart filling pressures during fluid resuscitation of patients with hypovolemic and septic shock. *Crit Care Med* 1983; **11**: 165–9.

9. Davis JW, Shackford SR, Holbrook TL. Base deficit as a sensitive indicator of compensated shock and tissue oxygen utilization. *Surg Gynaecol Obstet* 1991; **173**: 473–8.

10. American College of Physicians. Practice strategies for elective red blood cell transfusion. *Ann Intern Med* 1992; **116**: 403–6.

11. Consensus Conference. Perioperative red blood cell transfusion. *JAMA* 1988; **260**: 2700–3.

12. Levy PS, Chavez RP, Crystal GJ et al. Oxygen extraction ratio: a valid indication of transfusion need in limited coronary vascular reserve. *J Trauma* 1992; **32**: 769–74.

13. Griffel MI, Kaufman BS. Pharmacology of colloids and crystalloids. *Crit Care Clin* 1992; **8**: 235–54.

14. Kaminski MV, Haase TJ. Albumin and colloid osmotic pressure: implications for fluid resuscitation. *Crit Care Clin* 1992; **8**: 311–22.

15. Sutin KM, Ruskin KJ, Kaufman BS. Intra-

venous fluid therapy in neurological injury. *Crit Care Clin* 1992; **8**: 367–408.

16. Lowery BD, Cloutier CT, Carey LC. Electrolyte solutions in resuscitation of human hemorrhagic shock. *Surg Gynaecol Obstet* 1971; **131**: 273–9.

17. Griffith CA. The family of Ringer's solutions. *J Nat Intravenous Ther Assoc* 1986; **9**: 480–3.

18. *American Association of Blood Banks Technical Manual*. Arlington, VA: American Association of Blood Banks, 1990.

19. Talpers SS, Romberger DJ, Bunce SB et al. Nutritionally associated increased carbon dioxide production. *Chest* 1992; **102**: 551–5.

20. Gunther B, Jauch W, Hartl W et al. Low-dose glucose infusions in patients who have undergone surgery. *Arch Surg* 1987; **122**: 765–71.

21. DeGoute CS, Ray MJ, Manchon M et al. Intraoperative glucose infusion and blood lactate: endocrine and metabolic relationships during abdominal aortic surgery. *Anesthesiology* 1989; **71**: 355–61.

22. Sieber FE, Traystman RJ. Special issues: glucose and the brain. *Crit Care Med* 1992; **20**: 104–14.

23. Doweiko JP, Nompleggi DJ. Role of albumin in human physiology and pathophysiology. *J Parenter Enter Nutr* 1991; **15**: 207–11.

24. Guthrie RD, Hines C. Use of albumin in the critically ill patient. *Am J Gastroenterol* 1991; **86**: 255–63.

25. Nearman HS, Herman ML. Toxic effects of colloids in the intensive care unit. *Crit Care Clin* 1991; **7**: 713–23.

26. Kapiotis S, Quehenberger P, Eichler HG et al. Effect of hydroxyethyl starch on the activity of blood coagulation and fibrinolysis in healthy volunteers: comparison with albumin. *Crit Care Med* 1994; **22**: 606–12.

27. Waxman K, Holness R, Tominaga G et al. Hemodynamic and oxygen transport effects of pentastarch in burn resuscitation. *Ann Surg* 1989; **209**: 341–5.

28. Strauss RG, Stansfield C, Henriksen RA et al.

Pentastarch may cause fewer effects on coagulation than hetastarch. *Transfusion* 1988; **28**: 257–61.

29. Drumi W, Polzleitner D, Laggner AN et al. Dextran-40, acute renal failure, and elevated plasma oncotic pressure. *N Engl J Med* 1988; **318**: 352–4.

30. Collier FA, Bartlett RM, Bingham DL et al. The replacement of sodium choride in surgical patients. *Ann Surg* 1938; **108**: 769–75.

31. Blalock A. *Principles of Surgical Care, Shock and Other Problems*. St Louis, MO: CV Mosby, 1940.

32. Moyer CA. *Fluid Balance*. Chicago: Year Book, 1954.

33. Shires GT. *Care of the Trauma Patient*. New York: McGraw-Hill, 1967.

34. Shires GT, Carrico CT, Cohn D. The role of the extracellular fluid in shock. *Int Anesthesiol Clin* 1964; **2**: 435–42.

35. Shires GT, Coln D, Carrico J et al. Fluid therapy in hemorrhagic shock. *Arch Surg* 1964; **88**: 688–94.

36. Shires GT, Williams J, Brown F. Acute changes in extracellular fluids associated with major surgical procedures. *Ann Surg* 1961; **154**: 803–9.

37. Herbst CA. Simultaneous distribution rate and dilution volume of bromide-82 and thiocyanate in fluid overload. *Ann Surg* 1974; **179**: 200–8.

38. Appel Pl, Shoemaker WC. Fluid therapy in adult respiratory failure. *Crit Care Med* 1981; **9**: 862–90.

39. Baek SM, Makabali GG, Bryan-Brown CW et al. Plasma expansion in surgical patients with high CVP: the relationship of pressure and cardiorespiratory changes. *Surgery* 1975; **78**: 304–11.

40. Nees JE, Hauser CJ, Shippy C et al. Comparison of cardiorespiratory effects of crystalline hemoglobin, whole blood, albumin, and Ringer's lactate in the resuscitation of hemorrhagic shock in dogs. *Surgery* 1978; **83**: 639–46.

41. Dahn MS, Lucas CE, Ledgerwood AM et al. Negative inotropic effect of albumin resuscitation for shock. *Surgery* 1979; **86**: 235–41.

42. Lucas CE, Ledgerwood AM, Higgins RF et al. Impaired pulmonary function after albumin resuscitation from shock. *J Trauma* 1980; **20**: 446–51.

43. Lucas CE, Ledgerwood AM, Higgins RF et al. Impaired salt and water excretion after albumin resuscitation for hypovolemic shock. *Surgery* 1979; **86**: 544–9.

44. Lucas CE, Ledgerwood AM, Mammen EF. Altered coagulation protein content after albumin resuscitation. *Ann Surg* 1982; **196**: 198–202.

45. Faillace DF, Ledgerwood AM, Lucas CE et al. Immunoglobulin changes after varied resuscitation regimens. *J Trauma* 1982; **22**: 1–5.

46. Lowe RJ, Moss GS, Jilek J et al. Crystalloid vs. colloid in the etiology of pulmonary failure after trauma: a randomized trial in man. *Surgery* 1977; **81**: 676–83.

47. Moss GS, Lowe RJ, Jilek J et al. Colloid or crystalloid in the resuscitation of hemorrhagic shock: a controlled clinical trial. *Surgery* 1981; **89**: 434–8.

48. Rackow EC, Falk JL, Fein A et al. Fluid resuscitation in circulatory shock; a comparison of the cardiorespiratory effects of albumin, hetastarch and saline solutions in patients with hypovolemic and septic shock. *Crit Care Med* 1983; **11**: 839–50.

49. Twigley AJ, Hillman KM. The end of the crystalloid era? A new approach to perioperative fluid administration. *Anaesthesia* 1985; **40**: 860–71.

50. Shoemaker WC, Schluter M, Hopkins JA et al. Comparison of the relative effectiveness of colloids and crystalloids in emergency resuscitation. *Am J Surg* 1981; **142**: 73–81.

51. Shoemaker WC, Hauser CJ. Critique of crystalloid versus colloid therapy in shock and shock lung. *Crit Care Med* 1979; **7**: 117.

52. Hankeln K, Radel C, Beez M et al. Comparison of hydroxyethyl starch and lactated

Ringer's solution on hemodynamics and oxygen transport of critically ill patients in prospective cross-over studies. *Crit Care Med* 1989; **17**: 133–5.

53. Choi PT, Yip G, Quinonez MD et al. Crystalloids vs. colloids in fluid resuscitation: a systemic review. *Crit Care Med* 1999; **27**: 200–10.

54. McClelland DB. Human albumin solutions. *BMJ* 1990; **300**: 35–7.

55. Goldwasser P, Feldman J. Association of serum albumin and mortality risk. *J Clin Epidemiol* 1997; **50**: 693–703.

56. Cochrane Injuries Group. Human albumin administration in critically ill patients: systematic review of randomised controlled trials. *BMJ* 1998; **317**: 235–40.

57. Soni N. Wonderful albumin? *BMJ* 1995; **310**: 887–8.

58. Fleck A, Raines G, Hawker F et al. Increased vascular permeability: a major cause of hypoalbuminaemia in disease and injury. *Lancet* 1985; **i**: 781–4.

59. Mattox KL. Prehospital hypertonic saline-dextran infusion for post-traumatic hypotension: the USA Multicenter Trial. *Ann Surg* 1991; **213**: 482–6.

60. Vassar MJ, Fischer RP, O'Brien PE et al. A multicenter trial for resuscitation of injured patients with 7.5% sodium chloride. *Arch Surg* 1993; **128**: 1003–13.

61. Myers C. Fluid resuscitation. *Eur J Emerg Med* 1997; **4**: 224–32.

62. Duke BJ, Modin GW, Schecter WP et al. Transfusion significantly increases the risk for infection after splenic injury. *Arch Surg* 1993; **128**: 1125–32.

63. Shoemaker WC, Appel PL, Waxman K et al. Clinical trial of survivors' cardiorespiratory patterns as therapeutic goals in critically ill postoperative patients. *Crit Care Med* 1982; **10**: 398–403.

64. Brazzi L, Gattinoni L. Does optimizing oxygen transport improve outcome in intensive care patients? *Br J Anaesth* 1998; **81**(Suppl 1): 46–9.

65. Powers SR, Mannal R, Neclerio M et al. Physiological consequences of positive end-expiratory pressure (PEEP) ventilation. *Ann Surg* 1973; **178**: 265–72.

66. Bihari D, Smithes M, Gimson A et al. The effects of vasodilation with prostacyclin on oxygen delivery and uptake in critically ill patients. *N Engl J Med* 1987; **317**: 397–403.

67. Albert RK, Schrijen F, Poincelot F. Oxygen consumption and transport in stable patients with chronic obstructive pulmonary disease. *Am Rev Respir Dis* 1986; **134**: 678–82.

68. Mohsenifar Z, Jasper AC, Koerner SK. Relationship between oxygen uptake and oxygen delivery in patients with pulmonary hypertension. *Am Rev Respir Dis* 1988; **138**: 69–73.

69. Mohsenifar Z, Amin D, Jasper AC et al. Dependence of oxygen consumption on oxygen delivery in patients with chronic congestive heart failure. *Chest* 1987; **92**: 447–50.

70. Stratton HH, Feustel PJ, Newell JC. Regression of calculated variables in the presence of shared measurement error. *J Appl Physiol* 1987; **62**: 2083–93.

71. Phang PT, Rich T, Ronco J. A validation and comparison study of two metabolic monitors. *J Parenter Enter Nutr* 1990; **14**: 259–61.

72. Ronco J, Phang PT. Validation of an indirect calorimeter to measure oxygen consumption in the ranges seen in critically ill patients. *J Crit Care* 1991; **6**: 36–41.

73. Shoemaker WC, Chang P, Czer L et al. Cardiorespiratory monitoring in postoperative patients: I. prediction of outcome and severity of illness. *Crit Care Med* 1979; **7**: 237–42.

74. Shoemaker WC, Czer LS. Evaluation of the biological importance of various hemodynamic and oxygen transport variables: which variables should be monitored in postoperative shock? *Crit Care Med* 1979; **7**: 424–31.

75. Berlauk JF, Abrams JH, Gilmour IJ et al. Preoperative optimization of cardiovascular hemodynamics improves outcome in peripheral vascular surgery. A prospective randomized clinical trial. *Ann Surg* 1991; **214**: 289–97.

76. Boyd O, Grounds RM, Bennet ED. A randomized clinical trial of the effect of deliberate perioperative increase of oxygen delivery on mortality in high-risk surgical patients. *JAMA* 1993; **270**: 2699–707.

77. Bishop MH, Shoemaker WC, Appel PL et al. Prospective, randomized trial of survivors' values of cardiac index, oxygen delivery, and oxygen consumption as resuscitation endpoints in severe trauma. *J Trauma* 1995; **38**: 780–7.

78. Fleming A, Bishop M, Shoemaker W et al. Prospective trial of supranormal values as goals of resuscitation in severe trauma. *Arch Surg* 1992; **127**: 1175–9.

79. Yu M, Levy MM, Smith P et al. Effects of maximizing oxygen delivery on morbidity and mortality rates in critically ill patients: a prospective, randomized, controlled study. *Crit Care Med* 1993; **21**: 830–8.

80. Tuchschmidt J, Fried J, Astiz M et al. Elevation of cardiac output and oxygen delivery improves outcome in septic shock. *Chest* 1992; **102**: 216–20.

81. Gattinoni L, Brazzi L, Pelosi P et al. A trial of goal-orientated hemodynamic therapy in critically ill patients. *N Engl J Med* 1995; **333**: 1025–32.

82. Hayes MA, Timmins AC, Yau EH et al. Elevation of systemic oxygen delivery in the treatment of critically ill patients. *N Engl J Med* 1994; **330**: 1717–22.

83. Richard C. Tissue hypoxia. How to detect, how to correct, how to prevent? *Intens Care Med* 1996; **22**: 1250–7.

84. Dietrich KA, Conrad SA, Herbert CA et al. Cardiovascular and metabolic response to red blood cell transfusion in critically ill volume-resuscitated nonsurgical patients. *Crit Care Med* 1990; **18**: 940–4.

85. Czer LS, Shoemaker WC. Optimal hematocrit value in critically ill post-operative patients. *Surg Gynaecol Obstet* 1978; **147**: 363–8.

86. Gramm J, Smith S, Gamelli RL et al. Effect of transfusion on oxygen transport in critically ill patients. *Shock* 1996; **5**: 190–3.

87. Babineau TJ, Dzik WH, Borlase DC et al. Reevaluation of current transfusion practices in patients in surgical intensive care units. *Am J Surg* 1992; **164**: 22–5.

88. Heiss MM. Risk of allogeneic transfusions. *Br J Anaesth* 1998; **81**(Suppl 1): 16–19.

89. Heiss MM, Delanoff C. Immunmodulatorische wirkung der bluttransfusion and einfluß auf infektionsrate und tumorrezidiv. *Infusionsther Transfusionsmed* 1997; **24**: 20–31.

90. Lenhard V, Gemsa D, Opelz G. Transfusion-induced release of prostaglandin E_2 and its role in the activation of T-suppressor cells. *Transplant Proc* 1985; **17**: 2380–2.

91. Stephan RN, Kisala JM, Dean RE et al. Effect of blood transfusion on antigen presentation function and on interleukin-2 generation. *Arch Surg* 1988; **123**: 235–40.

92. Kalechman Y, Gafter U, Sobelman D et al. The effect of a single whole-blood transfusion on cytokine secretion. *J Clin Immunol* 1990; **10**: 99–105.

93. Ellis TM, Mohanakumar T, Muakkassa W et al. Influence of immunosuppressive therapy and blood transfusion on human T-cell subpopulations. *Transplant Proc* 1983; **15**: 1173–5.

94. Kaplan J, Sarnaik S, Gitlin J et al. Diminished helper/suppressor lymphocyte ratios and natural killer activity in recipients of repeated blood transfusions. *Blood* 1984; **64**: 308–10.

95. Waymack JP, McNeal N, Warden GD et al. Effect of blood transfusions on macrophage-lymphocyte interaction in an animal model. *Ann Surg* 1986; **204**: 681–5.

96. Fischer E, Lenhard V, Seifert P et al. Blood transfusion-induced suppression of cellular immunity in man. *Hum Immun* 1980; **3**: 187–94.

97. Pohanka E, Manfro RC, Oto C et al. Anti-idiotypic antibodies to HLA after donor-specific blood transfusion (DST). *Transplant Proc* 1989; **21**: 1806–9.

98. Smith MD, Williams JD, Coles GA et al. The effect of blood transfusion on T-suppressor

cells in renal dialysis patients. *Transplant Proc* 1981; **13**: 181–3.

99. MacLeod AM, Mason RJ, Stewart KN et al. Fc-receptor blocking antibodies develop after blood transfusions and correlate with good graft outcome. *Transplant Proc* 1983; **15**: 1019–21.

100. Starzl TE, Demetris AJ, Murase N et al. Cell migration, chimerism and graft acceptance. *Lancet* 1992; **339**: 1579–82.

101. Heiss MM, Mempel W, Delanoff CH et al. Blood transfusion-modulated tumour recurrence: First results of a randomized study of autologous vs. allogeneic blood transfusion in colorectal cancer surgery. *J Clin Oncol* 1994; **12**: 1859–67.

102. Houbiers JGA, Brand A, van de Watering LMG et al. Randomised controlled trial comparing transfusion of leucocyte-depleted or buffy-coat-depleted blood in surgery for colorectal cancer. *Lancet* 1994; **344**: 573–7.

103. Gould SA, Rice CL, Moss GS. The physiological basis of the use of blood and blood products. *Surg Annu* 1984; **16**: 13–21.

104. Wilkerson DK, Rosen AL, Gould SA et al. Oxygen extraction: a valid indicator of myocardial metabolism in anemia. *J Surg Res* 1987; **42**: 629–34.

105. Gould SA, Rosen AL, Sehgal RC et al. Oxygen extraction ratio: a physiological indicator of transfusion need. *Transfusion* 1983; **23**: 416.

106. Adams RC, Lundy JS. Anesthesia in cases of poor surgical risk: Some suggestions for decreasing the risk. *Surg Gynaecol Obstet* 1941; **71**: 1011–14.

107. Friedman BA, Burns TL, Shork MA. An analysis of blood transfusions of surgical patients by sex; a quest for the transfusion trigger. *Transfusion* 1980; **20**: 179–84.

108. Welch HG, Meehan KR, Goodnough LT. Prudent strategies for elective red blood cell transfusion. *Ann Intern Med* 1992; **116**: 393–402.

109. Zauder HL. Preoperative hemoglobin require-ments. *Anesthesiol Clin North Am* 1990; **8**: 471–80.

110. Audet AM, Goodnough LT. Practice strategies for elective red blood cell transfusion. *Ann Intern Med* 1992; **116**: 403–6.

111. Silberstein LE, Kruskall MS, Stehling MC et al. Strategies for the review of transfusion practices. *JAMA* 1989; **262**: 1993–7.

112. Consensus Conference: Perioperative Red Blood Cell Transfusion. *JAMA* 1988; **260**: 2700–3.

113. Stehling LC, Ellison N, Faust RJ et al. A survey of transfusion practices amongst anesthesiologists. *Vox Sang* 1987; **52**: 60–2.

114. Stehling LC. Preoperative blood ordering. *Int Anesthesiol Clin* 1982; **20**: 45–57.

115. Stehling L, Esposito B. An analysis of the appropriateness of intraoperative transfusion. *Anesth Analg* 1989; **68**(S1): S278.

116. Hebert PC, Wells G, Martin C et al. A Canadian survey of transfusion practices in critically ill patients. *Crit Care Med* 1998; **26**: 482–7.

117. Gutierrez G, Pohil RJ. Oxygen comsumption is linearly related to oxygen supply in critically ill patients. *J Crit Care* 1986; **1**: 45–53.

118. Shoemaker WC, Appel PL, Kram HB et al. Prospective trial of supranormal values of survivors as therapeutic goals in high-risk surgical patients. *Chest* 1988; **94**: 1176–86.

119. Yu M, Takanishi D, Myers SA et al. Frequency of mortality and myocardial infarction during maximizing oxygen delivery: a prospective, randomized trials. *Crit Care Med* 1995; **23**: 1025–32.

120. Hebert PC, Wells G, Tweeddale M et al. Does transfusion practice alter mortality in critically ill patients? *Am J Respir Crit Care Med* 1997; **155**: A20.

121. Carson JL, Duff A, Poses RM et al. Effect of anaemia and cardiovascular disease on surgical mortality and morbidity. *Lancet* 1996; **348**: 1055–60.

122. Herd TC, Dasmahapatra KS, Rush BF et al. Red blood cell deformability in human and

experimental sepsis. *Arch Surg* 1988; **123**: 217–20.

123. Langenfeld JE, Livingston DH, Machiedo GW. Red cell deformability is an early indicator of infection. *Surg* 1991; **110**: 398–404.

124. Baker CH, Wilmoth FR, Sutton ET. Reduced RBC versus plasma microvascular flow due to endotoxin. *Circul Shock* 1986; **29**: 127–39.

125. Mollitt DL, Poulos ND. The role of pentoxyfilline in endotoxin-induced alterations of red cell deformability and whole blood viscosity in the neonate. *J Pediatr Surg* 1991; **26**: 572–4.

126. Messmer KFW. Acceptable hematocrit levels in surgical patients. *World J Surg* 1987; **11**: 41–6.

127. Messmer K, Kreimeier U, Intaglietta M. Present state of intentional hemodilution. *Eur Surg Res* 1986; **18**: 254–63.

128. Messmer K, Sunder-Plassmann L, Klovekorn WP et al. Circulatory significance of hemodilution: rheological changes and limitations. *Adv Microcircul* 1972; **4**: 1–77.

129. Weisel RD, Charlesworth DC, Mickleborough LL et al. Limitations of blood conservation. *J Thorac Cardiovasc Surg* 1984; **88**: 26–38.

130. Johnson RG, Thurer RL, Kruskall MS et al. Comparison of two transfusion strategies after elective operations for myocardial revascularization. *J Thorac Cardiovasc Surg* 1992; **104**: 307–14.

131. Fortune JB, Feustel PJ, Saifi J et al. Influence of hematocrit on cardiopulmonary function after acute hemorrhage. *J Trauma* 1987; **27**: 243–9.

132. Hebert PC, Wells GA, Marshall JC et al. Transfusion requirements in critical care. A pilot study. *JAMA* 1995; **273**: 1439–44.

133. Blair SD, Janvrin SB, McCollum CN et al. Effect of early blood transfusion on gastrointestinal hemorrhage. *Br J Surg* 1986; **73**: 783–5.

134. Hebert PC, Wells G, Blajchman MA et al. A multicenter, randomised, controlled clinical trial of transfusion requirements in critical care. *N Engl J Med* 1999; **340**: 409–17.

10 Pharmacologic alternatives to blood

Lawrence Tim Goodnough

INTRODUCTION

Recombinant human erythropoietin (EPO) therapy has been approved for use in patients undergoing autologous blood donation (ABD) in Japan, the European Union, and Canada since 1993, 1994, and 1996, respectively, and is also approved for perisurgical adjuvant therapy in Canada, Australia, the USA and the European Union (Table 10.1). Intravenous iron preparations with better safety profiles are now available in the USA. Finally, considerable progress has been made in the development of artificial oxygen carriers in the last decade. The emergence of these pharmacologic alternatives to blood and their clinical application in transfusion medicine will be addressed in this chapter.

ERYTHROPOIETIN THERAPY

EPO therapy has been approved for use as a blood conservation intervention, beginning in 1989 for patients with medical anemia and in 1997 for surgical patients. The adoption of this strategy has been rapid in some settings (e.g. renal failure patients), progressive in others (e.g. cancer patients), and slow in others (e.g. surgical patients). At the same time, the risks of blood have declined substantially while the costs of blood have increased significantly. The evolution of new techniques such as acute normovolemic hemodilution and the novel erythropoiesis-stimulating protein (NESP, see below) bring new options for alternatives to allogeneic blood transfusion. EPO therapy, with or without autologous blood procurement, is undergoing new

Table 10.1 Approval of status of recombinant human erythropoietin therapy in surgical anemia

	USA	Canada	European Union*	Australia	Japan
Autologous blood donation	—	1996	1994	1996	1993
Surgery	1996[b]	1996	1998[c]	1996	—

[a]Approval dates for France, Germany, Italy, and the UK are the same as for other countries of the European Union.
[b]Non-cardiac, non-vascular surgery.
[c]Orthopedic surgery.

scrutiny as an alternative to blood transfusion – not only because of traditional concerns regarding blood risks, but also because of new blood inventory and cost considerations.

Current blood risks

The US blood supply is the safest it has ever been, owing to the evolution of a combination of donor education, donor screening, and new laboratory test procedures. Risks of transfusion-transmitted viral infections are extremely low – estimated in 1996 to be approximately one in 650 000 units for human immunodeficiency virus (HIV), one in 100 000 for hepatitis C virus (HCV), and one in 60 000 for hepatitis B virus (HBV).[1] More rigorous predonation screening has led to a rapid decline in prevalence of HIV and HCV in first-time blood donors at five US blood centers,[2] with HIV decreasing from 0.03% (1991–1992) to 0.02% (1993–1996) and HCV decreasing from 0.63% (1992) to 0.40% (1996), despite an increase in prevalence in the general population for both HIV (0.3% in 1992) and HCV (1.8% in 1988–1994). In 1999, introduction of nucleic acid amplification testing (NAT) for HIV and HCV further reduced the window period, which is the time between a potential blood donor infection and detectability by screening tests at time of donation, by 30–50%. The most significant risk of mortality from blood transfusion is now believed to be administrative error[1] resulting in an ABO mismatch between blood unit and transfusion recipient, with hemolysis (1 in 60 000) and death (1 in 600 000).

Yet, opinion surveys indicate that fully one-third of the public either disagrees or strongly disagrees with statements that 'the blood supply is safe' and that 'they would agree to accept blood transfusion if hospitalized'.[3] The search for ways to eliminate blood transfusions therefore continues,[4] despite the fact that, now, no alternative to blood can be proven to be as safe as blood.[5]

Current utilization of EPO therapy

Little is known about current utilization in the US of technologies or techniques to reduce allogeneic blood transfusion. A survey sent to 1000 US hospitals in 1997 reported on the use of such technologies (autologous blood procurement and/or pharmaceutical therapy in patients undergoing surgery).[6] Forty-three percent of respondents stated that EPO therapy was available, although only 11% stated that it was routinely (2%) or sometimes (9%) prescribed. The remainder stated that EPO was never (57%) or almost never (32%) used. Despite approval for perisurgical use of EPO therapy in the US in 1996, acceptance for its utilization as an alternative to blood transfusion has been slow, probably because of high costs and poor cost-effectiveness (more than $7 million per quality-adjusted life-year (QALY) saved).[7]

Clinical trials of EPO therapy

Patients donating autologous blood under standard conditions (i.e. one blood unit weekly[8,9]) have an inadequate response of endogenous erythropoietin to blood-loss anemia, suggesting a role for EPO therapy in facilitating autologous blood donation. This was confirmed[10,11] in a study comparing aggressive autologous blood donation (up to 6 units over a 3-week preoperative interval) with EPO therapy in patients undergoing orthopedic surgery. However, a subsequent clinical trial[12] in orthopedic patients demonstrated that for autologous blood donors who were not anemic (hematocrit >39%) at first donation, no clinical benefit (defined as reduced allogeneic blood exposure) was seen with EPO therapy when compared with aggressive autologous phlebotomy alone. Thus, for non-anemic patients, autologous blood donation remains an option if they can tolerate aggressive blood phlebotomy (i.e. up to 6 units over 3 weeks) and thereby achieve stimulation of erythropoiesis via their endogenous EPO response.[13]

For anemic (hematocrit ≤39%) autologous blood donors, a European clinical trial demonstrated that EPO therapy (300 or 600 u/kg intravenously in six doses) reduced exposure to allogeneic blood during orthopedic surgery when compared with placebo-treated patients.[14] However, this result was only achieved with concurrent administration of both intravenous and oral supplemental iron. A subsequent US trial with supplemental oral iron and EPO therapy (600 u/kg intravenously in six doses) could not demonstrate reduced allogeneic blood transfusions when compared with placebo-treated patients[15] – in large part because a substantial percentage of the patients either were severely anemic (hematocrit <33%) or were iron-deficient upon entry into the clinical trial.

Several studies have evaluated perisurgical EPO therapy in non-anemic orthopedic surgical patients without autologous blood procurement. Both a Canadian study[16] and two US studies[17,18] were able to show that EPO-treated (300 u/kg subcutaneously × 14 days, beginning 9 days preoperatively) patients had one half the rate of exposure (approximately 25%) to allogeneic blood as the placebo-treated patients (approximately 50%), despite mean initial hemoglobin levels that exceeded 130 g/l for patients in both studies. On the basis of these clinical trials, EPO therapy was approved for perisurgical use in Canada and the USA in 1996.

EPO therapy and erythropoietic response

An analysis of the relationship between EPO dose and the response in red blood cell (RBC) production[19] has demonstrated a good correlation (Figure 10.1). EPO-stimulated erythropoiesis is independent of age and gender,[20] and the variability in response among patients is in part due to iron-restricted erythropoiesis.[21] There is no evidence that surgery or EPO therapy affects the endogenous erythropoietic response to anemia, or the erythropoietic response to EPO.[22]

RBC expansion is seen, with an increase in reticulocyte count by day 3 of treatment in non-anemic patients treated with EPO who are iron-replete.[10] As illustrated in Figure 10.2, the equivalent of 1 blood unit is produced by day 7 and the equivalent of 5 blood units is produced over 28 days.[11] If 3–5 blood units are necessary in order to minimize allogeneic blood exposure in patients undergoing complex procedures such as orthopedic joint replacement surgery, the preoperative interval necessary for EPO-stimulated erythropoiesis can be estimated to be 3–4 weeks.

Normal individuals have been shown to have difficulty providing sufficient iron to support rates of erythropoiesis that are greater than three times basal.[23] A recent study confirmed that the maximum erythropoietic

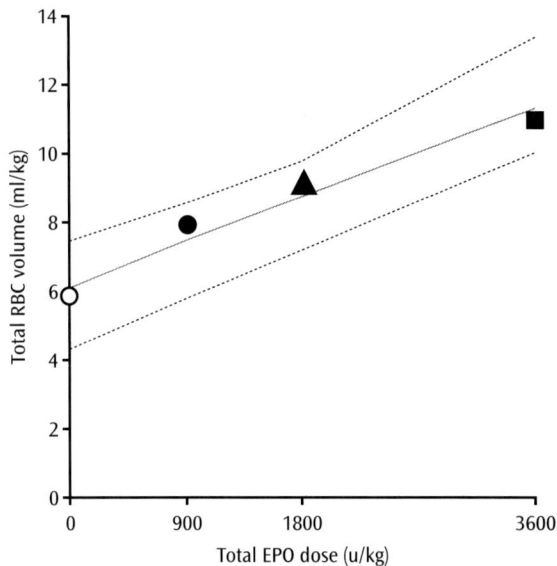

Figure 10.1
The dose–response relationship between total (cumulative) amount of erythropoietin (EPO) administered and the red blood cell (RBC) volume increase during the preoperative interval for patients treated intravenously with placebo, ○; 150 u/kg, ●; 300 u/kg, ▲; and 600 u/kg ■. The EPO dose is given in total (cumulative) units/kg of body weight for all six treatments combined over a period of 3 weeks; the increase in RBC volume is given in ml/kg body weight. The dashed lines indicate the 95% confidence interval. Reproduced by permission from Goodnough et al. *J Am Coll Surg* 1994; 179: 171–6.[19] © 1994 Journal of the American College of Surgeons.

has been estimated to increase by 6- to 8-fold over baseline RBC production with aggressive phlebotomy.[24] The term 'relative iron deficiency' has thus been termed by Finch[26] to occur in individuals when the iron stores are normal but the increased erythron iron requirements exceed the available supply of iron.

The results of a clinical trial of EPO therapy in patients undergoing total hip replacement surgery have been published recently. Feagan et al[27] conducted a multicenter randomized double-blinded study in 211 patients, comparing placebo with two EPO regimens administered as four weekly doses: 40 000 u ('standard'), equivalent to approximately 600 u/kg for a 70 kg patient) and 20 000 u (approximately 300 u/kg, or a 'low dose'). All patients received oral iron supplementation for at least 6 weeks before surgery. Both EPO regimens significantly reduced the need for allogeneic blood transfusion: 11.4% of patients in the standard-EPO-dose cohort and 22.8% of patients in the low-EPO-dose cohort, compared with 44.9% of patients receiving placebo. The incidence of thromboembolic events did not differ among the groups. A limitation in this study was the absence of a cost-effectiveness analysis.

The results have been published of another randomized non-placebo-controlled non-blinded trial of two EPO regimens (600 u/kg versus 300 u/kg) administered on preoperative days 14 and 7 in 200 men undergoing radical retropubic prostatectomy.[28] The mean increases in hematocrit (%) were 4.5 and 4.7, respectively, and the allogeneic exposure rates were 6% and 7%, respectively. These allogeneic exposure rates are comparable to the 9% seen with predonation of three autologous

response in the acute setting, seen in EPO-treated patients with measurable storage iron, is approximately four times the basal marrow RBC production.[21] Previous investigators have shown that conditions associated with enhanced plasma iron and transferrin saturation are necessary to produce a greater marrow response, such as in patients with hemochromatosis[24] or in patients supplemented with intravenous iron administration.[25] In hemochromatosis, marrow response

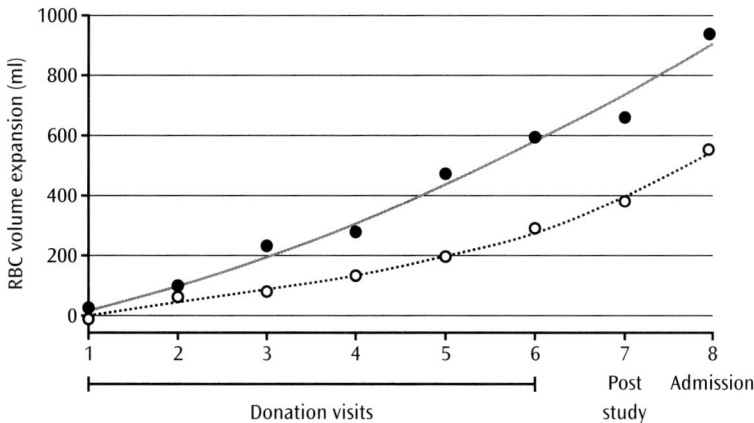

Figure 10.2
Red cell (RBC) production during autologous blood donation in 23 placebo-treated (open circles/dashed curve) and 21 EPO-treated (filled circles/full curve) patients. Data points represent calculated RBC production at donation visits 1–6, the post-study visit, and hospital admission. RBC production is indicated by a polynomial regression curve for each treatment group (n=44 at each point). The rate of RBC production can be derived for any preoperative interval. The mean cumulative interval since donation visit 1 was 3.5 days to visit 2, 7.2 days to visit 3, 10.6 days to visit 4, 14.2 days to visit 5, 17.6 days to visit 6, 20.9 days to visit 7 (poststudy visit), and 26.3 days to visit 8 (hospital admission). Reproduced by permission from Goodnough LT et al, *Transfusion* 1992; 32: 441–5.[11] © 1992 Blackwell Science Ltd.

blood units in a previous study by the same group. The calculated EPO costs per patient were $1218 and $656, respectively, which the authors feel may be justified if patient time and loss of work for autologous blood donation (as the alternative) is taken into account.

Economic considerations

The costs associated with EPO therapy and the potential impact of reimbursement policies are important issues in the setting of surgical anemia, as has been the case in medical anemia.[29,30] Costs associated with EPO therapy may be lowered by strategies that improve the dose–response relationship. One study[31] demonstrated that four weekly injections of subcutaneous EPO (600 u/kg) was

less costly but just as effective as a daily dose of EPO (300 u/kg for 14 doses). A similar regimen (300 u/kg × 6 over 3 weeks) has been recommended for administration of EPO in surgery.[32] However, an economic analysis of EPO therapy in orthopedic surgery concluded that with these doses, EPO therapy was not cost-effective.[33] One report demonstrated erythropoietic responses with a subcutaneous EPO dosage as low as 100 u/kg administered weekly, although clinical outcomes were not studied.[34] These regimens remain expensive,[35] and when unaccompanied by autologous blood procurement are still associated with an allogeneic exposure rate of 16–25%.[16–18] A review of randomized trials concluded that the optimal dose of perioperative EPO therapy remains to be established.[36] Nevertheless, the superiority of EPO therapy compared with autologous blood donation in reducing allogeneic blood exposure during total joint replacement procedures was confirmed in a multicenter study.[37]

Emerging Issues

An intriguing demonstration of an effect of EPO additional to its central role in erythropoiesis is that EPO crosses the blood–brain barrier and exerts a neuroprotective effect in animal models of experimental brain injury.[38] Similar to its regulation in the peripheral circulation, EPO within the central nervous system is inducible by hypoxia. Systemically administered EPO therapy has been shown to function in a neuroprotective manner in animal models of focal brain ischemia, concussive brain injury, experimental autoimmune encephalitis (EAE), and kainate-induced seizures.[38] The mechanism by which EPO serves as a neuroprotectant is unclear. One hypothesis is that it could rescue cells from death through modulation of aptoptosis – a role well defined in erythropoiesis and since extended to neuron-like cells in vitro. Important clinical implications are the potential benefits of improving cognition in the elderly and of protecting cognition in patients receiving chemotherapy, who have been demonstrated to have impaired cognitive function.[39]

Another important development is the development and characterization of a novel erythropoiesis-stimulating protein (NESP). NESP is a genetically engineered molecule that is biochemically distinct from recombinant human erythropoietin (rhEPO), containing additional carbohydrate and sialic acid moieties, that prolong its serum half-life and thus increase its in vivo biologic activity.[40] In pharmacokinetic studies in patients with renal disease, NESP was shown to have a threefold longer half-life than EPO after intravenous administration (25.3 hours versus 8.5 hours, respectively). Subcutaneous administration extended the half-life of NESP to 48.8 hours. NESP license application for treatment of renal anemia has been filed worldwide.

NESP has recently completed clinical trials in patients with cancer.[41,42] In one trial,[41] the feasibility of reduced dose frequency with NESP compared with EPO was demonstrated, comparing weekly NESP versus thrice-weekly EPO (according to current labeling indications), and comparing every-other-week and even every-third-week NESP versus weekly EPO (according to current prevailing practice in oncology). This trial also demonstrated a dose-dependent relationship between NESP and multiple measures of efficacy, including the proportion of patients responding (defined as an increase in hemoglobin to more than 2 g/l) to NESP. In a worldwide (non-USA) trial of NESP in cancer patients not receiving chemotherapy, up to 83% of patients responded to once-weekly subcutaneous administration of NESP.[42] NESP was well tolerated in all trials, and there was no evidence of antibody formation.

IRON THERAPY

In circumstances with significant ongoing iron losses, oral administration of iron does not provide enough to correct the iron-deficient erythropoiesis, and intravenous iron therapy should be considered. Renal dialysis patients have such blood losses, and the role of intravenous iron therapy has been best defined in clinical trials achieving target hematocrit levels in this setting. Addressing iron deficiency with intravenous iron therapy allows correction of anemia along with utilization of lower EPO dosage.[43] Another role for intravenous iron therapy is in the arena of bloodless medicine and bloodless surgery programs for patients who refuse blood transfusions on the basis of religious beliefs. Common clinical settings here include pregnancy[44] and patients with dysfunctional uterine bleeding who are scheduled for hysterectomy.[45]

Intravenous iron therapy has been closely scrutinized for risks and adverse events. Imferon (Iron Dextran BP) is an iron preparation previously associated with a 0.6% risk of life threatening anaphylactoid reactions and a 1.7% risk of severe delayed reactions that were serum-sickness-like and characterized by fever, arthragias, and myalgias.[46] An increased incidence of delayed reactions of up to 30% and severe reactions of 5.3% was subsequently described;[47] this product was eventually withdrawn from use.

InFed (Iron Dextran USP, Stein Farm Corp, Florham Park, NJ) is currently approved for parenteral (intramuscular or intravenous) use, with widespread intravenous administration in renal dialysis patients. Clinical studies have shown that InFed administered intravenously during the dialysis procedure was associated with clinically significant adverse reactions in 4.7% of patients, of which 0.7% were serious or life-threatening, and another 1.75% were characterized as anaphylactoid reactions.[48] The prevalence of these reactions does not appear to differ among patients receiving low-dose

(100 mg) or higher-dose (250–500 mg) infusions.[49] A review has reported 196 allergic/anaphylaxis cases with the use of iron dextran in the USA between 1976 and 1996, of which 31 (15.8%) were fatal.[50]

Safety aspects of parenteral iron in patients with end-stage renal disease for iron dextran, ferric gluconate, and iron saccharate have been scrutinized.[51] Iron saccharate is a preparation (available in Europe but not in the USA) for which allergic reactions are very rare. Possible adverse effects include a metallic taste, arthralgia, chest pain, and brochospasm.[51-53]

Ferric gluconate (Ferrlecit, Schein Pharm Corp, Florham Park, NJ) was approved for use in the USA in February 1999 as an intravenous iron preparation in renal dialysis patients.[54] The rate of allergic reactions (3.3 episodes per million doses) appears to be lower than that of iron dextran (8.7 episodes per million doses), and the safety profile of iron gluconate is substantially better; in the period 1976–1996, among 74 adverse events reported as severe, there were no deaths.[50] Adverse events that have been reported to be associated with ferric gluconate include hypotension, rash, chest or abdominal pain, with an incidence of less than 5%.[55] Another potential adverse effect of intravenous iron therapy is a clinical syndrome of acute iron toxicity (nausea, facial reddening, and hypotension), which has been attributed to oversaturation (>100%) of transferrin. This has been described with rapid infusion of ferric gluconate (62.5–125 mg within 30 minutes) in a study of 20 dialysis patients.[56] However, the existence of this effect has been disputed – two laboratory assays for measurement of serum iron yield misleading results for transferrin saturation if performed within 24 hours after infusion.[57] Serious reactions, including one hypotensive event, were reported in only three (1.3%) of 226 patients undergoing renal dialysis while treated with ferric gluconate in one European study.[58]

Previous studies[59] have indicated that the increased erythropoietic effect (4.5–5.5 times basal) of intravenous iron dextran (with an estimated half-life of 60 hours) is transient, lasting 7–10 days, after which the iron is sequestered in the reticuloendothelial system and erythropoiesis returns to 2.5–3.5 times normal.[60] Intravenous iron therapy may optimally be administered at intervals of 1–2 weeks.

A dose–response relationship of EPO and erythropoiesis that is affected favorably by iron supplementation has important implications for EPO dosage,[29] especially if the cost of therapy is taken into account. Current recommended EPO dosage to be administered in patients scheduled for elective surgery range from 1800 u/kg[32] to 4200 u/kg total dosage,[17,31] which for a 70 kg patient would cost $1300–3000.[30] However, an economic analysis of EPO therapy in patients undergoing orthopedic surgery concluded that, even with the lower currently recommended (1800 u/kg) total dosage, EPO therapy is not cost-effective.[33] Intravenous iron may potentiate the erythropoietic response in the setting of EPO therapy by improving iron-restricted erythropoiesis induced by EPO.[61] Current indications for intravenous iron therapy, along with opportunities for research, are listed in Table 10.2.

PLATELET GROWTH FACTORS

Owing to the biological nature of platelet products, the need for available donors, and the problems associated with platelet use, there is a growing role for pharmacological approaches to thrombocytopenia. At this time, treatment options include interleukin-11(IL-11), c-Mpl ligands, and c-Mpl mimetics. A variety of cytokines have been evaluated in attempts to identify an agent that would effectively treat chemotherapy-induced or other hypoproliferative thrombocytopenias.[62] Of these, only IL-11 has been approved by the

Table 10.2 Current status of intravenous iron therapy		
Beneficial	**No benefit**	**Investigational**
• Anemia of renal failure, with or without erythropoietin therapy • Patients with ongoing blood loss • Jehovah's Witness patients with iron deficiency, blood loss, or both	• Autologous blood donation in patients with or without iron deficiency	• Blood loss, iron deficiency, and EPO therapy • Anemia of chronic disease and EPO therapy • Perisurgical anemia, with or without EPO therapy

US Food and Drug Administration (FDA). Other cytokines remain under investigation for in vivo and ex vivo indications.

Interleukin-11

IL-11 is a cytokine with multiple effects on hematopoietic and non-hematopoietic cells. In vivo, it stimulates megakaryocytic maturation and produces an increase in circulating platelets. Following experimental myeloablation, mice treated with IL-11 exhibited accelerated recovery of trilinear hematopoiesis.[63] However, IL-11 does not appear to be essential for hematopoiesis, since adult mice with targeted mutations of the IL-11 receptor show normal hematopoiesis.[64] Furthermore, the residual megakaryocytopoiesis seen in c-Mpl-deficient mice does not appear to depend on the presence of IL-11.[65] These studies indicate that IL-11 plays an important, but secondary, role in megakaryocytopoiesis and platelet regulation.

The safety and efficacy of recombinant human IL-11 (rhIL-11) for the treatment of severe chemotherapy-induced thrombocytopenia was evaluated in a multicenter placebo-controlled trial.[66] Patients were randomized to either placebo or rhIL-11 (doses of 25 or 50 µg/kg/day subcutaneously, once daily for 14–21 days, beginning 1 day after chemotherapy). Of the patients receiving rhIL-11 at a dose of 50 µg/kg/day, 30% required no platelet transfusions, versus 4% in the placebo-treated group ($p < 0.05$). Adverse effects following rhIL-11 treatment included significant fatigue and edema as well as atrial arrhythmias and syncope. Although the activity of rhIL-11 in this study was modest and the effects of treatment just reached statistical significance, rhIL-11 was the first cytokine to show efficacy in this setting.

C-Mpl ligands

Thrombopoietin is the hematopoietic growth factor responsible for megakaryocytic growth, development, and platelet production. While its existence had been postulated for almost half a century, it was not until the early 1990s that real progress was made in identifying this elusive factor. Vigon et al[67] cloned the human homologue of the v-*mpl* oncogene transduced in the myeloproliferative leukemia retrovirus and described its striking similarities to members of the hematopoietic growth receptor superfamily. c-*mpl* knockout mice have approximately a 90% reduction in platelet count as a result of a reduction in megakaryocyte progenitors and a decrease in megakaryocyte ploidy.[67,68] In 1994, cloning of the gene for the c-Mpl ligand led to the identification of thrombopoietin.[69,70] Thrombopoietin promotes the full spectrum of megakaryocyte growth and development.[71] Two forms of recombinant thrombopoietin were developed for human studies: pegylated recombinant human megakaryocyte growth and development factor (PEG–rHuMGDF) and recombinant human thrombopoietin (rhTPO).

Pegylated megakaryocyte growth and development factor

Recombinant human megakaryocyte growth and development factor (rHuMGDF) consists of the N-terminal 163 amino acids of thrombopoietin (TPO). The molecule has been covalently linked to polyethylene glycol (PEG) to extend its half-life. PEG–rHuMGDF has been studied in myelosuppression,[72] and in platelet mobilization in normal donors.[73,74]

Owing to the reported development of neutralizing antibodies in patients[75] and normal subjects receiving repetitive doses, PEG–rHuMGDF has been withdrawn from clinical trials.

Recombinant human thrombopoietin

rhTPO is the full-length glycosylated molecule produced in genetically modified human cell lines. In clinical trials, it has been shown to attenuate the thrombocytopenia associated with cancer therapy, reduce the need for platelet transfusions, and (in combination with granulocyte colony-stimulating factor (G-CSF)) to improve the mobilization of peripheral blood stem cells.[76] To date, one in 400 patients receiving rhTPO has been reported to develop a transient, low-titer antibody that was partially inhibitory on bioassay.[77]

c-Mpl ligand mimetics

Additional pharmacological agents that mimic the activities of TPO at the c-Mpl receptor can be designed. GW395058 is a potent pegylated peptide human TPO receptor agonist[78] and is currently under investigation in preclinical studies for the treatment of thrombocytopenia. Another approach to agent development has been the synthesis of a monoclonal antibody (BAH-1) with agonist activity to the human c-Mpl receptor.[79] The eventual role of c-Mpl ligand mimetics awaits further development of these and other compounds.

Artificial oxygen carriers

In recent years, there has been increasing interest in the development of red cell substitutes.[80,81] Efforts have included the development of cell-free hemoglobin solutions that approximate the same oxygen-carrying and oxygen-delivery capacity as cellular hemoglobin, and the development of perfluorocarbon emulsions (as synthetic oxygen carriers). The hemoglobin solutions are polymerized or crosslinked (or both) to maximize the length of time in which they are in circulation and to minimize nephrotoxicity. The potential advantages of such products include a prolonged shelf life, the fact that they can be stored at room temperature, universal biocompatibility because ABO blood group testing is not necessary, and the fact that such products are subjected to viral inactivation procedures.[82] Their disadvantages include potential interference with the results of laboratory tests,[83] their relatively short time in circulation (24–48 hours), and the fact that perflurocarbons require a high inspired oxygen concentration (nearly 100%) to be effective.[82] Moreover, a recent study evaluating oxygen delivery after the administration of clinically relevant doses of a hemoglobin solution to anesthetized surgical patients[84] demonstrated that the ability of the hemoglobin-based oxygen carrier to increase oxygen delivery was limited by its vasoactivity. The vasoactive effect of hemoglobin solutions is thought to be a direct effect of the free hemoglobin, because free hemoglobin has a different affinity for or proximity to nitric oxide than cellular hemoglobin.[85] This binding increased blood pressure substantially in one study,[84] and may have been causally related to the discontinuation of one hemoglobin solution in another clinical trial.[86]

The two principal indications for the red cell substitutes currently under clinical investigation are in patients with acute trauma and patients who are undergoing surgery, with or without acute normovolemic hemodilution. The rationale for the use of red cell substitutes with hemodilution is several-fold: (i) the cellular hemoglobin collected during hemodilution would be used to replace the hemoglobin solution or other synthetic oxygen carrier as it is eliminated; (ii) the use of a red cell substitute would permit more aggressive hemodilution with lower targeted cellular hemoglobin levels than would otherwise be tolerated; and (iii) a red cell substitute could serve as a replacement fluid during blood loss.[87] However, patients with pre-existing anemia can be expected to derive only limited benefit from this approach, because the amount of autologous cellular hemoglobin is low to begin with.[87] A multinational prospective, randomized study[88] evaluated the use of perflubron, a perflurocarbon solution, to augment acute normovolemic hemodilution during orthopedic surgery. The investigators found that perflubron combined with 100% oxygen was more effective than autologous blood in reversing physiological transfusion triggers in patients undergoing orthopedic surgery. They concluded that this blood-conservation technique may represent a safe, temporary alternative to conventional blood transfusion. Because of the small sample size of the study, the efficacy of perflubron in eliminating allogeneic blood exposure was not demonstrated, and additional large clinical trials will be needed to evaluate its efficacy. At present, several of these 'blood substitute' products are in various stages of clinical development. If approved by the FDA, they would most likely be used in military and trauma patients and massive surgical blood loss settings. The role of these substances in other arenas will, most likely, be determined by issues related to blood inventory and costs, rather than the safety of the blood supply.

CONCLUSIONS

The evolution of new technologies such as NESP and artificial oxygen carriers bring new options for alternatives to allogeneic blood transfusion. EPO therapy, with or without autologous blood procurement, is undergoing new scrutiny as an alternative to blood transfusion, not only because of traditional concerns regarding blood risks but also because of new blood inventory and cost considerations.

REFERENCES

1. Goodnough LT, Brecher ME, Kanter MH, Aubuchon JP. Transfusion medicine. Part 1: Blood transfusion. *N Engl J Med* 1999; **340**: 439–47.
2. Glynn SA, Kleinman SH, Schreiber GB et al. Trends in incidence and prevalence of major transfusion-transmissible viral infections in US blood donors, 1991 to 1996. *JAMA* 2000; **284**: 229–35.
3. Finucane ML, Slovic P, Mertz CK. Public perception of the risk of blood transfusion. *Transfusion* 2000; **40**: 1017–22.
4. Spahn DR, Casutt M. Eliminating blood transfusions. *Anesthesiology* 2000; **93**: 242–55.
5. Klein HG. The prospect of red cell substitutes. *N Engl J Med* 2000; **342**: 1666–8.
6. Hutchinson AB, Fergusson D, Graham ID et al. Utilization of technologies to reduce allogeneic blood transfusion in the United States. *Transfusion Med* 2001; **11**: 79–85.
7. Marchetta M, Barosi G. Cost-effectiveness of epoetin and autologous blood donation in reducing allogeneic blood transfusions in coronary artery bypass graft surgery. *Transfusion* 2000; **40**: 673–81.

8. Goodnough LT, Brittenham G. Limitations of the erythropoietic response to serial phlebotomy: implications for autologous blood donor programs. *J Lab Clin Med* 1990; **115**: 28–35.

9. Kickler TS, Spivak JL. Effect of repeated whole blood donations on serum immunoreactive erythropoietin levels in autologous donors. *JAMA* 1988; **260**: 65–7.

10. Goodnough LT, Rudick S, Price TH et al. Increased collection of autologous blood preoperatively with recombinant human erythropoietin therapy. *N Engl J Med* 1989; **321**: 1163–7.

11. Goodnough LT, Price TH, Rudnick S. Preoperative red blood cell production in patients undergoing aggressive autologous blood phlebotomy with and without erythropoietin therapy. *Transfusion* 1992; **32**: 441–5.

12. Goodnough LT, Price TH and the EPO Study Group. A phase III trial of recombinant human erythropoietin therapy in non-anemic orthopaedic patients subjected to aggressive autologous blood phlebotomy: dose, response, toxicity, and efficacy. *Transfusion* 1994; **34**: 66–71.

13. Goodnough LT, Brecher ME, Kanter MH, AuBuchon JB. Autologous blood procurement. Transfusion medicine, Part II. Blood conservation. *N Engl J Med* 1999; **340**: 525–33. *Vox Sang* 1996; **71**: 133–41.

14. Mercuriali F, Zanella A, Barosi G et al. Use erythropoietin to increase the volume of autologous blood donated by orthopaedic patients. *Transfusion* 1993; **33**: 55.

15. Price TH, Goodnough LT, Vogler W et al. The effect of recombinant erythropoietin administration on the efficacy of autologous blood donation in patients with low hematocrits. *Transfusion* 1996; **36**: 29–36.

16. Canadian orthopedic perioperative erythropoietin study group. Effectiveness of perioperative recombinant human erythropoietin in elective hip replacement. *Lancet* 1993; **341**: 1227–32.

17. Faris PM, Ritter MA, Abels RI. The effects of recombinant human erythropoietin on perioperative transfusion requirements in patients undergoing major orthopaedic surgery. *J Bone Joint Surg* 1996; **78A**: 62–72.

18. de Andrade JR, Jove M, Landon G et al. Baseline hemoglobin as a predictor of risk of transfusion and response to epoetin alpha in orthopedic surgery patients. *Am J Orthop* 1996: **25**: 533–42.

19. Goodnough LT, Verbrugge D, Marcus RE, Goldberg V. The effect of patient size and dose of recombinant human erythropoietin therapy on red blood cell expansion. *J Am Coll Surg* 1994; **179**; 171–6.

20. Goodnough LT, Price TH, Parvin CA. The endogenous erythropoietin response and the erythropoietic response to blood loss anemia: the effects of age and gender. *J Lab Clin Med* 1995; **126**: 57–64.

21. Goodnough LT, Marcus RE. Erythropoiesis in patients stimulated with erythropoietin: the relevance of storage iron. *Vox Sang* 1998; **75**: 128–33.

22. Goodnough LT, Price TH, Parvin CA et al. Erythropoietin response to anaemia is not altered by surgery or recombinant human erythropoietin therapy. *Br J Haematol* 1994; **87**: 695–9.

23. Coleman PH, Stevens AR, Dodge HT, Finch CA. Rate of blood regeneration after blood loss. *Arch Intern Med* 1953; **92**: 341–8.

24. Crosby WH. Treatment of hemochromatosis by energetic phlebotomy. One patient's response to getting 55 liters of blood in 11 months. *Br J Haematol* 1958; **4**: 82–8.

25. Goodnough LT, Merkel K. The use of parenteral iron and recombinant human erythropoietin therapy to stimulate erythropoiesis in patients undergoing repair of hip fracture. *Int J Hematol* 1996; **1**: 163–6.

26. Finch CA. Erythropoiesis, erythropoietin, and iron. *Blood* 1982; **60**: 1241–6.

27. Feagan BG, Wong CJ, Lau CY et al. Transfusion practice in elective orthopaedic surgery. *Transfusion Med* 2001; **11**: 87–95.

28. Feagan BG, Wong CJ, Kirkley A et al. Erythropoietin with iron supplementation to prevent allogeneic blood transfusion in total hip joint arthroplasty. *Ann Intern Med* 2000; **133**: 845–54.

29. Goodnough LT, Monk TG, Andriole GL. Erythropoietin therapy. *N Engl J Med* 1997; **336**: 933–8.

30. Doolittle RF. Biotechnology – the enormous cost of success. *N Engl J Med* 1991; **324**: 360–2.

31. Goldberg MA, McCutchen JW, Jove M et al. A safety and efficacy comparison study of two dosing regimens of erythropoietin alpha in patients undergoing major orthopedic surgery. *Am J Orthop* 1996; **25**: 544–52.

32. Messmer K. Consensus statement: Using epoietin alfa to decrease the risk of allogeneic blood transfusion in the surgical setting. *Semin Hematol* 1999; **33**: 73–80.

33. Coyle D, Lee KM, Ferguson DA, Laupacis A. Economic analysis of erythropoietin use in orthopaedic surgery. *Transfusion Med* 1999: **9**: 21–39.

34. Sans T, Bofill C, Joven J et al. Effectiveness of very low doses of subcutaneous recombinant human erythropoietin in facilitating autologous blood donation before orthopedic surgery. *Transfusion* 1996; **36**: 822–6.

35. Erslev AJ. Erythropoietin. *N Engl J Med* 1991; **324**: 1339–44.

36. Laupacis A, Fergusson D. Erythropoietin to minimize perioperative blood transfusion: a systematic review of randomized trials. *Transfusion Med* 1998; **8**: 309–17.

37. Stowell CP, Chandler H, Jove M et al. An open-label, randomized study to compare the safety and efficacy of perioperative epoietin alpha with preoperative autologous blood donation in total joint arthroplasty. *Orthopedics* 1999; **22**:S105–12.

38. Brines ML, Ghezzi P, Keenan S et al. Erythropoietin crosses the blood–brain barrier to protect against experimental brain injury. *Proc Natl Acad Sci USA* 2000; **97**: 10526–31.

39. Brezden CB. Cognitive function in breast cancer patients receiving adjuvant chemotherapy. *J Clin Oncol* 2000; **18**: 2695–2701.

40. Egrie JC, Browne JK. Development and characterization of novel erythropoiesis stimulating protein (NESP). *Br J Cancer* 2001; **84**(Suppl 1): 3–10.

41. Glaspy J, Jadeja JS, Justice G et al. A dose-finding and safety study of novel erythropoiesis stimulating protein (NESP) for the treatment of anaemia in patients receiving multicycle chemotherapy. *Br J Cancer* 2001; **84**(Suppl 1): 17–23.

42. Smith RE, Jaiyesimi IA, Meza LA et al. Novel erythropoiesis stimulating protein (NESP) for the treatment of anaemia of chronic disease associated with cancer. *Br J Cancer* 2001; **84**(Suppl 1): 24–30.

43. Muirhead M, Bargman J, Burgess E et al. Evidence-based recommendations for the clinical use of recombinant human erythropoietin. *Am J Kidney Dis* 1995; **26**: S1–24

44. Kaisi M, Ngwalle EWK, Runyoro DE, Rogers J. Evaluation and tolerance of response to iron dextran (Imferon) administered by total dose infusion to pregnant women with iron deficiency anemia. *Int J Gynecol Obstet* 1988; **26**: 235–43.

45. Mays T, Mays T. Intravenous iron dextran therapy in the treatment of anemia occuring in surgical, gynecologic, and obstetric patients. *Surg Gynecol Obstet* 1976; **143**: 381–4.

46. Hamstra RD, Block MH, Schocket AL. Intravenous iron dextran in clinical medicine. *JAMA* 1980; **243**: 1726–31.

47. Woodman J, Shaw RJ, Shipman AJ, Edwards AM, A surveillance program on a long-established product: Imferon (Iron Dextran BP). *Pharmaceut Med* 1987; **1**: 289–93.

48. Fishbane S, Ungureanu VD, Maeska JK et al. The safety of intravenous iron dextran in hemodialysis patients. *Am J Kidney Dis* 1996; **28**: 529–34.

49. Auerbach M, Winchester J, Wahab A et al. A randomized trial of three iron dextran infusion methods for anemia in EPO-treated dialysis patients. *Am J Kidney Dis* 1998; **31**: 81–6.

50. Faich G, Strobos J. Sodium ferric gluconate complex in sucrose: safer intravenous iron therapy than iron dextran. *Am J Kidney Dis* 1999; **33**: 464–70.

51. Sunder-Plassmann G, Horl WH. Safety aspects of parenteral iron in patients with end stage renal disease. *Drug Safety* 1997; **17**: 241–50.

52. Silverberg DS, Blum M, Peer G et al. Intravenous ferric saccharate as an iron supplementation in dialysis patients. *Nephron* 1996; **72**: 413–19.

53. Sunder-Plassmann G, Horl WH. Importance of iron supply for erythropoietin therapy. *Nephrol Dial Transplant* 1995; **10**: 2070–6.

54. Nissenson AR, Lindsay RM, Swan S et al. Sodium ferric gluconate complex in sucrose is safe and effective in hemodialysis patients: North American Trial. *Am J Kidney Dis* 1999; **33**: 471–82.

55. Calvar C, Mata D, Alonso C et al. Intravenous administration of iron gluconate during haemodialysis. *Nephrol Dial Transplant* 1997; **12**: 574–5.

56. Zanen AL, Adriaansen HJ, Van Bommel EFH et al. 'Over saturation' of transferrin after intravenous ferric gluconate (Ferlecit) in haemodialysis patients. *Nephrol Dial Transplant* 1996; **11**: 820–4.

57. Seligman PA, Schleicher RB. Comparison of methods used to measure serum iron in the presence of iron gluconate or iron dextran. *Clin Chem* 1999; **45**: 898–901.

58. Pascual J, Teruel JL, Liano F et al. Serious adverse reactions after intravenous ferric gluconate. *Nephrol Dial Transplant* 1992; **7**: 271–6.

59. Hillman RS, Henderson PA. Control of marrow production by the level of iron supply. *J Clin Invest* 1969; **48**: 454–60.

60. Henderson PA, Hillman RS. Characteristics of iron dextran utilization in man. *Blood* 1969; **34**: 357–75.

61. Goodnough LT, Skikne B, Brugnara C. Erythropoietin, iron, and erythropoiesis. *Blood* 2000; **96**: 823–33.

62. Archimbaud E, Thomas X. Thrombopoietic factors potentially useful in the treatment of acute leukemia. *Leuk Res* 1998; **22**: 1155–64.

63. Goldman SJ. Preclinical biology of interleukin 11: a multifunctional hematopoietic cytokine with potent thrombopoietic activity. *Stem Cells* 1995; **13**: 462–71.

64. Nandurkar HH, Robb L, Tarlinton D et al. Adult mice with targeted mutation of the interleukin-11 receptor (IL11Ra) display normal hematopoiesis. *Blood* 1997; **90**: 2148–59.

65. Gainsford T, Nandurkar H, Metcalf D et al. The residual megakaryocyte and platelet production in c-Mpl-deficient mice is not dependent on the actions of interleukin-6, interleukin-11, or leukemia inhibitory factor. *Blood* 2000; **95**: 528–34.

66. Tepler I, Elias L, Smith JW II et al. A randomized placebo-controlled trial of recombinant human interleukin-11 in cancer patients with severe thrombocytopenia due to chemotherapy. *Blood* 1996; **87**: 3607–14.

67. Vigon I, Mornon J-P, Cocault L et al. Molecular cloning and characterization of *MPL*, the human homolog of the v-*mpl* oncogene: identification of a member of the hematopoietic growth factor receptor superfamily. *Proc Nat Acad Sci USA* 1992; **89**: 5640–4.

68. Gurney AL, Carver-Moore K, de Sauvage FJ et al. Thrombocytopenia in c-mpl-deficient mice. *Science* 1994; **65**: 1445–7.

69. de Sauvage FJ, Hass PE, Spencer SD et al. Stimulation of megakaryocytopoiesis and thrombopoiesis by the c-Mpl ligand. *Nature* 1994; **369**: 533–8.

70. Lok S, Kaushansky K, Holly RD et al. Cloning and expression of murine thrombopoietin cDNA and stimulation of platelet production in vivo. *Nature* 1994; **369**: 565–8.

71. Choi ES, Hokom MM, Chen JL et al. The role of megakaryocyte growth and development factor in terminal stages of thrombopoiesis. *Br J Haematol* 1996; **95**: 227–33.

72. Fanucchi M, Glaspy J, Crawford J et al. Effects of polyethylene glycol-conjugated recombinant human megakaryocyte growth and development factor on platelet counts after chemotherapy for lung cancer. *N Engl J Med* 1997; **336**: 404–9.

73. Kuter DJ, Goodnough LT, Roma J et al. Thrombopoietin therapy increases platelet yields in normal platelet donors. *Blood* 2001; **98**: 1339–45.

74. Goodnough LT, Kuter DJ, McCullough J et al. Prophylactic transfusions from normal apheresis platelet donors undergoing treatment with thrombopoietin. *Blood* 2001; **98**: 1346–51.

75. Li J, Xia Y, Bertino A et al. Characterization of an anti-thrombopoietin antibody that developed in a cancer patient following the injection of PEG-rHuMGPF. *Blood* 1999; **94**: 51A.

76. Somlo G, Sniecinski I, ter Veer A et al. Recombinant human thrombopoietin in combination with granulocyte colony-stimulating factor enhances mobilization of peripheral blood progenitor cells, increases peripheral blood platelet concentration, and accelerates hematopoietic recovery following high-dose chemotherapy. *Blood* 1999; **93**: 2798–806.

77. Vadhan-Raj S, Verschraegen CF, Bueso-Ramos C et al. Recombinant human thrombopoietin attenuates carboplatin-induced severe thrombocytopenia and the need for platelet transfusions in patients with gynecologic cancer. *Ann Intern Med* 2000; **132**: 364–8.

78. de Serres M, Ellis B, Dillberger JE et al. Immunogenicity of thrombopoietin mimetic peptide GW395058 in BALB/c mice and New Zealand white rabbits: evaluation of the potential for thrombopoietin neutralizing antibody production in man. *Stem Cells* 1999; **17**: 203–9.

79. Deng B, Banu N, Malloy B et al. An agonist murine monoclonal antibody to the human c-Mpl receptor stimulates megakaryocytopoiesis. *Blood* 1998; **92**: 1981–8.

80. Winslow RM. Blood substitutes – a moving target. *Nat Med* 1995; **1**: 1212–15.

81. Stowell CP, Levin J, Spiess BD, Winslow RM. Progress in the development of blood substitutes. *Transfusion* 2001; **41**: 287–99.

82. Scott MG, Kucik DF, Goodnough LT, Monk TG. Blood substitutes: evolution and future applications. *Clin Chem* 1997; **43**: 1724–31.

83. Ma Z, Monk TG, Goodnough LT et al. Effect of hemoglobin- and perflubron-based oxygen carriers on common clinical laboratory tests. *Clin Chem* 1997; **43**: 1732–7.

84. Kasper SM, Grune F, Walter M et al. The effects of increased doses of bovine hemoglobin on hemodynamics and oxygen transport in patients undergoing preoperative hemodilution for elective abdominal aortic surgery. *Anesth Analg* 1998; **87**: 284–91.

85. Loscalzo J. Nitritc oxide binding and the adverse effects of cell-free hemoglobins: What makes us different from earth worms? *J Lab Clin Med* 1997; **129**: 580–3.

86. Sloan EP, Koenigsberg M, Gens D et al. Diaspirin cross-linked hemoglobin (DCL-Hgb) in the treatment of severe traumatic hemorrhagic shock. *JAMA* 1999; **282**: 1857–64.

87. Brecher ME, Goodnough LT, Monk T. The value of oxygen-carrying solutions in the operative setting, as determined by mathematical modeling. *Transfusion* 1999; **39**: 396–102.

88. Spahn DR, van Brempt R, Theilmeier G et al. Perfusion emulsion delays blood transfusions in orthopedic surgery. *Anesthesiology* 1999; **91**: 1195–208.

11 Congenital and acquired disorders of coagulation

Jeanne M Lusher, Roshni Kulkarni

HEREDITARY COAGULATION DISORDERS

The haemophilias

Haemophilia A (factor VIII (FVIII) deficiency) and haemophilia B (factor IX (FIX) deficiency) are X-linked disorders of blood coagulation, and thus affect males almost exclusively. They are clinically indistinguishable, with both being characterized by bleeding into joints, muscles, and other soft tissues. Coagulation screening tests will reveal a prolonged activated thromboplastin time (APTT) in both, while the prothrombin time (PT) will be normal for age. The two types of haemophilia can be distinguished by performing FVIII and FIX assays. Since affected individuals lack FVIII (or FIX) at birth, occasional newborns have intracranial and/or extracranial haemorrhages, and many will have excessive bleeding with circumcision or other invasive procedures.

While haemophilia A and B are categorized as hereditary disorders, approximately one-third of affected newborns have no family history of haemophilia, the disorder having resulted from spontaneous mutation in the FVIII (or FIX) gene.[1,2] Hundreds of mutations in the FVIII and FIX genes that result in haemophilia have been described.[1,2] In severe haemophilia A, roughly 45% of affected individuals have the 'inversion mutation'[3,4] (commonly referred to as the 'flip-tip' mutation, since one of the long arms of the X chromosome is folded back on itself). The inversion mutation can be detected by Southern blot using a blood sample, or using fetal or chorionic villus cells. In families with no family history of haemophilia A who have an affected infant, it has been shown that the inversion mutation often occurred first in the infant's maternal grandfather.[4]

There are different degrees of severity of haemophilia, although affected members of the same kindred will have the same gene defect and the same degree of severity. Severe haemophilia is characterized by 1% or less FVIII or FIX activity, and spontaneous bleeding into joints and soft tissues. Moderate haemophilia is defined by a FVIII or FIX level of between 1% and 5%, with most bleeding resulting from trauma. Mild haemophilia is characterized by a FVIII or FIX level from 5% to 30%, and bleeding episodes resulting from significant trauma or surgery. (One unit (U) of FVIII or FIX is the amount present in 1 ml of pooled normal human plasma.)

Treatment of haemophilia A and haemophilia B

Treatment consists of giving an adequate amount of the clotting factor that is lacking or abnormal. Depending on the location and the extent of bleeding, different dosages are often used (see below in the section on 'Dosage and administration'). Dosage calculations and intervals between doses differ for hemophilia

A and B, because of the different distributions, recoveries, and half-lives of FVIII and FIX once infused.

Acute joint bleeding, intramuscular bleeding, head injury, or abdominal bleeding in an infant, child, or adult with haemophilia should be treated *immediately*! The aim is to increase the patient's FVIII (or FIX) level to a safe range to stop bleeding.

Just prior to any surgical procedure, invasive dentistry, or lumbar puncture, the patient's FVIII (or FIX) level should be increased to a safe range by infusing FVIII or FIX (or desmopressin in the case of mild haemophilia A) (see the section on 'Dosage and administration').

At regional comprehensive haemophilia treatment centres, the education of patients and their parents is of extreme importance. This includes an understanding of the disease and its potential complications, when to treat, how to calculate dosage, etc. Most patients are on home treatment, having been taught how and when to self-infuse (or infuse their child), how to complete treatment logs, and when to call the centre (e.g. for serious bleeding episodes or bleeding episodes that fail to respond to treatment).

Haemophilia A

Haemophilia A is more common than haemophilia B, accounting for approximately 80–85% of cases of haemophilia. Various types of products are licensed and available for treating or preventing bleeding. These include plasma-derived FVIII concentrates (viral-attenuation methods include pasteurization, solvent–detergent treatment, immuno-affinity purification, and nanofiltration) of varying degrees of purity (as defined by the specific activity of FVIII in the final product, excluding albumin added as a stabilizer to the final product), recombinant (r) FVIII concentrates, and desmopressin.

Plasma-derived FVIII concentrates

Various brands of plasma-derived FVIII concentrates are licensed and available in different countries. A fairly current listing of these is available on the World Federation of Hemophilia website (www.wfh.org). It should be noted that it is difficult to maintain a current listing, since pharmaceutical companies change names, and products change or are modified. The US National Hemophilia Foundation's (NHF) Medical and Scientific Advisory Council (MASAC) maintains listings of plasma-derived and rFVIII and FIX products for patients with and without inhibitors that are licensed in the USA. These appear on the NHF website (www. hemophilia.org), and are updated every 6 months. The most current listings appear in Tables 11.1–11.11.

There have been no reported instances of transmission of HIV or hepatitis viruses with products licensed for use in the USA, Canada, and European countries for over a decade; however, even with current techniques for donor screening and viral attenuation of products, there is still a slight risk of transmission of non-lipid-enveloped viruses such as hepatitis A and human parvovirus B19.[5–7]

Recombinant FVIII products

In 1984 scientists at Genentech (Berkeley, CA), and Genetics Institute (Cambridge, MA) simultaneously announced the successful cloning of the FVIII gene and the expression of its product, human FVIII.[8–10] Following purification and scale-up, pre-licensure

Table 11.1 Recombinant FVIII products licensed in the USA

Product name	Manufacturer	Method of viral depletion or inactivation	Stabilizer	Human or animal protein used in culture medium	Specific activity of final product (U FVIII/mg total protein)	Hepatitis safety studies in humans with this product?
Bioclate	Baxter (distributed by Aventis Behring)	Immunoaffinity chromatography	Human albumin	Bovine	1.65–19	Yes
Helixate FS	Bayer (distributed by Aventis Behring)	Immunoaffinity chromatography	Sucrose	Human	4000[a]	Yes
Kogenate FS	Bayer	Immunoaffinity chromatography	Sucrose	Human	4000[a]	Yes
Recombinate	Baxter	Immunoaffinity chromatography	Human albumin	Bovine	1.65–19	Yes
ReFacto	Pharmacia & Upjohn AB (Stockholm) (distributed by Genetics Institute)	1. Immunoaffinity chromatography 2. Solvent–detergent (TNBP and Triton X-100)	Sucrose	Human albumin	11 200–15 500	Yes

[a] Valid as long as the product is kept under refrigeration as recommended by the manufacturer.

Table 11.2 Immunoaffinity-purified FVIII products derived from human plasma licenced in the USA

Product name	Manufacturer	Method of viral depletion or inactivation	Specific activity of final product (U FVIII/mg total protein)	Hepatitis safety studies in humans with this product?	Hepatitis safety studies in humans with another product, but similar viral-inactivation method?
Hemofil M	Baxter	1. Immunoaffinity chromatography 2. Solvent–detergent (TNBP and Triton X-100)	2–15	Yes	No
Monarc-M	Manufactured by Baxter for American Red Cross (ARC) from ARC-collected plasma (distributed by ARC)	1. Immunoaffinity chromatography 2. Solvent–detergent (TNBP and octoxynol 9)	2–15	No	Yes
Monoclate-P	Aventis Behring	1. Immunoaffinity chromatography 2. Pasteurization (60°C, 10h)	5–10	Yes	Yes

Table 11.3 FVIII products containing von Willebrand factor and derived from human plasma licensed in the USA

Product name	Manufacturer	Method of viral inactivation	Specific activity of final product (U FVIII/mg total protein)	Hepatitis safety studies in humans with this product?	Hepatitis safety studies in humans with another product, but similar viral-inactivation method?	FDA approved for von Willebrand disease?
Alphanate SD	Alpha	1. Affinity chromatography 2. Solvent–detergent (TNBP and polysorbate 80) 3. Dry heat (80°C, 72 h)	8–30	No	Yes	No
Humate-P	Aventis Behring GmbH (Marburg, Germany)	1. Pasteurization (60°C, 10 h)	1–2	Yes	No	Yes
Koate-DVI	Eayer	1. Solvent–detergent (TNBP and polysorbate 80) 2. Dry heat (80°C, 72 h)	9–22	No	Yes	No

Table 11.4 Porcine FVIII product licensed in the USA[a]

Product name	Manufacturer	Method of viral inactivation	Specific activity of final product (U FVIII/mg total protein)	Hepatitis safety studies in humans with this product?	Hepatitis safety studies in humans with another product, but similar viral-inactivation method?
Hyate : C	Ipsen, Inc., Wales	None (but no report of transmission of any viruses to humans)	>50	No	Yes

[a]For use in patients with inhibitors to human FVIII

Table 11.5 Recombinant FIX product licensed in the USA

Product name	Manufacturer	Method of viral depletion or inactivation	Stabilizer	Human or animal protein used in culture medium?	Specific activity (U FIX/mg total protein)	Hepatitis safety studies in humans with this product?
BeneFIX	Wyeth-Genetics Institute	1. Affinity chromatography 2. Ultrafiltration	Sucrose	None	≥200	Yes

Table 11.6 FIX products derived from human plasma licensed in the USA

Product name	Manufacturer	Method of viral depletion or inactivation	Specific activity of final product (U FIX/mg total protein)	Hepatitis safety studies in humans with this product?	Hepatitis safety studies in humans with another product, but similar viral-inactivation method
AlphaNine SD	Alpha	1. Dual-affinity chromatography 2. Solvent–detergent (TNBP and polysorbate 80) 3. Nanofiltration (viral filter)	229 ± 23	Yes	Yes
Mononine	Aventis Behring	1. Immunoaffinity chromatography 2. Sodium thiocyanate 3. Ultrafiltration	>160	Yes	No

Table 11.7 Frothrombin complex concentrates containing FII, FVII, FIX, FX and derived from human plasma licensed in the USA[a]

Product name	Manufacturer	Method of viral inactivation	Specific activity of final product (U FIX/mg total protein)	Hepatitis safety studies in humans with this product?	Hepatitis safety studies in humans with another product, but similar viral-inactivation method?
Bebulin VH	Baxter (Vienna)	Vapour heat (10h, 60°C, 1190 mbar pressure plus 1h, 80°C, 1375 mbar)	2	Yes	No
Konyne 80	Bayer	Dry heat (80°C, 72 h)	1.25	No	Yes
Profilnine SD	Alpha	Solvent–detergent (TNBP and polysorbate 80)	4.5	No	Yes
Proplex-T	Baxter	Dry heat (60°C, 144 h)	3.9	No	No

[a]For use in patients with deficiencies of FII, FVII, or FX; note that content varies from lot to lot and product to product.

Table 11.8 Anti-inhibitor coagulation complex (activated prothrombin complex concentrates) derived from human plasma licensed in the USA[a]

Product name	Manufacturer	Method of viral depletion or inactivation	Specific activity of final product (U factor/mg total protein)	Hepatitis safety studies in humans with this product?	Hepatitis safety studies in humans with another product, but similar viral-inactivation method?
Autoplex-T	Baxter (distributed by Nabi)	Dry heat (60°C, 144 h)	5	No	No
FEIBA-VH	Baxter–Hyland Immuno	Vapour heat (10 h, 60°C, 1190 mbar plus 1 h, 80°C, 1375 mbar)	0.8	Yes	Yes

[a]For use in patients with inhibitors to FVIII or FIX. These products contain approximately equal unitages of FVIII/FIX bypassing activity, and prothrombin complex factors, II, IX and X.

Table 11.9 Recombinant FVlla product licensed in the USA

Product name	Manufacturer	Method of viral depletion or inactivation	Stabilizer	Human or animal protein used in culture medium	Hepatitis safety studies in humans with this product?
NovoSeven	Novo Nordisk (Bagsvaerd, Denmark)	Affinity chromatography	Mannitol	Bovine	Yes

Table 11.10 Desmopressin formulations useful in disorders of haemostasis licensed in the USA

Product name	Manufacturer	Formulation	Recommended dosage and administration
DDAVP injection	Ferring AB (Malmö, Sweden) (distributed by Aventis Pharma)	For parenteral use (intravenous or subcutaneous), 4 µg/ml in a 10 ml vial	1. 0.3 µg/kg, mixed in 30 ml normal saline solution, infused slowly over 30 min intraveously 2. 0.4 µg/kg subcutaneously. Maximum dose 24 µg/kg once every 24 h May repeat after 24 hours
Stimate nasal spray for bleeding	Ferring AB (Malmö, Sweden) (distributed by Aventis Behring)	Nasal spray, 1.5 mg/ml. The metered-dose pump delivers 0.1 ml (150 µg) per actuation. The bottle contains 2.5 ml, with a spray pump capable of delivering twenty-five 150 µg doses or twelve 300 µg doses	In patients weighing <50 kg, one spray in one nostril delivers 150 µg. For those weighing >50 kg, give one spray in *each nostril* (total dose 300 µg). May repeat after 24 hours

Table 11.11 Fresh-frozen plasma products licensed in the USA

Product name	Manufacturer	Method of viral depletion or inactivation	Pool size, No. of donor units
Donor Retested Fresh Frozen Plasma	Community Blood Banks (not ARC) (distributed by Community Blood Banks)	Donors must test negative on second donation in order for first donation to be released	1
Plas + SD	Vitex from plasma collected by American Red Cross (distributed by ARC)	Solvent–detergent (TNBP and Triton X-100)	2500

clinical trials in persons with haemophilia began in 1987. Two rFVIII products have been licensed by the US Food and Drug Administration (FDA: Recombinate (Baxter, Glendale, CA) in 1992 and Kogenate (Bayer Corporation, West Haven, CT) in early 1993. These same two products have also been sold by Centeon (King of Prussia, PA) (now Aventis-Behring), under different trade names (Tables 11.1–11.4).

Because of the size and complexity of the FVIII gene and the complexities of expression of FVIII, mammalian cells must be used. rFVIII is produced in well-characterized hamster cell lines – Recombinate and ReFacto in Chinese hamster ovary (CHO) cells and Kogenate in baby hamster kidney (BHK) cells.

The original (so-called 'first-generation') rFVIII products contained pasteurized human serum albumin (HSA) which was used in the culture medium and was added as a stabilizer. While HSA has an excellent track record of viral safety, there was concern over the fact that albumin made up most of the final formulation of the rFVIII concentrates. Thus, the newest rFVIII preparations do not contain albumin. ('Second-generation' products are not stabilized with HSA, while 'third-generation' products have none in the culture medium either.)

Genetics Institute's B-domain-deleted (BDD) rFVIII, ReFacto, is a truncated FVIII molecule that lacks the middle section (B domain). This much smaller molecule is secreted more efficiently by CHO cells. The currently licensed version (licensed by the US FDA in 2000, and earlier in Europe) contains no added HSA, but HSA is used in the culture medium. A newer version of ReFacto (currently in pre-licensure clinical trials), contains

no albumin. Similarly, as of April 2002, Recombinate, which is completely albumin-free, is in pre-licensure clinicals trials in persons with haemophilia A.

While each of these rFVIII products have proven to be effective and safe, it should be noted that there is an assay-discrepancy problem with BDDrFVIII (ReFacto). (This appears to result from marked differences in the phospholipid requirement in APTT based assays of BDDrFVIII compared with other FVIII preparations.) Following infusion of this product, standard one-stage FVIII assays of patient samples give values that are roughly 50% less than chromogenic assay values, and 50% less than calculated expected values.[11,12] Nonetheless, infusions using usual dosage calculations have generally been effective in controlling or preventing bleeding. The manufacturer currently recommends that a ReFacto standard be used in performing one-stage FVIII assays on patient samples following infusion of BDDrFVIII, in order to deal with the assay discrepancy. (Vials of this ReFacto standard are distributed by George King Biomedical in the USA.)

The main advantage of the rFVIII preparations is that of viral safety. Overall, recombinant clotting factor concentrates appear to be the safest form of treatment. While recombinant technology would seem to offer unlimited supply, at present, worldwide demands for rFVIII far exceed supply. The main disadvantage of recombinant products is their cost. These products are generally more costly than their plasma-derived alternatives.

Desmopressin (1-deamino-8-D-arginine vasopressin, DDAVP)

Desmopressin is the treatment of choice for

persons with mild haemophilia A, for carrier females who have very low levels of FVIII, and for persons with von Willebrand disease, type 1 (see below). This synthetic agent comes in several formulations, for intravenous, subcutaneous, and intranasal use.[13] While the drug is generally given intravenously for in-hospital use, the highly concentrated intranasal spray (Stimate nasal spray; Table 11.10) is ideal for home and outpatient use. The drug results in a rapid rise in von Willebrand factor and FVIII, by effecting their rapid release from storage sites. (It is ineffective in severe haemophilia A, since there is no FVIII in body stores to be released). The recommended intravenous dosage is 0.3 µg/kg body weight (maximum dose 20 µg); doses can be repeated at 12- to 24-hour intervals if necessary. However, it should be noted that most persons with mild haemophilia A will have a diminishing response (tachyphylaxis) with frequent repetitive doses. If this occurs, and there is a continued need for higher FVIII levels, one should switch to a FVIII concentrate.

An initial intravenous dose of desmopressin of 0.3 µg/kg effects an average threefold increase (range 2- to 12-fold) in FVIII over baseline values. The magnitude of response is generally reproducible in individuals (i.e., if a person with mild haemophilia A has a fourfold increase in FVIII on one occasion, he will probably have a fourfold increase if given the drug again a few weeks later).

Side-effects of desmopressin are generally minor (facial flushing and a feeling of facial warmth). However, the drug is a potent antidiuretic agent. Thus, there is a risk of hyponatraemia and water intoxication (which may be manifest by convulsions), especially if the patient is given large amounts of hypotonic fluids. (It is recommended that fluids be somewhat restricted for 18 hours post desmopressin, and that one monitor fluids and electrolytes in postoperative patients.) In view of a greater propensity to fluid balance problems in the very young and the elderly, desmopressin should be used with caution (or not at all) in children under 2 years of age, and in persons over 70. Additionally, in view of sporadic reports of coronary or cerebrovascular thrombosis associated with the use of desmopressin, it seems appropriate to avoid using it in those known to have risk factors for such complications.[14]

For intranasal use for haemostatic purposes, a highly concentrated intranasal spray (from a multidose spray bottle with metered dose pump) should be employed. The intranasal dosage of desmopressin is 15 times the intravenous dosage. The recommended dose is one spray (in one nostril) for patients weighing less than 50 kg, and two sprays (one in each nostril) for those heavier than this. As with the intravenous form, patients should be cautioned about the risk of fluid overload and advised to limit fluid intake for 12–18 hours post Stimate nasal spray.

Dosage and administration of FVIII concentrates

Dosage depends on the site and severity of bleeding (Table 11.12) and the desired circulating level of FVIII. To calculate dosage, one should keep in mind that the infusion of 1 U/kg body weight will increase the patient's FVIII level by 0.02 U/ml (2%). Thus, the FVIII dosage in U/kg equals the desired FVIII level divided by 2. If additional doses are needed,

Table 11.12 Dosage guidelines for treatment of bleeding in severe and moderately severe hemophilia A and B without inhibitors[a]

Type of bleeding	Desired factor level (%)	FVIII dose (IU/kg)[b]	FIX dose (IU/kg)[b,c]	Duration of treatment (days)	Ancillary treatment[d]
Persistent or profuse epistaxis	20–30	10–15	20–30	1–2	Local pressure
Oral mucosal bleeding (including tongue/mouth lacerations)	20–30	10–15	20–30	1–2	Avoidance of trauma that would dislodge clot; antifibrinolytic agent for 7–10 days; nil by mouth; sedation in small children with tongue laceration
Acute haemarthrosis	30–50	15–25	30–50	1–3	Non-weight-bearing on affected joint
Intramuscular haemorrhage	30–50	15–25	30–50	2–5	Non-weight-bearing
Iliopsoas or other retroperitoneal bleeding	30–50	15–25	30–50	3–10	Bed rest
Retropharyngeal bleeding	40–50	20–25	40–50	3–4	Antifibrinolytic agent for 7–10 days
Intracranial haemorrhage	80–100	40–50	80–100	10–14 [e,f]	
Surgery	80–100	40–50	80–100	10–14[c] (shorter duration for minor procedures)	
Gastrointestinal bleeding	30–50	15–25	30–50	2–3	Increased oral or intravenous fluids (avoid antifibrinolytic agents[f])
Persistent painless gross haematuria[g]	30–50	15–25	30–50	1–2	

[a] Reprinted (with slight modifications) from Lusher JM, Treatment of congenital coagulopathies. In: *Transfusion Therapy, Clinical Principles and Practice* (Mintz PD, ed). Bethesda, MD: AABB Press, 1999: 97–128.
[b] After calculating dosage, give to nearest vial without discarding clotting factor (unless a PCC is being used).
[c] Note that dosage calculations for rFIX differ (see text).
[d] Approximately 25% of HIV infected hemophiliacs have had some degree of thrombocytopenia. If severe, zidovudine or other agents such as intravenous immunoglobin may be helpful in increasing the platelet count.
[e] Continuous infusion is preferable in order to avoid dangerously low trough levels. Following a bolus dose, FVIII or FIX is given at a dose of 3–4 U/kg/h, with subsequent dosing dependent on circulating plasma level.
[f] This should be followed with a 6 to 12 month period of prophylaxis when feasible, in order to prevent recurrent intracranial haemorrage.
[g] Painless, spontaneous gross haematuria generally requires no treatment (other than increasing fluid intake to maintain renal output). If it persists more than 3–4 days, however, treat with clotting factor.

these are generally given at 12 to 24 hour intervals (the average half-life of FVIII, once infused, is 8–12 hours, but may be less in young children). FVIII can also be given by continuous infusion, which avoids peaks and troughs of FVIII levels. This is often used in postoperative patients, or in patients with severe bleeding episodes such as intracranial haemorrhage, major trauma, or compartment syndrome. Continuous infusion of FVIII can be done using a minipump; 1–5 IU/ml heparin may be used to prevent thrombophlebitis. The usual starting rate for continuous infusion is 3–4 IU/kg/h, with the rate being adjusted subsequently as indicated by the recipient's FVIII level.

Prophylactic use of FVIII

Prophylactic administration of FVIII is aimed at preventing joint bleeding and the development of chronic, progressive, debilitating joint disease. If acute haemarthroses are not treated promptly, blood accumulates in the joint space, resulting in irritation of the synovial membrane. This results in proliferation of vascular synovial tissue into the joint space. When this occurs, even routine use of the joint can lead to synovial trauma, and a vicious cycle of rebleeding occurs. Over time, greater synovial proliferation and thickening develops, and, finally, there is erosion of underlying cartilage and bone. Since this process often begins early in life in children with severe haemophilia, many physicians advocate beginning prophylaxis at 1 or 2 years of age (so-called 'primary prophylaxis'), before joint haemorrhages have occurred. This practice began in Sweden,[15] but is now used in several countries; in 1994, the US NHF's Medical and Scientific Advisory Council (MASAC) recommended that prophylaxis be considered optimal care for children with severe haemophliia A and B.[16] The recommended dosage of FVIII for prophylaxis is 25–40 IU/kg body weight given every other day (or at least three times per week), and that of FIX is 25–40 IU/kg twice weekly (in view of the longer half-life of FIX). When feasible, prophylaxis should be done by venipuncture. Doses should be given in the morning, so that peak levels occur during waking hours. If it is necessary to resort to a central line, one should discuss all potential complications, the need for a surgical procedure, and the need for education in the care and use of the line with the patient and/or caregiver.[16]

Inhibitors in haemophilia A – incidence, detection, and management

Inhibitor antibodies to FVIII develop in approximately 30% of persons with haemophilia A. Most appear early in life, after a median of 9–11 exposure days to FVIII.[17,18] Most are in persons with severe haemophilia, although some develop in moderately (or even mildly) affected individuals. Factors putting a haemophiliac at increased risk of inhibitor formation include certain defects in the FVIII gene causing the individual's haemophilia (large gene deletions, frameshift mutations, stop codons, etc.), race (African descent), and having a haemophilic brother who has an inhibitor.[17]

An inhibitor should be suspected if a patient's bleeding episode fails to respond to usual treatment with FVIII; however, most new inhibitors are now picked up by periodic testing for inhibitors. The assay most commonly used is the Bethesda assay;[19] in most coagulation laboratories, the cut-off between positive and negative is 0.6 Bethesda Units (BU), with values of 0.6 BU or higher indicating the presence of an inhibitor. In the case of a newly detected inhibitor, the patient is usually called back for a repeat inhibitor assay, and a FVIII recovery (normal recovery is a peak value of FVIII, following FVIII infusion, of 60% or more of that expected by calculation). Inhibitors are generally classified as being 'high-titre' ($\geqslant$5 BU), or 'low titre' (<5 BU). In the case of very low-level inhibitors (e.g. 0.7–1.5 BU), in order to separate true inhibitors from false negatives, it is recommended that one use the Nijmegen modification of the standard Bethesda assay, in which the normal substrate plasma is buffered to a pH of 7.4 and FVIII-deficient plasma is substituted for buffer in the control incubation mix.[20] An enzyme-linked immunosorbent assay (ELISA) performed on the sample in question may also be helpful in determining whether or not an inhbitor antibody is present.

Some low-titre inhibitors will disappear despite episodic treatment with FVIII,[17,21] while others persist. Occasional higher-titre inhibitors will also disappear spontaneously. Since bleeding episodes in patients with inhibitors respond poorly or not at all to FVIII, progressive joint and musculoskeletal disease can occur. Thus, many haemophilia treaters try an immune tolerance induction (ITI) regimen in an attempt to eradicate the inhibitor. ITI regimens most often consist of large daily doses of FVIII (50–150 IU/kg), the dose being chosen based on the patient's inhibitor titre.[21-23] Predictors of successful ITI include a historic maximum inhibitor titre of 50 BU or less, a low inhibitor level at the start of ITI, and duration of the inhibitor of less than 6 months. Most published reports indicate a 75–85% success rate with ITI.[17,21,22] However, it often takes many months. Also, many patients, once tolerized, are continued on prophylaxis with FVIII (25–40 IU/kg) given three times weekly; thus, it is difficult to determine if their inhibitor has really been eradicated.

Prior to an inhibitor patient being tolerized (i.e. before or during ITI), or if the patient chooses not to undergo or has failed ITI, bleeding episodes must be treated with another modality.[23] Choices include rFVIIa (NovoSeven; Table 11.9),[24] a 'bypassing agent' (Autoplex-T or FEIBA-VH; Table 11.8),[22] or porcine FVIII (Hyate : C; Table 11.4).[25] Each has advantages and disadvantages. The main advantage of rFVIIa is that it is a recombinant product and thus has an increased margin of viral safety. However, it has a very short half-life. Thus, if repeat doses are deemed necessary, they must be given every 2–3 hours. Also, the optimal dosage has not been determined (it may well be considerably higher than the 90 µg/kg recommended in the product's package insert), and there is no simple laboratory test for measuring efficacy in the recipient. The bypassing agents, FEIBA-VH and Autoplex-T, have the advantage of less frequent dosing and a longer track record of safe usage. They are also less expensive than rFVIIa and porcine FVIII. However, these products are not always effective, their precise mode of action in bypassing the need for FVIII (or FIX) remains unclear, and there is no readily available laboratory test for measuring efficacy in the recipient. Porcine FVIII is an option for persons whose FVIII inhibitors have little or no cross-reactivity to it. The main advantage of this product is that it is a FVIII preparation; thus, one can measure and follow the recipient's FVIII level. However, since it is a foreign-species protein, there is a possiblity of allergic reactions. Therefore most do not use this product for home treatment. Also, some patients develop inhibitors to porcine FVIII, rendering the product ineffective.[22]

Haemophilia B

Haemophilia B is less common than haemophilia A, accounting for 15–20% of cases of haemophilia. It is clinically indistinguishable from haemophilia A, and many of the principles of treatment are the same for both disorders. However, there are a few significant differences.[26] FIX is a much smaller molecule than is FVIII and distributes extravascularly; thus, dosage calcuation is different. For FIX, 1 IU/kg will result in an increase in circulating FIX of 1%. The half-life of FIX (approximately 18 hours) is longer than that of FVIII. The incidence of FIX inhibitors is 1–2%, which is considerably less than in haemophilia A. Approximately 40% of patients who develop FIX inihibitors also have allergic reactions (often severe) to any FIX-containing material. In haemophilia B patients who develop inhibitors, response to ITI regimens is approximately 50%, which is considerably less than the 80–85% response rate to ITI seen in haemophilia A. Desmopressin is not a treatment option for haemophilia B, since it increases FVIII and von Willebrand factor, but not FIX.

Table 11.13 Diagnostic laboratory tests for vWD
• APTT (often normal[a])
• Bleeding time (an insensitive screening test; many no longer use)
• vWF antigen assay (vWF : Ag)
• FVIII clotting activity (FVIII : C)
• Ristocetin cofactor activity (vWF : RCo)
• vWF multimer analysis (displays vWF protein on agarose gel; vWF multimers are separated by size)

[a] With most reagents, the APTT will be normal in vWD unless FVIII activity is less than 35%.

Plasma-derived FIX concentrates for haemophilia B

Products currently licensed for use in the USA are listed in Tables 11.5–11.8. Those available elsewhere can be found on the WFH website.

rFIX concentrate

Only one company (Wyeth-Genetics Institute) produces an rFIX concentrate (BeneFix; Table 11.5).

FIX was cloned in the early 1980s, and prelicensure clinical trials with rFIX began in 1995. The product was licensed in the USA in 1997. The CHO cell line used in its manufacture is coinfected with a human rFIX cDNA expression plasmid and a cDNA expression plasmid that encodes an engineered form of the paired amino acid-cleaving enzyme (PACE), which improves the processing efficiency of profactor IX expressed in CHO cells.[27] No albumin, human plasma, animal plasma, or animal-derived protein are used in the manufacture or purificaiton of BeneFix. While a dose of plasma-derived FIX of 1 U/kg will raise the plasma FIX level by 0.01 U/ml (1%), lower recoveries (as low as 50% lower) are seen with rFIX (BeneFix). This difference in recovery results from a difference in the posttranslational modification, namely, the differences in sulfation of tyrosine 155 and phosphorylation of serine 158 (residues that play a role in the clearance of FIX). Therefore, one should check the patient's FIX recovery following the initial dose of BeneFix, or, use a larger dose of BeneFix than one would of a plasma-derived FIX product (calculated as recommended in the product package insert). However, it should be noted that there are wide variations in recovery among individuals, with infants and children having lower recoveries than adults.

Dosage and administration of FIX concentrates

As in haemophilia A, the dose of FIX to be given depends on the type and severity of the patient's bleeding (Table 11.12), and the desired FIX level. Since the 18-hour half-life of FIX is longer than that of FVIII, repeat dosing (if necessary) is generally given once daily.

FIX (both plasma-derived and recombinant) can also be given by continuous infusion. This is often used in intra- and postoperative patients, or for central nervous system haemorrhage – situations in which it is desirable to avoid dangerously low trough levels of FIX.

Prophylaxis with FIX concentrates is generally given at a dosage of 25–40 IU/kg, twice weekly.

Management of patients with FIX inhibitors

As noted above, ITI regimens are less effective in eradicating FIX inhibitors than FVIII inhibitors; nonetheless, ITI may be tried, generally using large daily doses of FIX alone. Although numbers of patients are small, reports from retrospective surveys and registries indicate that approximately 50% of FIX inhibitors can be eradicated or suppressed with ITI. The success rate is even less in those with severe allergic reactions, and some will develop nephrotic syndrome 8–9 months after beginning ITI.[28]

Therapeutic options for treating bleeding episodes in patients with FIX inhibitors include rFVIIa and activated prothrombin complex concentrates (FEIBA-VH or Autoplex-T). Advantages and disadvantages are the same as discussed under FVIII inhibitors. However, in the roughly 40% of FIX-inhibitor patients who have severe allergic reactions to any FIX-containing product (which includes FEIBA-VH and Autoplex-T), rFVIIa is the treatment of choice.[29]

While a dosage of 90 μg/kg is recommended in the package insert, as with FVIII inhibitors, the optimal dose of rFVIIa has not been established. However, repeat dosing, when indicated, should be given every 2–3 hours in view of the short half-life of rFVIIa. Continuous infusion is not recommended.

von Willebrand disease

von Willebrand disease (VWD) is the most common of the hereditary disorders of blood coagulation, affecting an estimated 1–1.5% of the population.[30] It is worldwide in distribution and affects all racial and ethnic groups. The gene for VWD is on chromosome 12.

Clinical severity varies considerably, and many affected individuals have very little bleeding unless challenged by surgery. This disorder was first described by Dr Erik von Willebrand of Helsinki, Finland, in 1926.[31] He studied a large kindred from the Åland Islands, many of whom had mucous membrane bleeding. Several family members died in childhood as a result of uncontrollable bleeding. Both males and females were affected, but bleeding was often more severe and problematic in young women, due to menorrhagia. von Willebrand found that affected individuals had normal numbers of platelets but prolonged bleeding times (BT). For some time thereafter, the diagnosis of VWD was based on the findings of mucous membrane bleeding, a normal platelet count with prolonged BT, and an autosomal dominant inheritance pattern. Now, however, our understanding of this disorder has greatly improved. It is now known that the basic underlying defect in VWD is in von Willebrand factor (VWF), a large, multimeric plasma glycoprotein that is synthesized in endothelial cells and megakaryocytes. VWF has two major functions. It serves as a 'bridge' between platelets and injury sites in the vessel wall, and forms a complex with FVIII, protecting the latter from rapid proteolytic degradation in the circulation.

VWF circulates as a series of multimers of increasing size, the largest having a molecular weight of 20 000 kDa. The multimers consist of protomers of about 500 kDa; each protomer is made up of two identical subunits of 220 kDa. This repeating structure provides a large number of binding sites, allowing vWF to serve as a bridge between platelets, and between platelets and injury sites in the vessel wall. The multimeric structure of VWF can be visualized by multimeric analysis; utilizing electrophoresis of plasma in SDS gels, and autoradiography, one can observe the variant structures of VWF.

Revised classification for VWD types[32] and abbreviations[33] have been recommended by the von Willebrand Subcommittee of the International Society of Thrombosis and Haemostasis (ISTH).

The diagnosis of VWD is made based on the patient's history, family history (autosomal dominant inheritance pattern), and a series of laboratory tests (Table 11.13). The ristocetin cofactor assay gives the closest approximation to VWF functional activity (although some prefer the collagen-binding assay for this purpose). Many things influence FVIII and VWF levels (adrenaline, ABO blood type,[34] hyperthyroidism, pregnancy, stress, etc.)

The most common form of VWD (accounting for approximately 80% of cases) is type 1. It is characterized by a prolonged BT and proportionately decreased levels of FVIII, VWF and VWF : Ag, and a normal multimeric structure of VWF. Affected individuals do not produce enough VWF, but what they do produce is structurally and functionally normal.

In the type 2 variants (which account for about 20% of cases), the haemostatically important higher MW forms of VWF are absent. Among the type 2 variants, the most common subtypes are 2A and 2B. In VWD type 2A, a genetic mutation in the A2 domain produces a VWF that is very susceptible to proteolysis. Affected individuals may have a normal or only slightly reduced levels of VWF and FVIII, lack the high- and intermediate-molecular-weight multimers of VWF, and generally have a mild to moderate bleeding tendency. In type 2B, missense mutations in the A1 domain result in a heightened affinity of VWF binding to platelets (platelet GP 1b/IX). The patient's VWF spontaneously binds to platelets and is unusually sensitive to the reagent ristocetin. Affected individuals often have some degree of thrombocytopenia due to in vivo platelet aggregation, and in vitro their platelets agglutinate with very low concentrations of ristocetin (enhanced ristocetin-induced platelet aggregation).

VWD type 2N (Normandy variant) is an uncommon variant in which the mutation in VWF prevents the binding of FVIII, but does not interfere with platelet adhesion. Unprotected FVIII is rapidly degraded in the circulation, resulting in low levels of FVIII, mimicking mild haemophilia A.[32,35]

In type 3 VWD, which is rare, individuals have inherited two genes for VWD (homozygous or doubly heterozygous). This is the most severe form of VWD, with very low or undetectable levels of VWF and FVIII. In addition to severe mucous membrane bleeding, affected persons often have bleeding into joints and muscles.

Treatment of vWD

Treatment depends on the type of VWD. Desmopressin is the treatment of choice for the most common form, VWD type 1, and may be of some benefit in type 2A. When given intravenously in the recommended dosage of 0.3 µg/kg, it will effect a rapid three-fold (range 2- to 10-fold) increase in VWF, and a transient shortening of the BT (and cessation of bleeding). If repeat doses are needed, they are generally given daily. Tachyphylaxis (diminishing response) is considerably less in VWD than in mild haemophilia.[36]

The effectiveness of desmopressin results from the rapid release of VWF (and FVIII) from storage sites. The drug will be ineffective in VWD type 3, since there is nothing in the stores to be released. It is generally thought to be contraindicated in VWD type 2B, since the VWF released will be abnormal, with a heightened affinity for platelets (thus, there is no beneficial effect on haemostasis, and a likelihood of in vivo platelet agglutination and a rapid drop in platelets).

There are several formulations of desmopressin for intravenous, subcutaneous, and intranasal use. The highly concentrated Stimate nasal spray (Table 11.10) is ideal for home or outpatient use. It results in an increase of VWF similar to that achieved with an intravenous dose of 0.2 µg/kg. The compression-metered spray pump delivers 0.1 ml (150 µg) per activation of the pump. The recommended dose is one spray (in one nostril) for children and adolescents less than 50 kg body weight, and two sprays (one in each nostril) for adults. The intranasal spray is very effective in most women with VWD type 1 who have menorrhagia (given at the onset of menses, with a second dose given the next day), and in persons with VWD type 1 pre-invasive dentistry, preoperatively, or pre contact sports (such as soccer).

For persons whose responses to desmopressin are not sufficient, or who are not candidates for desmopressin (e.g. those with type 2 or 3 VWD), one should use an intermediate purity, plasma-derived FVIII concentrate rich in the higher-molecular-weight multimers of VWF.[37,38] As of April 2002, the only such product that has been licensed for this indication (i.e. use in VWD) by the US Food and Drug Administration is Humate-P (Table

11.3). However, other products have also been used to treat bleeding in persons with type 2 or 3 VWD (e.g. AlphaNine SD; Table 11.6). Some products include the ristocetin cofactor (VWF : RCo) units on the label, while others list only the FVIII content.

For dosage calculation, for severe bleeding episodes or for surgical coverage, many use a FVIII dosage of 40–60 IU/kg, given twice daily.

Other agents that may be useful in treating bleeding in vWD

The antifibrinolytic agents ε-aminocaproic acid (EACA) and tranexamic acid are useful adjuncts in treating bleeding in the oral cavity. As in haemophilia A and B, and other hereditary disorders of blood coagulation, the usual dosage for EACA is 75 mg/kg/dose, given every 6 hours for 7–10 days. The usual dose of tranexamic acid is 25 mg/kg, given three times daily. For invasive dentistry, EACA or tranexamic acid should be started the evening before the procedure. Such drugs should be given in conjunction with an agent that will result in clot formation (e.g. desmopressin or an intermediate-purity, plasma-derived FVIII concentrate rich in the higher-molecular-weight multimers of VWF).

Oral contraceptive agents may also be helpful in alleviating menorrhagia in women with VWD. As is the case for all coagulopathies, individuals with VWD should avoid the use of aspirin, all aspirin-containing compounds, and other drugs known to interfere with platelet function.

Other inherited disorders of coagulation

Hereditary deficiencies of all the other coagulation factors have been described, but these are rare. These deficiency states are heterogenous, and not all affected families with a particular deficiency have the same degree of bleeding. For most of these rare disorders, no specific concentrates are licensed and readily available in the USA; however, for some of them, a concentrate is available through a pre-licensure clinical trial mechanism, or through off-label use. The treatment for most of these disorders is still fresh-frozen plasma (FFP) – either solvent–detergent treated FFP – or donor retested FFP – or cryoprecipitate. In most of these conditions, the level required to achieve haemostasis is low, and can be attained by plasma in a dosage of 10 ml/kg. Once bleeding has stopped, continued treatment is generally unnecessary. However, both plasma and cryoprecipitate have the disadvantages of potential bloodborne viral transmission, allergic reactions, and volume overload.

Bleeding in persons with congenital afibrinogenaemia or hypofibrinogenaemia should be treated with cryoprecipitate in a dosage of 4 bags/10 kg body weight (cryoprecipitate contains, on average, 200 mg of fibrinogen per bag, or 'unit'). Because of the long half-life of fibrinogen, additional doses, if necessary, are given every 3–4 days at a dosage of 2 bags/10 kg.

In hereditary deficiencies of FII (prothrombin), FVII, or FX, plasma or a prothrombin complex concentrate (PCC) can be used. For serious, life-threatening bleeding, a PCC should be used in order to attain higher levels. In the case of FVII deficiency, NovoSeven (Table 11.9) should be used – this is a very high-purity rFVIIa product, and high levels can be attained if needed. For FV deficiency, FFP should be used. Deficiencies of the 'contact factors', FXII (Hageman factor), prekallikrein (Fletcher factor), and HMW kininogen (Fitzgerald factor) are rarely associated with bleeding, and thus do not require treatment, even for surgery. In FXI deficiency (which is more common in persons of Ashkenazi Jewish descent), the bleeding tendency is usually mild. However, some affected individuals have epistaxis, excessive bruising, menorrhagia, and excessive bleeding with surgery. The half-life of transfused FXI is 60–80 hours. Although a plasma-derived FXI concentrate was produced in the UK, it is currently not being produced (because of concerns about new variant Creutzfeldt–Jakob disease. FFP, 10–20 ml/kg/day, usually provides sufficient FXI to maintain haemostasis in those affected individuals who bleed. The APTT, or a FXI assay can be used to monitor treatment.

Congenital deficiency of FXIII (fibrin-stabilizing factor) is a rare disorder, with autosomal recessive inheritance, that is characterized by umbilical stump bleeding in neonates, excessive bruising, and delayed wound healing. Epistaxis, gum bleeding, musculoskeletal bleeding, and severe intracranial haemorrhage have also been reported. Only homozygous individuals with no detectable levels of FXIII activity have bleeding manifestations. While routine coagulation screening tests (PT, APTT, and thrombin time) are normal, the diagnosis can be made by testing for clot solubility in 5 M urea (normal clots remain insoluble for 24 hours), or by assaying the patient's plasma for FXIII. Low concentrations of FXIII (0.01–0.05 U/ml of plasma) appear to be sufficient for adequate haemostasis. Although not yet licensed, Fibrogammin (Aventis-Behring) is available on a clinical-

trial basis for patients with severe FXIII deficiency. Because of the long half-life of FXIII, prophylactic dosing (250 U in children and 500 U in adults) is given once monthly. If this drug is not readily available, a single dose of plasma of 5–10 ml/kg will usually suffice for bleeding episodes.

ACQUIRED COAGULATION DISORDERS

Acquired coagulation disorders are abnormalities in blood coagulation secondary to a large number of disorders. In contrast to the inherited coagulation disorders, which are often characterized by a single-factor deficiency, acquired disorders are complex and associated with multiple haemostatic abnormalities, including thrombocytopenia, platelet function defects, and vascular abnormalities. Furthermore, there is poor correlation between severity of bleeding and laboratory tests. While no specific replacement therapy exists, treatment of the underlying disorder is sometimes helpful in ameliorating the bleeding. The following are the most common acquired bleeding disorders.

Vitamin K deficiency bleeding (VKDB)

The term VKDB is preferred to 'haemorrhagic disease of the Newborn' (HDN), since not all bleeding in the newborn is due to vitamin K (VK) deficiency and bleeding due to VKDB is not necessarily confined to the newborn.[39] The diagnosis is confirmed when bleeding is rapidly reversed following VK administration and other causes of coagulopathy such as disseminated intravascular coagulation (DIC), inherited coagulation disorders, and other causes have been excluded.

In the newborn, VKDB is classified into early, classical, and late, based on the age of presentation. *Early VKDB* is characterized by bleeding within the first 24 hours of life, and is due to maternal ingestion of medications such as anticonvulsants, warfarin, cephalosporins, rifampicin, and isoniazid. The incidence of VKBD in newborns of such mothers without VK supplementation is 6–12%.[40] *Classic VKDB* occurs between 1 and 7 days (mostly 3–5 days) of life, and is seen in breast-fed newborns with poor intake or delayed onset of feeding. Significant blood loss can occur from the gastrointestinal tract, puncture sites, umbilicus, intracranial haemorrhage (ICH) and widespread ecchymosis. *Late VKDB* occurs between 2 and 6 months of age. It is classically seen in breast-fed infants (low VK content) and in infants with underlying liver disease. It is associated with a high incidence of ICH (59%) and long-term morbidity and mortality (30%).[39,40]

Laboratory diagnosis of VKDB is established by a prolonged PT and APTT, and normal platelet counts, fibrinogen, FV and FVIII. Specific factor assays reveal deficiencies in VK-dependent factors (FII, FVII, FIX and FX) and an elevation of proteins induced by VK absence (PIVKA) – the non-carboxylated forms of VK-dependent factors.

Prevention of VKBD is accomplished by prophylactic administration of VK either as a single intramuscular dose of 0.5–1 mg or an oral dose of 2–4 mg at birth. The main disadvantages of oral prophylaxis are erratic gastrointestinal absorption, parental compliance, and short half-life. To increase the efficacy of oral VK prophylaxis, weekly dosing (1 mg weekly or 25–50 µg daily) for a longer interval (5 weeks–3 months) should be considered.

Newborns with suspected VKDB should be treated with subcutaneous (preferred route) or intravenous VK in doses ranging from 2–10 mg. The response to oral VK, as measured by correction of PT, is slower (6–8 hours) compared with parenteral VK (2–6 hours). Intravenous VK may be associated with haemolysis, and should be administered slowly (1 mg/min). The intramuscular route should be avoided because of pain and haematoma formation. Patients with life-threatening haemorrhage may benefit from FFP (10–20 ml/kg) or PCCs (50 U/kg) in addition to VK.[40]

Other causes of VKDB, which can occur at all ages, include diseases that interfere with the absorption of VK, such as biliary atresia, cystic fibrosis, and malabsorption syndromes (sprue, coeliac disease, ulcerative colitis, regional enteritis, and intestinal parasites such as ascariasis and idiopathic steatorrhoea). VK deficiency may also result from drugs such as warfarin and cholestyramine.[41]

For patients with bleeding manifestations, besides FFP, VK and tranexamic acid have been used. Reversal of warfarin anticoagulation is accomplished with oral or (more rapidly) with intravenous VK.[42,43] rFVIIa has been used successfully for the treatment of warfarin bleeding. Berntorp[44] reported successful reversal of warfarin anticoagulation in a 60-year-old woman with profuse epistaxis with 90 µg/kg of rFVIIa. High levels of VK-dependent coagulation factors were seen following rFVIIa administration.

Disseminated intravascular coagulation (DIC)

The subcommittee on DIC of the ISTH's Scientific and Standardization Committee (SSC) recently proposed the following definition:[45] 'DIC is an acquired syndrome characterized by intravascular activation of coagulation with loss of localization arising from different causes. It can originate from and cause damage to the microvasculature which if sufficiently severe can produce organ dysfunction.' The causes of DIC are multiple – the most common are listed in Table 11.14. DIC is encountered in 30–50% of patients with Gram-negative sepsis, in 50–70% of those with severe trauma, in 50% of obstetrical disorders, in 25% of giant haemangiomas, and in 10–15% of malignancies.[46,47] Multiple initiating pathways eventually lead to excess thrombin formation, with subsequent systemic fibrin formation. Impaired fibrinolysis and suppression of physiologic anticoagulation also play a pivotal role.

The major mechanisms involved in DIC are as follows. Endotoxin and cytokines (interleukin (IL)-6, IL-1, and tumour necrosis factor α (TNF-α)) increase tissue factor (TF) expression on the surface of perturbed endothelium, activated monocytes, and injured organs.[46,47] Endothelial injury also results, besides TF expression, in increased synthesis of plasminogen activator inhibitor-1 (PAI-1), decreased thrombomodulin expression, and exposure of blood to collagen, which promotes platelet adherence and aggregation. Coagulation is initiated by activation of FVII by TF and results in the generation of thrombin. Inhibition of cytokines by monoclonal anti-IL-6 and of TF by recombinant tissue factor pathway inhibitor (TFPI), as well as inhibition of FVIIa, have resulted in suppression of endotoxin generation of thrombin.[46,48] Although the intrinsic pathway contributes to vasodilatation and hypotension

Table 11.14 Common causes of disseminated intravascular coagulation (DIC)

- Sepsis (bacterial, viral, fungal, rickettsial, and protozoal infections)
- Obstetric causes:
  - Amniotic fluid embolism
  - Abruptio placentae
  - Dead fetus syndrome
  - Pre-eclampsia
- Trauma
- Vascular abnormalities:
  - Giant haemangiomas (Kasabach–Merritt syndrome)
  - Aortic aneurysm
- Malignancies: leukaemia and solid tumours
- Toxins and venoms
- Immunologic causes:
  - Transfusion reaction
  - Severe allergy
  - Graft rejection
  - Severe collagen vascular disease
- Miscellaneous:
  - Haemolytic–uremic syndrome
  - Thrombotic thrombocytopenic purpura
  - Infusion of prothrombin complex concentrates
  - Hypothermia and hyperthermia
  - Burns
- Newborn:
  - Meconium aspiration
  - Hyaline membrane disease
  - Purpura fulminans (homozygous protein C deficiency)

via the activation of FXII and the kallikrein–kinin system, it is not the primary pathway and its inhibition does not affect endotoxin activation of coagulation.

In DIC, all naturally occurring circulating anticoagulants such as antithrombin III (ATIII), protein C, protein S, and TFPI are decreased, further aggravating hypercoagulable states. A combination of decreased hepatic synthesis and cytokine dysregulation of thrombomodulin accounts for the decrease in circulating anticoagulants. Fibrinolysis mediated by plasmin is crucial in determining the clinical picture in DIC. In the initial stages, fibrinolysis is suppressed, and excess thrombin results in microvascular thrombosis and organ ischaemia. Thrombin induces release of tissue plasminogen activator (t-PA), which activates plasminogen to plasmin. The latter degrades primarily fibrin and to some extent fibrinogen, FV, FVIII, and FXIII. Excess plasmin generation coupled with inhibition of fibrin polymerization by fibrin(ogen) degradation products (fragments X, Y, D, and E) results in bleeding.[46,48]

Clinical manifestations

DIC can be acute or chronic. Acute DIC is often due to sepsis, trauma, obstetric disorders, purpura fulminans, liver diseases, and snake venom, whereas chronic DIC is encountered in cases of cancer, retained dead fetus syndrome, and liver disease. DIC can be overt or non-overt, depending on whether the hemostatic system is decompensated or compensated. Overt DIC can be 'controlled' when the process reverses when the predisposing condition is removed or stopped (e.g. abruptio placentae) or 'uncontrolled' when the DIC overrides the regulatory mechanisms (e.g. sepsis and trauma).[45] The consumptive coagu-

lopathy can be 'disseminated', as described in the above situations, or 'localized'. Localized consumptive coagulopathy occurs in haemangiomas, aortic aneurysm, and renal disease such as haemolytic–uraemic syndrome (HUS).

Acute DIC may present with signs of microvascular thrombosis or bleeding diathesis. Both manifestations are organ-specific. For instance, in the skin, necrosis, petechiae and ecchymoses may occur. Renal signs include oliguria, azotaemia and haematuria. Neurologic manifestations include delirium, coma or ICH. There may be massive gastrointestinal bleeding or pulmonary haemorrhage resembling acute respiratory distress syndrome (ARDS). Haemolytic anaemia and mucous membrane bleeding can also occur.[49,50] In sick newborns, DIC is often due to bacterial or viral sepsis, hyaline membrane disease, homozygous protein C deficiency, and meconium or amniotic fluid aspiration.[49]

DIC is commonly encountered in head trauma, and has been reported in 22.2% of children with severe head injury.[51,52] Coagulopathy, often secondary to parenchymal brain damage, occurs owing to the release of TF and phospholipid and cytokine damage of endothelium. Hymel et al[53] reported mild prolongation of PT and APTT in 54% and 24% of child abuse patients ($n = 101$), respectively, with parenchymal brain damage. In children with head trauma but without parenchymal brain damage ($n = 46$), 20% had prolonged PT and 27% had prolonged APTT. Factor assays were not reported in these patients.

Vascular disorders such as large aortic aneurysms or giant haemangiomas (Kasabach–Merritt syndrome, KMS) may be associated with thrombocytopenia and localized consumptive coagulopathy.[54] KMS, a vascular malformation, can be cutaneous or visceral, single or multiple, and can grow rapidly and produce local compression and haemorrhage. The thrombocytopenia in KMS is due to platelet trapping and is often severe; hypofibrinogenaemia is prominent and fibrin degradation products are elevated. Red cell fragmentation is evident on the peripheral smear. Treatment options include surgery (for single small tumours), corticosteroids, anticoagulants (low-dose heparin, ATIII concentrates) antiplatelet agents (aspirin ticlopidine), and antifibrinolytics.[54]

There is no specific test for the laboratory diagnosis of DIC. The most common abnormalities seen in DIC are thrombocytopenia (98% of cases) and elevated D-dimers (93%). PT is prolonged in 75% and APTT in approximately 60% of cases, and there may be a depletion of coagulation factors.[47] ATIII levels in the blood may be low and fibrinogen levels may be variable. Assays for detection of prothrombin activation such as fragment F_{1+2} or thrombin–antithrombin (TAT) complexes may not be widely available. Tests for assessment of fibrinolytic activity such as euglobulin lysis time and plasminogen may be helpful.

Management consists of prompt and vigorous treatment of the underlying disorder. Treatment of haemostatic abnormalities depends on the severity of the clinical manifestation. Supportive care for clinically significant bleeding may require packed cells, platelets, and FFP (10–20 ml/kg every 8–12 hours). Cryoprecipitate may be helpful in cases of hypofibrinogenaemia. The dose of cryoprecipitate is 1 bag/5 kg body weight (continued until fibrinogen is >75 mg/dl). Moscardó et al[55] successfully used rFVIIa in the treatment of severe intra-abdominal bleeding associated with DIC in a woman following caesarean section. Haemostasis was achieved using rFVIIa 90 µg/kg at 3-hourly intervals for nine doses. Although coagulation factor concentrates such as rFVIIa are a low-volume alternative to infusions of large volumes of plasma, their high cost may be a limiting factor.

Unfractionated heparin has been widely used in the treatment of DIC associated with clinically overt thromboembolism, purpura fulminans, and deposition of fibrin; its major drawback has been increased bleeding complications. The dose of heparin in adults is a 5000 U bolus followed by 1000 U/h (or 15–20 U/kg/h). In the presence of hypofibrinogenaemia and thrombocytopenia, a continuous infusion of low-dose heparin 5–10 U/kg/h or 300–500 U/h combined with platelet and FFP support may suffice.[50] In children, heparin is administered as a bolus of 75 U/kg over 10 minutes followed by a continuous infusion of 28 U/kg/h for infants younger than 1 year and 20 U/kg/h for children older than 1 year. The dose of heparin is adjusted to maintain an APTT of 60–85 seconds.

Low-molecular-weight heparin (LMWH) has also been used in DIC as an alternate to low-dose heparin for thromboprophylaxis. In a randomized clinical trial comparing unfractionated heparin with LMWH, although there was no difference in mortality, the LMWH group demonstrated improved bleeding symptoms and organ failure scores.[46] Recombinant hirudin (desiurdin), an ATIII-independent inhibitor of thrombin, may be more effective than heparin, but so far, no clinical trials regarding its use in DIC have been reported.[47,56]

ATIII is a natural anticoagulant, has potent anti-inflammatory properties, and may shorten the duration of DIC. ATIII concentrates have shown survival benefits in sepsis-induced DIC. A recent multicentre phase III trial, however, failed to confirm benefit of ATIII concentrates in adult sepsis.[57] Recombinant TFPI may block TF activity, and has shown promising results in animals.[58] It is currently in phase III studies in humans. A specific inhibitor of the ternary complex between TF, FVIIa, and FXa (recombinant nematode anticoagulant protein c2, rNAPc2) is also under clinical evaluation.[59,60]

Meningococcal septicaemia in association with purpura fulminans and acquired protein C deficiency has a mortality rate in excess of 50%. White et al[61] treated 36 patients (aged 3 months–72 years) with meningococcal septicaemia with protein C concentrates; death occurred in only 8% (3 of 36) as compared with the predicted mortality rate of 50%. The protein C concentrate used in this study was manufactured by monoclonal antibody purification of viral-inactivated PCC by Baxter Hyland-Immuno (Vienna). After an initial test dose (10 IU/kg intravenous over 10 minutes), a loading dose of 100 IU/kg followed by a continuous infusion of 10 IU/kg/h was administered. The dose was adjusted on a daily basis to maintain a plasma protein C level of 80–120 IU/ml. Protein C concentrates in severe meningococcal septicaemia was associated with a reduction in predicted morbidity and mortality.

Systemic fibrin(ogen)olysis

Physiologic fibrinolysis is a localized response to thrombosis, and is necessary for re-establishment of blood flow. Plasminogen is activated to plasmin, a serine protease, by t-PA, which is primarily located on the vascular endothelium and urokinase-plasminogen activator (u-PA), which is normally present in the urine. PAI-1 inhibits t-PA and u-PA, and is synthesized by the endothelium and liver. Once plasmin is formed, it degrades fibrin and fibrinogen to several fragments (E, X, D, and Y). Crosslinked fibrin is cleaved to D-dimers, which can be assayed in the laboratory and serve as a clinical marker for fibrinolysis. α_2-Antiplasmin inhibits plasmin. FXIII crosslinks α_2-antiplasmin to fibrin, making it more resistant to the action of plasmin.[49]

Spontaneous systemic fibrinolysis is a pathologic event associated with bleeding in which degradation of fibrin/fibrinogen occurs in the circulation. Excess fibrinolysis may occur as an 'inappropriate' response to DIC or may result from an inherited or acquired deficiency of fibrinolytic mechanism.

The most common cause of systemic fibrinolysis is liver disease. Plasminogen activator levels are increased owing to decreased clearance coupled with decreased production of PAI-1. Other causes include urogenital neoplasm (associated with increased secretion of urokinase), acute promyelocytic leukaemia (APL cells contain TF and plasminogen activator), primary amyloidosis, immediate puerperium, cardiopulmonary bypass, and inherited PAI-1 and α_2-antiplasmin deficiency. Iatrogenic causes include therapeutic administration of plasminogen activators (t-PA, strep tokinase, or urokinase).[62]

It is difficult to distinguish between DIC and primary fibrinolysis by laboratory tests; a normal platelet count coupled with a short clot lysis time may indicate fibrinolysis. Treatment consists of replacement of deficient haemostatic factors and heparin. The use of antifibrinolytics is hazardous, and may lead to further clotting and organ ischaemia.

Liver disease

The liver is the major site of synthesis of activators and inhibitors of coagulation and fibrinolysis, with the exception of vWF, FVIII, t-PA and u-PA. Haemorrhagic complications are common in patients with acute and chronic liver diseases and liver transplantation. Coagulopathies secondary to liver disease reflect failure of synthesis of coagulation proteins, poor clearance of activated factors, activation of coagulation and fibrinolytic systems, and loss of haemostatic proteins. Cholestasis often results in VK deficiency, and thrombocytopenia occurs because of splenic sequestration and increased clearance. Acute liver failure due to hepatitis (either infectious or drug-induced) may present with ecchymosis, epistaxis, petechiae, and gastrointestinal bleeding. Cirrhotic patients are at increased risk of bleeding with routine procedures such as dental extraction, liver biopsies, and central-line placements.[63]

Coagulation screening tests such as PT, APTT, and thrombin clotting time are usually prolonged in liver disease. Plasma levels of FV and FVII are decreased; FVIII levels are usually normal, and reflect extrahepatic synthesis. Fibrinogen levels are variable, and D-dimers are elevated in liver disease owing to decreased clearance and further aggravate platelet dysfunction. Secondary VK deficiency due to poor absorption because of cholestasis and DIC may further contribute to the coagulation abnormalities.[63,64]

FFP, VK, cryoprecipitate, and desmopressin are short-term haemostatic measures currently available for the treatment of bleeding for patients with liver disease. rFVIIa in doses ranging from 5–80 µg/kg has been found to be an effective haemostatic agent allowing for liver biopsies and other procedures in cirrhotic patients without the risk of systemic activation of coagulation.[65] Exchange transfusion combined with platelet transfusion may be effective in controlling bleeding in acute liver failure. The clinical benefits of desmopressin, ATIII, and antifibrinolytics remain uncertain.

Renal disease

Haemostatic defects in renal disease include platelet function abnormalities, endothelial cell dysfunction and abnormal platelet–vessel wall interaction. There appears to be no correlation between vWF and the platelet function abnormalities.[66] Plasma levels of vWF are increased, but its multimeric structure is normal. Uraemic bleeding in chronic renal failure is often due to associated platelet dysfunction, as evidenced by prolonged bleeding time, decreased adhesion, and defective aggregation and release. These defects are partially corrected by dialysis, and implicate circulating 'uraemic toxin' (guanidosuccinic acid, phenol, and phenolic acids) in the pathogenesis of the platelet function defect.[66,67] Furthermore, patients with renal disease are treated with a variety of drugs that may augment the platelet defect and provoke bleeding. These include aspirin (to prevent thrombosis of dialysis graft), heparin during haemodialysis, and non-steroidal anti-inflammatory drugs. Haematocrit plays a major role in primary haemostasis by influencing blood viscosity and platelet adhesion. The majority of patients with uraemia are anaemic. Raising the haematocrit above 30%, either by packed red cell transfusions or the use of erythropoietin, shortens and sometimes corrects the bleeding time.[67]

Clinical manifestations of bleeding in uraemic patients are mucosal (purpura and epistaxis) or gastrointestinal, and reflect abnormal primary haemostasis. Serious haemorrhages such as intracranial, retroperitoneal, and pulmonary may also occur and are often induced by heparin. Patients with uraemia have prolonged bleeding times but usually normal PT and APTT. There is no correlation between prolongation of bleeding time and clinical bleeding. PT or APTT may be abnormal because of concomitant heparin use or VK deficiency due to poor nutrition.

Treatment of bleeding episodes in uraemic patients consists of aggressive dialysis, the use of desmopressin, cryoprecipitate, estrogens, and progesterone and correction of anaemia by transfusions or erythropoietin.[67]

Thrombotic thrombocytopenic purpura (TTP) and haemolytic–uraemic syndrome (HUS)

TTP, first described by Moschcowitz, is characterized by fever, haemolytic anaemia, impaired renal and neurologic functions, and thrombocytopenia. The clinical features of HUS, as described by Gasser, include thrombocytopenia, haemolytic anaemia, and impaired renal function.[68] HUS is classified based on the presence or absence of prodromal diarrhoea as diarrhoea-positive (D+ HUS, which is more common in children) or diarrhoea-negative (D− HUS, which is more common in adults). Many consider TTP and HUS to be variants of the same disorder, although TTP usually occurs in adults and neurologic symptoms predominate, whereas HUS occurs mainly in children and is associated with symptoms of renal damage.[68] However, some cases of TTP can present with severe renal manifestations, and likewise patients with HUS may express extrarenal signs, making it difficult to distinguish the two. Epidemic HUS in children is associated with *Escherichia coli* 0157 : H7 infections, and is characterized by bloody diarrhoea and renal failure. More recently, some differences in the pathophysiology of TTP and HUS have begun to emerge. Furlan et al[69] reported deficient vWF-cleaving protease activity in TTP and normal activity in HUS. The deficient vWF-cleaving protease accounted for unusually large vWF multimers in the plasma that agglutinated circulating platelets under high shear stress and caused arteriolar thrombi. Non-familial TTP appeared to be due to an inhibitor of vWF-cleaving protease, whereas the familial form seemed to be caused by a constitutional deficiency of the protease enzyme. Other recent advances in the study of TTP–HUS have shown that plasma from D− HUS and idiopathic TTP induces apoptosis in microvasculature of many tissues. Some D− HUS patients have decreased serum complement levels owing to activation of alternative complement pathways.[68]

Treatment of HUS in children consists of supportive care. Adults with TTP are often treated with transfusion of FFP or plasma exchange using FFP, or cryoprecipitate-poor plasma (to avoid giving vWF). The survival with plasma exchange is 80%. Other treatment modalities with variable success have included corticosteroids, splenectomy, vincristine, antiplatelet agents such as aspirin, and dipyridamole.

Antiphospholipid antibody syndrome (APS)

APS is an autoimmune disorder due to antiphospholipid antibodies (APLA). The latter are autoantibodies (IgG, IgM, IgA, or a mixture) directed against phospholipid-bound plasma protein such as prothrombin and β_2-glycoprotein-I. APS can occur in healthy individuals (adults and children), and is often detected as an incidental finding on a routine preoperative screening.[70] It has been reported in a variety of clinical disorders, including autoimmune disorders such as primary antiphospholipid syndrome (PAPS), and systemic lupus erythematosis (SLE), malignancies, infections, drug-related disorders, neurologic disorders, liver disease, and sickle cell disease. Clinical manifestations of APS include thrombosis (arterial and venous), fetal loss, thrombocytopenia, and haemolytic anaemia and bleeding.[71] Approximately 30–40% of adults with APS present with thromboembolic events and 50% with mild thrombocytopenia; bleeding complications are rare.[70] Male et al[72] recently described the spectrum of APS in children: 84% (80 of 95) were asymptomatic, 10% had bleeding symptoms (purpura, bruising, gastrointestinal, epistaxis, and post-traumatic symptoms), 5% had thromboembolic events, and 1% had SLE. Transient hypoprothrombinaemia was seen in 8.5% (8 of 95) and 5 of 8 had bleeding symptoms. Thrombocytopenia (4%) and transient decreases in FIX (22%), FXI (13%), and FXII (29%) were also observed.

The diagnosis of APS is established by detection of lupus anticoagulant (LA) and anticardiolipin (aCL) antibodies. The presence of LA is made based on prolongation of phospholipid-dependent coagulation tests.[73] These include a prolonged APTT or dilute Russell viper venom test (DRVVT) that is not corrected with normal plasma.[74] ACL is determined by reactivity to cardiolipin in a solid-phase immunoassay. Clinical studies indicate that LA is a stronger risk factor for thrombosis than aCL.[70,74] Detection of LA helps to identify patients at risk of thrombosis, whereas measurement of aCL antibodies is of little value.

The treatment of APS is based on clinical manifestations. While thrombosis is a common manifestation, some patients may present with bleeding episodes due to hypoprothrombinaemia.[71,73] Asymptomatic patients with APS may need no treatment except during periods of prolonged immobilization. Patients with thrombosis and/or APS-associated fetal loss are candidates for antithrombotic therapy with LMWH or unfractionated heparin. Long-term oral anticoagulants and low-dose aspirin are often recommended for prevention of recurrent thrombosis. Monitoring of anticoagulation therapy by APTT is difficult and unreliable – hence, heparin assays by automated methodology, as well as prothrombin–proconvertin time and chromogenic FX assays are recommended. Besides anticoagulant therapy, immune-suppression with intravenous immunoglobulin (IVIG), corticosteroids, or cyclophosphamide are sometimes utilized to decrease antibody levels in symptomatic patients.

Acquired inhibitors of coagulation

Coagulation inhibitors are antibodies that inhibit the function of a specific coagulation factor by neutralizing it, or by promoting its rapid clearance, or by altering the clotting factor.[75] Coagulation inhibitors may occur as alloantibodies as a consequence of replacement therapy in patients with congenital factor deficiencies or as autoantibodies in patients with a previously normal coagulation. Alloantibodies to FVIII and FIX occur in 20–25% of cases of haemophilia A and 1–3% of haemophilia B.[22] They occur primarily in children. Autoantibodies to coagulation FI–FXIII, vWF, proteins C and S are rare, and occur in non-haemophilic individuals (mostly adults). They are seen in a variety of settings such as autoimmune disease (SLE, rheumatoid arthritis, and ulcerative colitis), liver disease, amyloidosis, and malignancies, and following the use of topical bovine thrombin and fibrin glue during surgery. Autoantibodies can also occur in the postpartum period and as a result of medications.[22]

Individuals with autoantibodies often present with severe rapidly expanding ecchymosis, mucous membrane bleeding such as epistaxis, gross haematuria, postoperative bleeding, and life-threatening haemorrhages; haemarthroses are rare. Non-haemophilic persons with FVIII autoantibody have a high mortality rate (15–22%) but may sometimes experience spontaneous remission.[22] Severe intracranial haemorrhage due to transplacental transfer of acquired FVIII inhibitor has been reported.[76]

Laboratory findings consist of an abnormal PT or APTT, and decreased or undetectable levels of clotting factors. Lack of correction on mixing studies (performed on a 1 : 1 mixture of patient's plasma and normal plasma) indicates the presence of a neutralizing antibody. Other indicators of inhibitors are a shortened plasma half-life of infused clotting factor, indicating rapid clearance.

Therapeutic approaches for inhibitor patients are based on the acuity of bleeding, and the potency and cross-reactivity of the inhibitor.[77] In haemophilias, the inhibitors may be transient or can be overcome by repeated or frequent infusions of higher than normal doses of factor concentrate. Treatment of bleeding episodes in high titre inhibitor patients (>5 BU) requires haemostatic agents that either do not cross-react (porcine FVIII) or bypass the need for FVIII or FIX.[78] These include PCCs, activated PCCs (aPCCs), and rFVIIa.[77,78] Dosing with these haemostatic agents is empiric, and there are no laboratory tests to monitor the effectiveness of treatment.

Temporary measures to stop bleeding in patients with acquired inhibitors include plasmapheresis and extracorporeal immuno-adsorption to decrease antibody titres[79] or immune suppression with steroids and IVIG.[80] rFVIIa has also been used in the management of amyloid-associated FX deficiency.[81]

Dilutional coagulopathy

Massive blood transfusion is defined as the administration of more than one blood volume (60–75 cm^3/kg) over 24 hours.[82] Such transfusions are usually administered in cases of trauma or haemorrhagic shock. They are complicated by dilutional coagulopathy, especially when replacement therapy consists of crystalloid, packed red cells, or hydroxyethyl-starch. Dilution of coagulation factors, platelet dysfunction, and impaired production of clotting factors because of tissue hypoxia due to hypotension may contribute to the 'diffuse coagulopathic bleeding'.[83] Treatment consists of transfusions of whole blood or FFP, platelets, and cryoprecipitate. More recently, rFVIIa has been used successfully as a low-volume alternative to FFP in achieving haemostasis in trauma patients.[83]

Cardiopulmonary bypass and extracorporeal membrane oxygenation (ECHMO)

Coagulation abnormalities in cardiopulmonary bypass (CPB) are multifactorial, resulting in intraoperative and postoperative bleeding. Dilutional coagulopathy coupled with a high concentration of heparin, platelet adhesion, thrombocytopenia, and systemic fibrinolysis all contribute to bleeding. During the first 15 minutes of bypass, the platelet count falls by 25–30% owing to exposure to the CPB devices. After initiation of CBP, plasminogen and α_2-antiplasmin levels fall, reflecting dilutional coagulopathy. During CPB, activation of fibrinolytic system occurs and D-dimer levels increase.[84] Administration of antifibrinolytics, prior to bypass, has significantly decreased blood loss. A similar reduction in blood loss was seen with aprotinin, a powerful inhibitor of α_2-antiplasmin and other serine proteases such as trypsin, kallikreins, and chymotrypsin.[85]

ECHMO is used in the treatment of life-threatening respiratory failure unresponsive to mechanical ventilation. It is used in newborns with respiratory failure, meconium aspiration syndrome, congenital diaphragmatic hernia, congenital heart disease repair, and persistent pulmonary hypertension.[86] It is also used in adults with cardiopulmonary failure. Heparinized venous blood is propelled through a membrane oxygenator for prolonged periods, warmed to body temperature, and returned to either the venous or the arterial system. Bleeding, thromboembolic events, hypoxia and exposure to blood products are potential complications of ECHMO.[87] Intracranial haemorrhages are of particular concern, and mediastinal haemorrhage occurs in 30% of cases of cardiac ECHMO. Activation of the haemostatic system, fibrinolysis, platelet adhesion with ensuing thrombocytopenia, and heparinization all contribute to the bleeding and thrombosis seen in these patients.[87] The role of antifibrinolytics and protease inhibitors in newborns undergoing ECHMO needs to be investigated further.

REFERENCES

1. Giannelli F, Green PM, Sommer SS et al. Haemophilia B. Database of point mutations and short additions and deletions. 8th Edition. *Nucleic Acids Res* 1998; **26**: 265–8.
2. Peake I. The molecular basis of haemophilia A. *Haemophilia* 1998; **4**: 346–9.
3. Lakich D, Kazazian HH Jr., Antonarakis SE, Gitschier J. Inversions disrupting the factor VIII gene are a common cause of severe hemophilia A. *Nat Genet* 1993; **5**: 238–41.
4. Rossiter JP, Young M, Kimberland ML et al. Factor VIII gene inversions causing severe hemophilia A originate almost exclusively in male germ cells. *Hum Mol Genet* 1994; **3**: 1035–9.
5. Lee CA. Transfusion-transmitted disease. *Baillière's Clin Haematol* 1996; **9**: 369–94.
6. Azzi A, Ciappi S, Zakrzewska K et al. Human parvovirus B19 infection in hemophiliacs first infused with two high-purity virally attenu-

ated factor VIII concentrates. *Am J Hematol* 1992; **39**: 228–30.

7. Mannucci PM, Gdovin S, Gringeri A et al. Transmission of hepatitis A to patients with hemophilia by factor VIII concentrates treated with organic solvent and detergent to inactivate viruses. *Ann Intern Med* 1994; **120**: 1–7.

8. Vehar GA, Keyt B, Eaton D et al. Structure of human factor VIII. *Nature* 1984; **312**: 337–42.

9. Toole JT, Knopf JL, Wozney JM et al. Molecular cloning of a cDNA encoding human antihemophilic factor. *Nature* 1984; **312**: 342–7.

10. Wood WI, Capon DJ, Simonsen CC et al. Expression of active human factor VIII from recombinant DNA clones. *Nature* 1984; **312**: 330–7.

11. Mikaelsson M, Oswaldsson Y, Sandberg H. Influences of phospholipids on the assessment of factor VIII activity. *Haemophilia* 1998; **4**: 646–50.

12. Sandberg H, Almstedt A, Brandt J et al. Structural and functional characteristics of the B-domain deleted recombinant factor VIII protein, r-VIII SQ. *Thromb Haemost* 2001; **85**: 93–100.

13. Nilsson I, Lethagen S. Current status of DDAVP formulations and their use. In: *Hemophilia and von Willebrand's Disease in the 1990's* (Lusher JM, Kessler CM, eds). Amsterdam: Excerpta Medica, 1991: 443–53.

14. Lusher JM. Myocardial infarction and stroke: Is the risk increased by desmopressin? In: *Desmopressin in Bleeding Disorders.* (Mariani G, Mannucci PM, Cattaneo, eds). New York: Plenum Press, 1993: 347–53.

15. Nilsson IM, Berntorp E, Lofqvist T et al. Twenty-five years experience of prophylactic treatment in severe haemophilia A and B. *J Intern Med* 1992; **232**: 25–32.

16. National Hemophilia Foundation. Medical and Scientific Advisory Council (MASAC) recommendations concerning prophylaxis.

Medical Bulletin 193, Chapter Advisory 197. New York: The National Hemophilia Foundation, 1994.

17. Lusher JM. Natural history of inhibitors in severe haemophilia A and B: incidence and prevalence. In: *Inhibitors in Patients with Haemophilia* (Rodriguez-Merchan EC, Lee CA, eds). Blackwell Publ., 2002 (in press).

18. Scharrer I, Bray GL, Neutzling O. Incidence of inhibitors in haemophilia A patients: a review of recent studies of recombinant and plasma-derived factor VIII concentrates. *Haemophilia* 1999; **5**: 145–54.

19. Kasper CK, Aledort LM, Counts RB et al. A more uniform measurement of factor VIII inhibitors. *Thromb Diath Haemorrh* 1975; **34**: 869–72.

20. Verbruggen B, Novakova I, Wessels H et al. The Nijmegen modification of the Bethesda assay for factor VIII inhibitors: improved specificity and reliability. *Thromb Haemost* 1995; **73**: 247–51.

21. Lusher JM. Treatment of congenital coagulopathies. In: *Transfusion Therapy: Clinical Principles and Practice.* (Mintz PD, ed). Bethesda, MD: AABB Press, 1999: 97–128.

22. Lusher JM. Inhibitor antibodies to factor VIII and factor IX: management. *Semin Thromb Haemost* 2000; **26**: 179–88.

23. Lusher JM. Inhibitors in young boys with hemophilia A and B. *Baillière's Clin Haematol* 2000; **13**: 457–68.

24. Hedner U, Ingerslev J. Clinical use of recombinant FVIIa. *Transfus Sci* 1998; **19**: 163–76.

25. Kernoff PBA. Porcine factor VIII: preparation and use in treatment of inhibitor patients. *Progr Clin Biol Res* 1984; **150**: 207–24.

26. High KA. Factor IX. Molecular structure, epitopes, and mutations associated with inhibitor formation. In: *Inhibitors to Coagulation Factors* (Aledort L, Hoyer L, Lusher J et al, eds). New York: Plenum Press, 1995: 79–86.

27. White GCII, Beebe A, Nielsen B. Recombinant factor IX. *Thromb Haemost* 1997; **78**: 261–5.

28. Ewenstein B, Takemoto C, Warrier I et al. Nephrotic syndrome as a complication of immune tolerance in hemophilia B. *Blood* 1997; **89**: 1115–16.

29. Warrier I, Ewenstein B, Koerper MA et al. Factor VIII inhibitors and anaphylaxis in haemophilia B. *J Pediatr Hematol Oncol* 1997; **19**: 23–7.

30. Rodeghiero F, Castaman G, Dini E. Epidemiologic investigation of the prevalence of von Willebrand's disease. *Blood* 1987; **69**: 454.

31. von Willebrand EA. Hereditar pseudohemofili. *Finska Lak Handl* 1926; **68**: 87.

32. Sadler JE, Matshshita T, Dong Z et al. Molecular mechanism and classification of von Willebrand disease. *Thromb Haemost* 1995; **74**: 161–6.

33. Mazurier C, Rodeghiero F. Recommended abbreviations for von Willebrand factor and its activities. *Thromb Haemost* 2001; **86**: 712.

34. Gill GC, Endres-Brooks J, Bauer PJ et al. The effect of ABO blood group on the diagnosis of von Willebrand disease. *Blood* 1987; **69**: 1691–5.

35. Gaucher C, Jorieux S, Mercier B et al. The 'Normandy' variant of von Willebrand's disease: characterization of a point mutation in the von Willebrand factor gene. *Blood* 1991; **77**: 1937–41.

36. Montgomery RR, Gill GC, Scott JP. Hemophilia and von Willebrand disease. In: *Nathan and Oski's Hematology of Infancy and Childhood*, 5th edn. (Nathan DG, Oski SH, eds). Philadelphia: WB Saunders, 1998: 1631–59.

37. Rodeghiero F, Castaman G, Mannucci PM. Clinical indications for desmopressin (DDAVP) in congenital and acquired von Willebrand disease. *Blood Rev* 1991; **5**: 155–61.

38. Rodeghiero F, Castaman G, Meyer D, Mannucci PM. Replacement therapy with virus-inactivated plasma concentrates in von Willebrand disease. *Vox Sang* 1992; **2**: 193–9.

39. Andrew M and Brooker LA. Hemostatic disorders in the newborns. In: *Avery's Diseases of the Newborn*, 7th edn. (Taeusch HW, Ballard RA, eds). Philadelphia: WB Saunders, 1998: 1045–79.

40. Sutor AH, von Kries R, Cornelissen EA et al. Vitamin K deficiency bleeding (VKDB) in infancy. ISTH Pediatric/Perinatal Subcommittee. International Society on Thrombosis and Haemostasis. *Thromb Haemost* 1999; **8**: 456–61.

41. Andrew M, Monagle M. Hemorrhagic and thromboembolic complications during infancy and childhood. In: *Hemostasis and Thrombosis: Basic Principles and Clinical Practice.* (Colman RW, Hirsh J, Marder VJ et al, eds). Philadelphia: Lippincott Williams & Wilkins, 2001: 1053–70.

42. Hung A, Singh S, Tait RC. A prospective randomized study to determine the optimal dose of intravenous vitamin K in reversal of over-warfarinization. *Br J Haematol* 2000; **109**: 537–9.

43. Watson HG, Baglin T, Laidlaw SL et al. A comparison of the efficacy and rate of response to oral and intravenous vitamin K in reversal of over-anticoagulation with warfarin. *Br J Haematol* 2001; **115**: 145–9.

44. Berntorp E. Recombinant factor VIIa in the treatment of warfarin bleeding. *Semin Thromb Hemost* 2000; **26**: 433–5.

45. Taylor Jr FB, Toh CH, Hoots KW et al. Scientific and Standardization Committee Communications: Towards a definition, clinical and laboratory criteria, and a scoring system for disseminated intravascular coagulation: On Behalf of the Scientific Subcommittee on Disseminated Intravascular Coagulation (DIC) of the International Society on Thrombosis and Haemostasis. http://www.med.unc.edu/isth/ssccomm.htm.

46. Levi M, ten Cate H. Disseminated intravascular coagulation. *N Engl J Med.* 1999; **341**: 586–92.

47. Levi M, de Jonge E, van der Poll T, ten Cate H. Disseminated intravascular coagulation. *Thromb Haemost* 1999; **82**: 695–705.

48. ten Cate H, Timmerman JJ, Levi M. The pathophysiology of disseminated intravascular coagulation. *Thromb Haemost* 1999; **82**: 713–17.

49. Edstorm CS, Christensen RD, Andrew M. Developmental aspect of blood hemostasis and disorders of coagulation and fibrinolysis in the neonatal period. In: *Hematologic Problems of the Neonate* (Christensen RD, ed). Philadelphia: WB Saunders, 2000: 239–71.

50. Levi M, de Jonge E. Current management of disseminated intravascular coagulation. *Hosp Pract* 2000; **35**: 59–66.

51. Chiaretti A, Pezzotti P, Mestrovic J et al. The influence of hemocoagulative disorders on the outcome of children with head injury. *Pediatr Neurosurg* 2001; **34**: 131–7.

52. Vora A, Markis M. An approach to investigation of easy bruising. *Arch Dis Child.* 2001; **84**: 488–91.

53. Hymel KP, Abshire TC, Luckey DW, Jenny C. Coagulopathy in pediatric abusive head trauma. *Pediatrics* 1997; **99**: 371–5.

54. Hall GA. Kasabach-Merritt Syndrome: pathogenesis and management. *Br J Haematol* 2001; **112**: 851–62.

55. Moscardó F, Pérez F, de la Rubia J et al. Successful treatment of severe intra-abdominal bleeding associated with disseminated intravascular coagulation using recombinant activated factor VII. *Br J Haematol* 2001; **114**: 174–6.

56. Miyake Y, Yokota K, Fujishima Y, Sukamoto T. The effects of danaparoid, dalteparin and heparin on tissue factor-induced experimental disseminated intravascular coagulation and bleeding time in the rat. *Blood Coagul Fibrinolysis* 2001; **12**: 349–57.

57. Krishnagopalan S, Phillip DR. Innovative therapies for sepsis. *Biodrugs* 2001; **15**: 645–54.

58. Creasey AA, Reinhart K. Tissue factor pathway inhibitor activity in severe sepsis. *Crit Care Med* 2001; **29**: 126–9.

59. Levi M, de Jonge E, van der Poll T. Rationale for restoration of physiological anticoagulant pathways in patients with sepsis and disseminated intravascular coagulation. *Crit Care Med* 2001; **29**: 90–4.

60. Levi M, de Jonge E, van der Poll T, ten Cate H. Novel approaches to the management of disseminated intravascular coagulation. *Crit Care Med* 2000; **28**: 20–4.

61. White B, Livingstone W, Murphy C et al. An open-label study of the role of adjuvant hemostatic support with protein C replacement therapy in purpura fulminans-associated meningococcemia. *Blood* 2000; **96**: 3719–24.

62. Alan BM, Grosset ABM, Rodgers GM. Acquired coagulation disorders. In: *Wintrobe's Clinical Hematology*, 10th edn. (Lee GL, Foerster J, Lukens J et al, eds) Baltimore, MD: Lippincott Williams & Wilkins, 1999: 1733–80.

63. Rapaport SI. Coagulation problems in liver disease *Blood Coagul Fibrinolysis* 2000; **11**: 69–74.

64. DeLoughery TG. Management of bleeding with uremia and liver disease. *Curr Opin Hematol* 1999; **6**: 329–33.

65. Bernstein D. Effectiveness of the recombinant factor VIIa in patients with the coagulopathy of advanced child's B and C cirrhosis. *Semin Thromb Hemost* 2000; **26**: 437–8.

66. Casonato A, Pontara E, Vertolli UP et al. Plasma and platelet von Willebrand factor abnormalities in patients with uremia: lack of correlation with uremic bleeding. *Clin Appl Thromb Hemost* 2001; **7**: 81–6.

67. Weigert AL and Schafer AI. Uremic bleeding: pathogenesis and therapy. *Curr Opin Hematol* 1998; **316**: 94–104.

68. Liu J, Hutzler M, Li C, Pechet L. Thrombotic thrombocytopenic purpura (TTP) and hemolytic uremic syndrome (HUS): the new thinking. *J Thromb Thrombolysis* 2001; **11**: 261–72.

69. Furlan M, Robles R, Galbusera M et al. von Willebrand factor-cleaving protease in

thrombotic thrombocytopenic purpura and the hemolytic-uremic syndrome. *N Engl J Med* 1998; **339**: 1578–84.

70. Arnout J. Antiphospholipid syndrome: diagnostic aspects of lupus anticoagulant. *Thromb Haemost* 2001; **86**: 83–91.

71. Schmugge M, Tolle S, Marbet GA et al. Gingival bleeding, epistaxis and haematoma three days after gastroenteritis: the haemorrhagic lupus anticoagulant syndrome. *Eur J Pediatr* 2001; **160**: 43–6.

72. Male C, Lechner K, Eichinger S et al. Clinical significance of lupus anticoagulants in children. *J Pediatr* 1999; **134**: 199–205.

73. Guerin J, Smith O, White B et al. Antibodies to prothrombin in antiphospholipid syndrome and inflammatory disorders. *Br J Haematol* 1998; **102**: 896–902.

74. Greaves M, Cohen H, MacHin SJ, Mackie I. Guidelines on the investigation and management of the antiphospholipid syndrome. *Br J Haematol* 2000; **109**: 704–15.

75. Macik BG, Crow P. Acquired autoantibodies to coagulation factors. *Curr Opin Hematol* 1999; **6**: 323–8.

76. Ries M, Wolfel D, Maier-Brandt B. Severe intracranial hemorrhage in a newborn infant with transplacental transfer of an acquired factor VII:C inhibitor. *J Pediatr* 1995; **127**: 649–50.

77. Kessler CM. New products for managing inhibitors to coagulation factors: a focus on recombinant factor VIIa concentrate. *Curr Opin Hematol* 2000; **7**: 408–13.

78. Penner JA. Management of haemophilia in patients with high-titer inhibitors: focus on the evolution of activated prothrombin complex concentrate AUTOPLEX T. *Haemophilia* 1999; **5**: 1–9.

79. Jansen M, Schmaldienst S, Banyai S et al. Treatment of coagulation inhibitors with extracorporeal immunoadsorption (Ig-Therasorb). *Br J Haematol* 2001; **112**: 91–7.

80. Robbins D, Kulkarni R, Gera R et al. Successful treatment of high titer inhibitors in mild hemophilia A with avoidance of factor VIII and immunosuppressive therapy. *Am J Hematol* 2001; **68**: 184–8.

81. Boggio L, Green D. Recombinant human factor VIIa in the management of amyloid-associated factor X deficiency. *Br J Haematol* 2001; **112**: 1074–5.

82. Goskowicz R. Perioperative use of anticoagulants and thrombolytics. The complications of massive blood transfusion. *Anesthesiol Clin North Am* 1999; **17**: 959–78.

83. Martinowitz U, Kenet G, Segal E et al. Recombinant activated factor VII for adjunctive hemorrhage control in trauma. *J Trauma* 2001; **51**: 431–9.

84. Bevan DH. Cardiac bypass haemostasis: putting blood through the mill. *Br J Haematol* 1999; **104**: 208–19.

85. Munoz JJ, Birkmeyer NJ, Birkmeyer JD et al. Is epsilon-aminocaproic acid as effective as aprotinin in reducing bleeding with cardiac surgery? A meta-analysis. *Circulation* 1999; **99**: 81–9.

86. Somme S, Liu DC. New trends in extracorporeal membrane oxygenation in newborn pulmonary diseases. *Artificial Organs* 2001; **25**: 633–7.

87. Muntean W. Coagulation and anticoagulation in extracorporeal membrane oxygenation. *Artificial Organs* 1999; **23**: 979–83.

12 Therapeutic apheresis

Mark E Brecher

INTRODUCTION

In 1914, Abel, Rowntree and Turner[1] coined the term plasmaphaeresis (from the Greek word *aphairesis* – a withdrawal). Their early experiments were for the relief of symptoms following bilateral nephrectomy in dogs. Although these experiments were associated with deaths (due to apparent overbleeding and hemorrhage), the improvement in the clinical condition of the animals successfully treated was 'marked'. The term apheresis has since been generalized to refer to the separation of blood into its components, removing one component, and returning the remainder. Thus, leukapheresis means the removal of leukocytes and erythrocytapheresis means the removal of erythrocytes. Alternative terminologies such as plasma exchange and red cell exchange are frequently used interchangeably for plasmapheresis and erythrocytapheresis, respectively. Some authors have suggested that the term 'plasma exchange' or therapeutic plasma exchange be reserved for low-volume procedures involving no more then 500–600 ml of plasma and plasmapheresis for large-volume procedures; however, these terms are frequently used interchangeably. Hemapheresis is also used as a broad term encompassing all apheresis procedures.

Despite the success of early experiments in animals, there was little clinical enthusiasm for the selective removal of blood components, since the technique was perceived as being cumbersome and time-consuming. It was not until the 1950s that the first human therapeutic application of such techniques was reported for the treatment of hyperviscosity syndrome, and it was only after cell separators became available in the 1970s that apheresis began to emerge as a standard of care for a variety of diseases.[2–6] This chapter serves as an introduction both to the science underlying apheresis therapy and to the clinical application of this technology.

OVERVIEW OF TECHNOLOGY

Apheresis instrumentation allows the separation of selected blood components (plasma, platelets, granulocytes, mononuclear cells, and red blood cells) and return of the remaining components to the patient. The selected components may be either treated and returned to the patient or disposed. Anticoagulation with citrate alone or in combination with heparin allows for the extracorporeal flow of blood through a one-time-use disposable sterile pathway. Flow rates of 30–150 ml/min from either central or peripheral venous access generally allow for the processing of one to two blood volumes in one to four hours.[7] The methodology of separation of blood components is by centrifugation or filtration, and the processing of blood may be either continuous or intermittent.

Differential centrifugation

Differential centrifugation has historically been the technology principally used in apheresis. With differential centrifugation, blood enters a rotating bowl, chamber, or tubular rotor, or a belt-shaped channel, and as the blood settles in the centrifugal field, blood components layer out based on relative density. The densest cells are the red blood cells, which are concentrated in the area where the gravitational forces are greatest, followed by granulocytes, mononuclear cells (including lymphocytes and peripheral blood progenitor cells), platelets, and plasma.

With *intermittent flow* (discontinuous flow), whole blood is processed in batches. With each cycle, the centrifuge device is filled; separation occurs until the red cell component fills the separation container. Then, collection of whole blood is temporally suspended as the chamber is emptied. The centrifuge chambers that are most commonly employed are modifications of the Latham bowl (Figure 12.1). This conically shaped chamber has a rotating seal through which blood enters the bottom and rises between two conical surfaces. The centrifugal forces cause a vertical interface between red blood cells (the outside layer) and plasma (the inside layer). *Continuous-flow* separators enable removal of components of different densities without interruption of processing. Use of continuous flow allows for smaller extracorporeal blood volumes and more rapid blood processing.

Filtration

Filtration-based systems allow for the separation of plasma from cellular elements.

Hollow-fiber systems consist of a bundle of narrow hollow fibers with perforations along their surfaces contained within a larger outer cylinder. As whole blood enters, the plasma passes through the pores along the fibers, leaving a more concentrated cell suspension to exit the fibers; plasma is collected from the outer enclosing cylinder. Similarly, flat-plate membrane systems allow whole blood to pass between two membranes, with plasma passing through the pores to be collected separately from the cellular elements. A second column with smaller pore sizes can be added. Cascade filtration (or double filtration) describes the arrangement of two or more columns of different pore size in series. Large molecules such as low-density lipoproteins can be preferentially removed from plasma while allowing the reinfusion of smaller molecules that one would not want to non-selectively remove (such as high-density lipoproteins).[8]

Following removal of a selected component, the component can be further treated or processed and returned to the patient.

Affinity adsorption apheresis

Affinity adsorption apheresis involves the selective extraction of immunologic or non-immunologic substances from the circulation by means of a column, with the benefit of returning non-extracted proteins, such as clotting factors, to the patient. The column contains a sorbent or ligand attached to a carrier (sepharose or silica) to which patient plasma is exposed. Such columns include the *Staphylococcus* protein A columns, which adsorb immune complexes and immunoglobulins via their Fc portion (with greatest affinity for IgG subclasses 1, 2, and 4, and lower

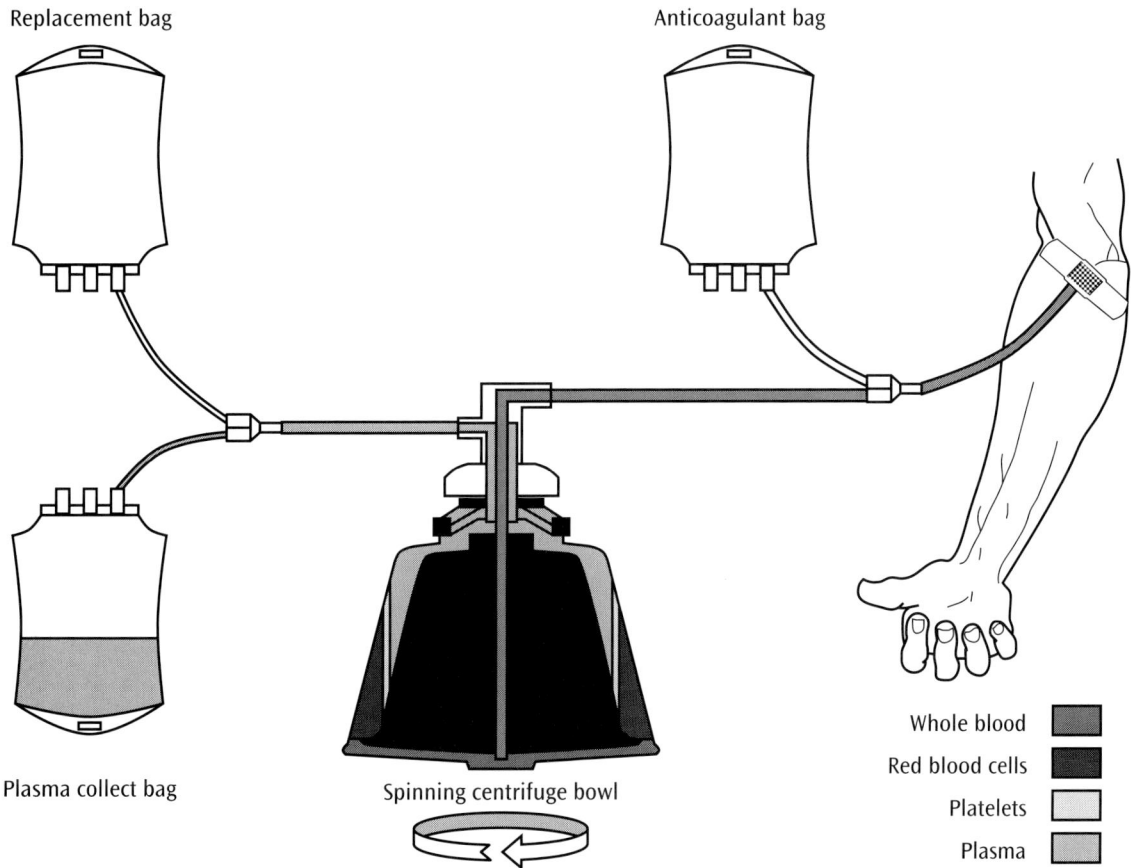

Figure 12.1
Simplified representation of an intermittent-flow plasma exchange. Whole blood enters the Latham bowl through a central channel, is dispersed at the bottom of the bowl, and then rises between two concentric conical surfaces. The centrifugal force causes the plasma, platelet-rich plasma, and red blood cells to form vertical layers. As more whole blood enters the bowl, plasma, being of lowest density begins to exit the top of the bowl to the plasma collect bag as the red blood cell layer widens. When the bowl is filled with red cells, the centrifuge is paused, the pumps are reversed, and the red blood cells are reinfused to the patient.

affinity for IgG3, IgM, and IgA).[9] The use of such columns invokes an immunomodulation that is presently poorly understood. They are approved for clinical use in the USA for the treatment of idiopathic thrombocytopenic purpura (ITP) and, most recently, refractory

rheumatoid arthritis. However, they have been used anecdotally to treat a variety of other immune-mediated medical conditions, such as clotting factor inhibitors, platelet refractoriness, and autoimmune neutropenia. Alternatively, affinity adsorption columns composed of dextran sulfate cellulose columns are used for the removal of low-density lipoproteins.

Photopheresis

In photopheresis, circulating lymphocytes are harvested and exposed to ultraviolet A light in the presence of a photoactive psoralen (8-methoxypsoralen) and then reinfused into the patient. Photopheresis is effective in the treatment of cutaneous T-cell lymphoma (Sézary syndrome), where there is evidence that the treated cells stimulate an autologous suppressor response that targets the malignant T-cell clone or similar clones.[10]

KINETICS OF APHERESIS THERAPY

Models of apheresis removal of a blood component (or a solute of interest) typically assume that the component or solute being removed is neither synthesized nor degraded substantially during the procedure, that it remains within the intravascular compartment, and that there is instantaneous mixing. Such assumptions are largely valid for solutes located predominantly within the intravascular space, such as IgM (76% within the intravascular space) or red cells, but apply less well to solutes such as IgG, IgA, IgM, and albumin, which have intravascular distributions of approximately 45%, 42%, 76%, and 40% respectively.[11]

For continuous-flow plasma exchange, the removal of plasma or solute can be described by the same differential equation that applies to isovolemic hemodilution:

$$\frac{dS}{dV_{ex}} = -\frac{S}{PV}$$

where S = solute concentration, V_{ex} = volume exchanged, and PV = plasma volume. This equation can be integrated and rearranged to yield the following:

$$\text{fraction remaining} = \frac{S_f}{S_i} = e^{-V_{ex}/PV}$$

where S_i is the initial solute concentration and S_f is the final solute concentration. Alternatively, the volume to be removed to achieve a specific fraction of a solute is given by the following equation:

$$V_{ex} = PV \ln\left(\frac{S_i}{S_f}\right)$$

For intermittent-flow exchange, if the replacement is given after the removal of the plasma, then, after N repetitions of removal, the remaining fraction of the solute in question is given by the following equation:

$$\text{fraction remaining} = \left(\frac{\text{plasma volume} - \text{volume removed}}{\text{plasma volume}}\right)^N$$

If the replacement is given before the removal of the plasma, then, after N repetitions of plasma removal, the remaining fraction of the analyte in question is given by the following equation:

$$\text{fraction remaining} = \left(\frac{\text{plasma volume}}{\text{plasma volume} + \text{volume removed}}\right)^N$$

Because of the initial hemodilution that occurs if the replacement is given before the removal of the plasma, for each cycle of plasma removal, the fraction remaining is less than if the replacement had only been given after each repetition of plasma removal.

A comparison of continuous- versus intermittent-flow exchange and the percent removal is illustrated in Figure 12.2.

Calculations for red cell exchanges are only somewhat more complicated. For example, given a sickle cell patient with a blood volume of 5000 ml and a hematocrit of 0.32, if it is assumed that the patient has 100% hemoglobin S (HbS) and that the therapeutic goal is to decrease the percent HbS to 30% while maintaining the patient's hemat-

ocrit at 0.32, the amount of blood that must be processed is given by:

$$V_{ex} = 5000 \text{ ml} \times \ln\left(\frac{100\%}{30\%}\right) = 6020 \text{ ml}$$

(assuming a continuous-flow exchange). The volume of red cells needed for replacement in order to maintain the patient's hematocrit at 0.32 throughout the procedure is:

$$6020 \text{ ml} \times 0.32 = 1926 \text{ ml}$$

If it is assumed that a typical allogeneic unit contains 200 ml of red cells, then 10 units (1926 ml/200 ml per unit = 9.6 units) would be required.

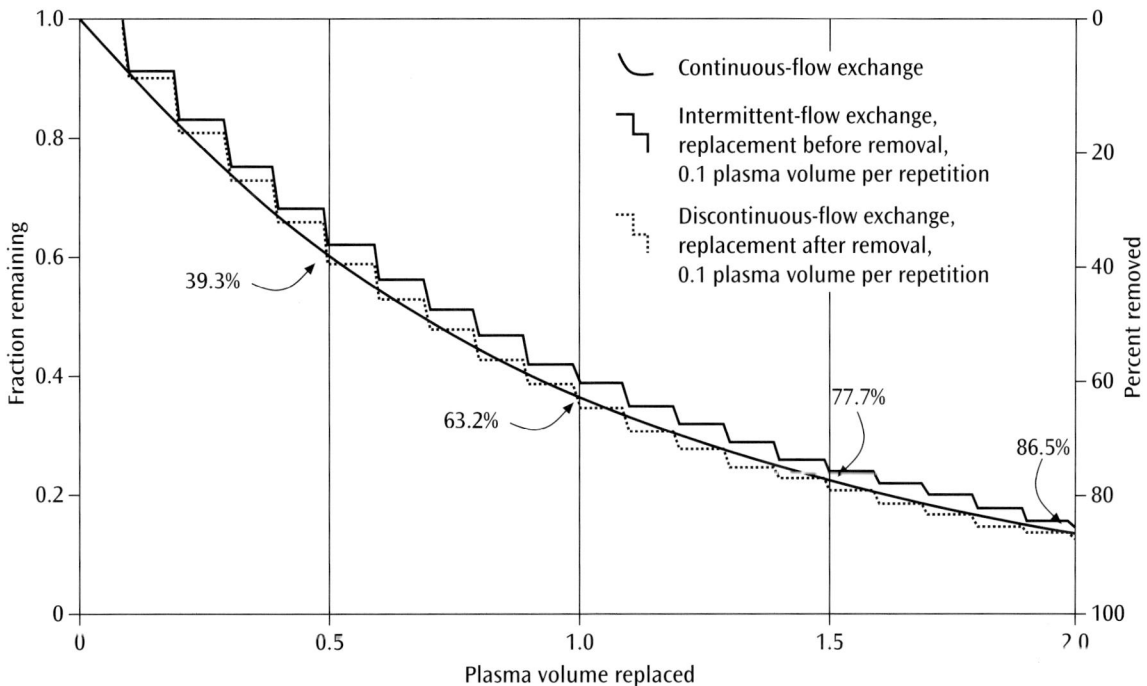

Figure 12.2
Theoretical fraction of plasma remaining following plasma exchange for continuous- and intermittent-flow separation. The exchange of 0.5, 1, 1.5, and 2 plasma volumes would be associated with the removal of 39.3%, 63.2%, 77.7% and 86.5% of plasma.

CHOICE OF REPLACEMENT SOLUTIONS FOR PLASMA EXCHANGE

Following the introduction of cell separators for plasma exchange some three decades ago, it was common practice to replace plasma removed with stored allogeneic plasma. Unfortunately, this early use of plasma led to unacceptable rates of viral contamination (particularly hepatitis) and citrate toxicity. As large amounts of plasma protein were being removed, it seemed reasonable to replace the removed human plasma protein with human-derived plasma protein in the form of 5% albumin (which is ≥96% pure albumin) or plasma protein fraction (≥83% pure albumin). These replacement solutions largely resolved the problems of disease transmission and citrate toxicity. Subsequently, the introduction of partial saline replacement was integrated into many program's replacement regimens.[12,13] In recent years, market recalls (due to Creutzfeld–Jacob disease or bacterial contamination) decreased availability, rising costs, recognition of drug interactions with albumin (i.e. angiotensin-converting enzyme (ACE) inhibitors) and a fear of disease transmission have led several groups to the use of colloidal starches (hydroxethylstarches, HES) as partial or full replacement for plasma during plasma exchange.[14–19] One regimen currently in use includes 3% HES (6% hetastarch diluted one-to-one with 0.9% saline) at 110% replacement for the initial replacement, followed by a final liter of replacement with 5% albumin at 100% replacement.[18] Alternatively, 10% pentastarch employed for the first half of the colloid replacement followed by 5% albumin has also been a successful replacement strategy.[19] In some cases, 25% albumin has been diluted to 5% albumin for use as replacement. Hemolysis has occurred when hypotonic solutions have been used as a diluent. 25% albumin should be diluted with 0.9% saline.[20–22]

In specific clinical settings, patients may require replacement of a specific plasma protein (such as von Willebrand factor metalloproteinase in thrombotic thrombocytopenic purpura; see below) or clotting factors in patients at increased risk for bleeding (e.g Goodpasture's syndrome with pulmonary hemorrhage). In such cases, plasma or modified plasma (such as solvent–detergent-treated plasma or cryoreduced plasma supernatant) may be indicated as full or partial replacement.

INDICATIONS FOR THERAPEUTIC APHERESIS

Hemapheresis therapy is used for a vast variety of clinical indications. Ideally, such indications are based on objective evidence of efficacy provided by published clinical and basic research. Unfortunately, such studies frequently do not exist for a variety of diseases for which apheresis has been advocated. In 1985, the American Medical Association convened a panel of experts to review the efficacy of plasmapheresis. Indications were categorized as follows:[23]

(i)   standard therapy, acceptable but not mandatory;
(ii) available evidence tends to favor efficacy – conventional therapy usually tried first;
(iii) inadequately tested at this time;
(iv) no demonstrated value in controlled trials.

Since then, these guidelines have been both updated and expanded (to include other apheresis techniques in addition to plasmapheresis) by the American Association of Blood Banks (1992, 1993, and 1994), the American Society for Apheresis (1986, 1993, and 2000), and the American Academy of Neurology (1996).[24–28] A compilation of these more recent guidelines is presented in Table 12.1. The relative fractions of therapeutic hemapheresis procedures by type is illustrated in Figure 12.3.[29]

Although a complete and in-depth review of all the indications for therapeutic hemapheresis is beyond the scope of this introductory chapter, brief summaries for several of the more common diseases for which routine or emergent requests for hemapheresis are provided below. More extensive reviews of the literature over a much greater range of diseases are available.[30]

Inflammatory demyelinating polyradiculoneuropathies (IDP)

Acute inflammatory demyelinating polyradiculoneuropathy (AIDP), or Guillain–Barré syndrome, is characterized by a generalized weakness with distal paresthesias progressing over several days. The peripheral nerve demyelination is mediated by an antibody that appears to be stimulated by a preceding infection. *Campylobacter jejuni* infection is seen in up to 40% of AIDP cases.[31] The annual incidence of disease is 1 in 50 000, and 10–23% of patients may require ventilatory support.[32] Five percent of patients die as a consequence of the disease, 5–15% are chronically disabled, and up to 10% relapse.[32]

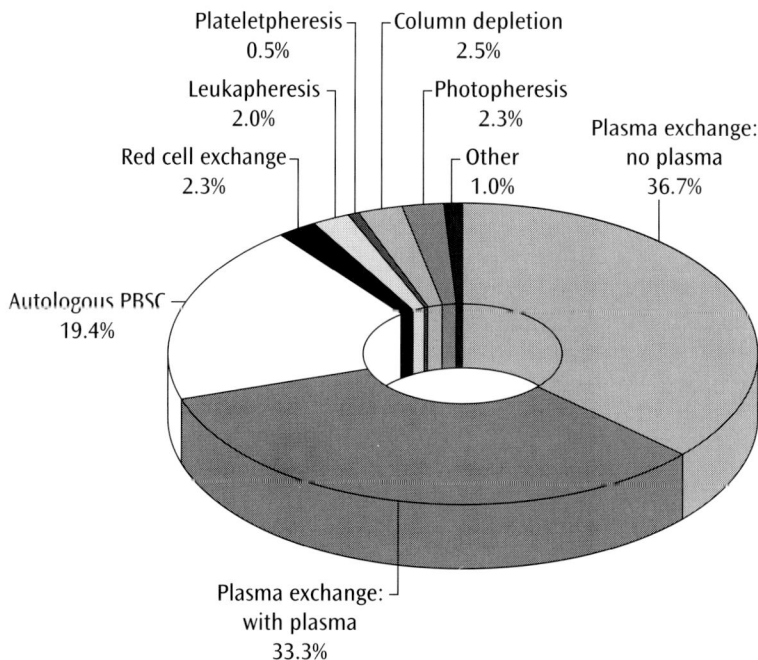

Figure 12.3
Relative frequency of therapeutic procedures by type, based on data from 18 institutions in the USA encompassing 3421 procedures.[29] PBSC, peripheral blood stem cells.

Plateletpheresis 0.5%
Column depletion 2.5%
Leukapheresis 2.0%
Photopheresis 2.3%
Red cell exchange 2.3%
Other 1.0%
Plasma exchange: no plasma 36.7%
Autologous PBSC 19.4%
Plasma exchange: with plasma 33.3%

Table 12.1 Guidelines for therapeutic hemapheresis: American Society for Apheresis (ASFA), American Association of Blood Banks (AABB), and American Academy of Neurology (AAN)

Disease	Procedure	ASFA 2000[a]	AABB 1994[a]	AAN 1996[b]
Neurologic disorders				
Chronic inflammatory demyelinating polyradiculoneuropathy (CIDP)	Plasma exchange	I	I	Established
Acute inflammatory demyelinating polyradiculoneuropathy (AIDP, Guillain–Barré syndrome)	Plasma exchange	I	I	Established
Myasthenia gravis	Plasma exchange	I	I	Established
Lambert–Eaton myasthenic syndrome	Plasma exchange	II		Possibly useful
Multiple sclerosis:				
Acute fulminant CNS demyelination/ relapsing or progressive	Plasma exchange	II/III	III	Possibly useful
Paraneoplastic neurologic syndromes	Plasma exchange	III		No role
	Immunoadsorption	III		
Paraproteinemic polyneuropathies:				
Demyelinating polyneuropathy with IgG/IgA	Plasma exchange	I		Established
	Immunoadsorption	III		
Polyneuropathy with IgM (± Waldenström's macroglobulinemia)	Plasma exchange	II		Investigational
	Immunoadsorption	III		
Cryoglobulinemia with polyneuropathy	Plasma exchange	II		Investigational
Multiple myeloma with polyneuropathy	Plasma exchange	III		
POEMS syndrome	Plasma exchange	III		
Systemic (AL) amyloidosis	Plasma exchange	IV		
Inflammatory myopathies:				
Polymyositis or dermatomyositis	Plasma exchange	III	IV	
	Leukocytapheresis	IV		
Inclusion-body myositis	Plasma exchange	III		
	Leukocytapheresis	IV		
Rasmussen's encephalitis	Plasma exchange	III	III	
Stiff-man syndrome	Plasma exchange	III		Investigational
Sydenham's chorea /pediatric autoimmune neuropsychiatric disorders associated with streptococcal infections (PANDAS)	Plasma exchange	II		

Table 12.1 continued				
Disease	Procedure	ASFA 2000[a]	AABB 1994[a]	AAN 1996[b]
Hematological diseases				
ABO-incompatible hematopoietic stem cell transplant	Plasma exchange (recipient)	II	III	
Erythrocytosis/polycythemia vera	Erythrocytapheresis	II		
Leukocytosis and thrombocytosis	Cytapheresis	I	I	
Thrombotic thrombocytopenic purpura (TTP)	Plasma exchange	I	I	
Post-transfusion purpura	Plasma exchange	I	I	
Sickle cell diseases	Red cell exchange	I	I	
Myeloma/paraproteins/hyperviscosity	Plasma exchange	II	I	
Myeloma/acute renal failure	Plasma exchange	II		
Coagulation factor inhibitors	Plasma exchange	II	III	
Aplastic anemia/pure red cell aplasia	Plasma exchange	III		
Cutaneous T-cell lymphoma	Photopheresis	I	II	
	Leukapheresis	III	II	
Hemolytic disease of the newborn	Plasma exchange	III		
Platelet alloimmunization and refractoriness	Plasma exchange	III		
	Immunoadsorption	III		
Malaria/babesiosis	Red cell exchange	III	II	
Renal and metabolic diseases				
Anti-glomerular-basement-membrane antibody disease (Goodpasture's syndrome)	Plasma exchange	I	I	
Rapidly progressive glomerulonephritis	Plasma exchange	II	II	
Hemolytic–uremic syndrome	Plasma exchange	III	II	
Renal transplantation:				
Rejection	Plasma exchange	IV	IV	
Presenstitization	Plasma exchange	III		
Recurrent focal glomerulosclerosis	Plasma exchange	III		
Heart transplant rejection	Plasma exchange	III		
	Photopheresis	III		

Table 12.1 continued

Disease	Procedure	ASFA 2000[a]	AABB 1994[a]	AAN 1996[b]
Acute hepatic failure	Plasma exchange	III	IV	
Familial hypercholesterolemia	Selective adsorption	I	I	
	Plasma exchange	II	I	
Overdose poisoning	Plasma exchange	III		
Phytanic acid storage disease	Plasma exchange	I	I	Investigational
Autoimmune and rheumatic diseases				
Cryoglobulinemia	Plasma exchange	II	I	
Idiopathic thromboctyopenic purpura	Immunoadsorption	II		
Raynaud's phenomenon	Plasma exchange	III		
Vasculitis	Plasma exchange	III		
Autoimmune hemolytic anemia	Plasma exchange	III		
Rheumatoid arthritis	Immunoadsorption	II		
	Lympho-plasmapheresis	II		
	Plasma exchange	IV		
Scleroderma/progressive systemic sclerosis	Plasma exchange	III		
Systemic lupus erythematosus	Plasma exchange	III		

[a]Category I, standard acceptable therapy; category II, sufficient evidence to suggest efficacy, usually as adjunctive or supportive therapy; category III, inconclusive evidence of efficacy or uncertain risk/benefit ratio; category IV, lack of efficacy in controlled trials.
[b]Established, accepted as appropriate; possibly useful, given current knowledge, this appears appropriate; investigational, insufficient evidence to determine appropriateness, and warrants further study.

In patients with severe disease treated with supportive care, the median time to unassisted walking is 111 days, and recovery to full strength by one year is only seen in 52% of patients.[33,34] Multiple randomized studies have demonstrated accelerated recovery with plasma exchange therapy.[33–35] With severely affected patients, the time to reach unassisted walking is shortened by 32–72 days, and for those patients requiring ventilatory support after initiation of therapy the median time to extubation was reduced from 48 days to 24 days.[33–35] The recommended therapy is five or six plasma exchanges over 10–14 days initiated within 14 days of the onset of symptoms. Interestingly, initiation of therapy once a patient has required ventilatory support for several days has been reported to have little benefit.[35] This may reflect that the time of most active disease, for which plasma exchange might have been effective, had already passed.

Recently, the use of intravenous immunoglobulin (IVIG) has been studied as an alternative or as an adjuvant therapy for AIDP. In the largest study to date, 383 adult patients with severe disease were enrolled within the first 2 weeks after the onset of symptoms into one of three treatment arms that compared plasma exchange, IVIG, and plasma exchange followed by IVIG.[36] Plasma exchange and IVIG had equivalent efficacy, and the combination of plasma exchange followed by IVIG did not confer a significant advantage.[36] It has been argued that, given the equivalent therapeutic benefit and comparable cost of IVIG versus plasma exchange therapy, IVIG, having a greater convenience of administration, may be the preferred therapy.

Chronic inflammatory demyelinating polyradiculoneuropathy (CIDP) describes a somewhat heterogenous group of neurologic disorders characterized by a progressive or relapsing multifocal sensorimotor peripheral nerve demyelination (in 6–20% of cases, only sensory or motor nerves are involved) developing over at least 2 months. Patients are typically hypo- or areflexic in all four extremities. Like AIDP, the demyelination is thought to involve a humorally mediated autoimmunity directed against peripheral nerve myelin. Unlike AIDP, patients with CIDP frequently show some response to corticosteroid therapy. Small randomized studies of plasma exchange have shown clinical improvement in 33–80% of patients.[37,38] Improvement is usually noted within 3–6 days of initiating therapy; however, relapse within 1–2 weeks following therapy has been reported in two-thirds of patients. The use of IVIG has also been shown to be effective in CIDP, and in the one small (20 patients) prospective trial of plasma exchange versus IVIG, there was no significant difference in effect.[39] Similarly, a large retrospective study of plasma exchange and IVIG for CIDP (33 patients in the plasma exchange group, and 21 in the IVIG group) found similar responses to therapy.[40] As with AIDP, given the equivalent therapeutic benefit and comparable cost of IVIG versus plasma exchange, since IVIG has a greater convenience of administration and less morbidity, it may be the preferred therapy. If plasma exchange is used, a course of four to six exchanges over 2 weeks followed by a taper as needed to achieve a stable response has been recommended.

Myasthenia gravis

Myasthenia gravis is characterized by variable weakness of voluntary (striated) muscle. Autoantibodies, which are demonstrable in the majority of patients, compete with the neurotransmitter acetylcholine for the acetylcholine receptors in postsynaptic membranes of the neuromuscular junction. These antibodies cause steric hindrance of acetylcholine binding and lead to receptor destruction by inducing endocytosis and complement activation.[41,42]

Therapy consists of (1) the use of cholinesterase inhibitors (pyridostigmine bromide or neostigmine bromide), which prolong the availability of acetylcholine at the neuromuscular junction, and (2) immunosuppression with corticosteroids or other immunosuppresive agents. Plasma exchange is frequently employed for acute severe myasthenia gravis or in preparation for thymectomy to acutely decrease circulating autoantibody. Unfortunately, not all patients respond to plasma exchange, and clinical improvement with plasma exchange is not immediate and typically requires several days to become apparent. In one study of 70 patients with severe myasthenia gravis receiving concomitant immunosuppression, clinical improvement was seen within 7 days in 70% of patients after receiving two plasma exchanges over 2 days.[43] Alternatively, plasma exchange can be used as an adjunctive therapy for chronic immunosuppression.

IVIG is also thought to be of benefit in some myasthenic patients. In a randomized trial of 87 patients (41 treated with plasma exchange and 46 treated with IVIG), the median time to response was 9 days in the plasma exchange group and 15 days in the IVIG group ($p = 0.14$).[44] Although this study suggests a possible superiority of plasma exchange over IVIG, the study did not have sufficient power to distinguish a 50% difference in improvement.

Hematology/oncology

The therapeutic applications of apheresis techniques for the acute treatment of hematologic or oncologic clinical presentations are as varied as the underlying diseases that fall into this category. Therefore, depending on the underlying process, the use of plasma exchange, red cell exchange, cytoreduction, or immunoadsorption may be indicated.

Thrombotic thrombocytopenic purpura (TTP)/hemolytic–uremic syndrome (HUS)

The presentation of TTP is classically described by a clinical pentad of (i) microangiopathic hemolytic anemia (MAHA), (ii) thrombocytopenia; (iii) renal failure, (iv) fever, and (v) mental status changes. In practice, the presence of thrombocytopenia ($<100 \times 10^9/l$) and an elevated lactate dehydrogenase (LDH > 1000 units/l, a manifestation of systemic ischemia and hemolysis) *in the absence of another likely cause* is sufficient to make the diagnosis.[45,46] Although this disease was once associated with a mortality rate in excess of 80%, following the introduction of daily plasma exchange the mortality rate has been reduced to 10–20%.

It has been shown that TTP is associated with an acquired (IgG-mediated) or inherent deficiency of a metalloproteinase that cleaves von Willebrand factor (vWF) multimers.[47,48] Decreased levels of this enzyme result in elevated high-molecular-weight vWF multimers, which have an increased affinity for platelet glycoproteins Ib and IIb/IIa, causing excessive platelet aggregation. This understanding of the pathophysiology provides a rationale for the use of plasma exchange, with removal of the metalloproteinase antibody and concomitant replacement of the deficient metalloproteinase enzyme. A variety of replacement solutions have been successfully employed, including complete replacement with FFP, cryo-poor plasma, and solvent–detergent-treated plasma.[49–51] The use of cryo-poor plasma or solvent–detergent-treated plasma is thought to offer an advantage, since vWF levels are decreased in these products. Alternatively, the use of albumin for the first half of the replacement, followed by plasma, has also been shown to be effective.[52] The use of a combination of albumin and plasma may be of particular advantage in the case of limited supplies of ABO-compatible plasma, such as with a group AB patient or in patients prone to allergic reactions to plasma. Typically, daily plasma exchanges are performed until the platelet concentration is greater than $150 \times 10^9/l$ and the LDH levels are normal or near-normal for 2 days. In general, 50% of patients respond by 8 days and an additional 20% within 2 weeks.[52] Relapses or exacerbations occur in 30–60% of survivors, and typically respond to re-initiation of therapy.

Hyperviscosity

Hyperviscosity can result from the over production of immunoglobulins (paraproteins) by malignant plasma cells in multiple myeloma (IgD, IgG, IgA, or IgE) or Waldenström's macroglobulinemia (IgM). Hyperviscosity can cause a reduction in blood flow to the brain, resulting in symptoms of headache, vertigo, somnolence, or obtundation. Sludging may also effect the pulmonary circulation, and in combination with the intravascular volume expansion seen with paraproteinemias may result in right-sided heart failure. Bleeding may be a consequence of paraprotein binding to platelets and clotting factors, interfering with their function. The serum viscosity relative to water normally ranges from 1.4 to 1.8. Most patients remain aymptomatic until their relative serum viscosity is in the 4–8 range.[53]

Although viscosity rises with increasing amounts of paraprotein, there is considerable variation from patient to patient, and small increases in the paraprotein level can result in disproportionate increases in viscosity. Symptomatic hyperviscosity is seen in approximately 50% of Waldenström's macroglobulinemia patients but in less than 5% of multiple myeloma patients.[54] In general, symptoms are typically alleviated with one or two plasma exchanges. Therapy of the primary disorder is essential for long-term control of this condition.

Sickle cell anemia

Sickle cell anemia is an inherited abnormality of hemoglobin synthesis resulting in the formation of hemoglobin S (HbS) instead of hemoglobin A (HbA). Clinical disease is seen in patients who are homozygous for HbS or in heterozygotes in combination with an alternative abnormal gene combination (e.g. HbS or β-thalassemia). The homozygous S genotype is seen in 1 in 625 Black newborns in the USA.[55] HbS polymerization and aggregation can lead to irreversible erythrocyte membrane alteration, resulting in a crescent-shaped 'sickle cell'. Episodes of severe sickling are periodic and are associated with increased blood viscosity, leading to sludging, microthrombi, and tissue ischemia – described as a 'crisis'. Most crises are transient, presenting as musculoskeletal, abdominal, or thoracic painful presentations. In some cases, depending on the degree of sludging and the location of vascular sequestration may lead to irreversible organ dysfunction (e.g. priapism or retinopathy) or may actually be life-threatening when the sludging involve the central nervous system, pulmonary, or hepatic vessels. In such cases, emergent reduction of the percent of HbS with HbA erythrocytes may be organ- or life-saving. Automated red cell exchanges are generally preferred to manual exchanges in this setting, since they are more controlled and rapid. Care must be exercised to avoid inadvertently increasing the blood viscosity by raising the hemoglobin to too high a level. General guidelines for acute therapy are to achieve a hematocrit no higher than 0.30–0.35 and a proportion of HbA to greater than 60%. Continuous-flow cell separators are often preferred, since gelation of blood has been seen in the processing bowls of non-continuous-flow cell separators.[56]

In the setting of previous stroke or in children at high risk for stroke (with abnormal transcranial Doppler ultrasonography) and in some patients with frequent debilitating pain crises, the use of chronic prophylactic transfusions to suppress HbS to less than 30% is thought to be beneficial. The advantage of an automated exchange compared with simple transfusion is better control of target hematocrits and proportion of HbA, less risk of iron overload (since HbS red cells are removed as HbA cells are infused) and a smaller requirement for transfused red cells (and the concomitant number of donor exposures). All red cells transfused in this setting should be HbS negative; in some centers, partial erythrocyte phenotype matching (e.g. for C, E, and K) is employed to minimize alloimmunization in this chronically transfused population.

Extreme leukocytosis and extreme thrombocytosis

Blood hyperviscosity and leukostasis can occur with extreme leukocytosis. Although extreme leukocytosis can be seen in a variety of leukemias, symptomatic leukostasis is generally only seen with acute myeloid leukemias (AML), where the elevated leukocytes are principally monocytic, myelomonocytic, or myelocytic blasts. This likely reflects the large size, lack of deformibility, and the 'stickiness' of such myelocytic or moncytic blasts. Patients typically present with central nervous system or pulmonary symptoms, manifested as dizziness, headache, somnolence, obtundation, or shortness of breath (similar to the hyperviscosity presentation seen with elevated paraproteins). Leukostasis can lead to either tissue ischemia secondary to vasocclusion or bleeding secondary to vascular tumor cell infiltration or possibly a reperfusion injury. Patients are typically asymptomatic until the peripheral cell count exceeds $100 \times 10^9/l$ (leukocrit > 0.20) or a blast count of $50 \times 10^9/l$.[57] Regardless of the leukocyte or blast count, patients with pulmonary or central nervous system symptoms require emergent cytoreduction, which typically results in rapid clinical improvement. One large-volume cytoreduction (two blood volumes processed) will typically reduce the leukocyte count by 30–50%. Unfortunately, the reduction is transient, since the bulk of the tumor burden is extravascular and rapidly re-equilibrates into the intravascular space. Therefore, more than one cytoreduction is typically required until more definitive control of the leukocytosis by chemotherapy can be achieved.

In some cases, the rapid lysis of tumor cells by chemotherapy (the tumor lysis syndrome) can lead to a variety of metabolic aberrations, including hyperuricemia, hyperkalemia, hyperphosphatemia, and hypocalcemia. To minimize the effects of this syndrome, some centers routinely cytoreduce patients with extreme leukocytosis regardless of symptoms. However, the benefits of cytoreduction in this setting have never been studied in a controlled fashion, and this therapy fails to address the bulk of the tumor burden which is located extravascularly.

Management of chronic leukemias such as chronic myeloid leukemia (CML) and chronic lymphocytic leukemia (CLL) with repeated cytoreductions has been attempted.[58,59] However, cytoreduction does not alter the course of these diseases, and cytoreductions in this setting are no longer performed. In certain specific situations, such as a pregnant patient with CML, where the risk of teratogenicity associated with chemotherapy may be considered an unacceptable risk, repeated cytoreductions have been employed.[60]

Extreme thrombocytosis with platelets counts typically greater than $100 \times 10^9/l$ can be seen in CML, essential thrombocythemia (ET), and polycythemia vera (PV). In most cases, patients are asymptomatic, even with extreme thrombocytosis. However, symptoms of thrombosis secondary to platelet aggregation and thrombosis or bleeding due to platelet dysfunction or reperfusion injury can be seen in these clonal disorders (but not in reactive thrombocytosis). As with extreme leukocytosis, symptomatic patients are treated regardless of the actual count, and respond readily to cytoreduction. A single large-volume cytoreduction results in a transient 30–50% reduction in the platelet count, but may need to be repeated until more definitive control of the thrombocytosis by chemotherapy can be achieved.

Use of apheresis in renal transplantation

In the context of renal transplantation, apheresis is generally considered in one of the following three settings: (i) reduction of circulating antibodies that would preclude transplantation; (ii) the treatment of post-transplant rejection, and (iii) the treatment of post-transplant recurrent disease.

Preformed antibodies to HLA specificities resulting from prior transplants, pregnancies, or transfusions places a patient at high risk of hyperacute rejection. The presence of such antibodies detected in a HLA-antibody screen (panel-reactive antibodies) or an HLA cross-match generally precludes the possibility of a transplant. However, the removal of anti-HLA antibodies by plasma exchange with concurrent immunosuppression (to abrogate antibody rebound) has been used to successfully transplant 53 of 60 alloimmunized patients in three series.[61–63] Similar protocols have been used to successfully transplant kidneys across ABO barriers.[64,65]

Historically, much of the interest in the use of apheresis in renal transplantation has been for the treatment of graft rejection. Kidney graft rejection is generally divided into hyperacute (immediate), acute (days to weeks), and delayed (weeks to months) post transplantation. Hyeracute rejection is thought to be humorally mediated, while delayed rejection is generally felt to be predominantly cell-mediated, and therefore any benefit from plasma exchange would be expected to be demonstrable with early rejection. Multiple controlled studies have failed to demonstrate any significant improvements in graft survival.[66–69] In view of the risks, expense, and lack of efficacy in multiple controlled trials, plasma exchange for rejection is not recommended.

Following transplantation, the initial underlying disease, such as focal segmental glomerulosclerosis (FSGS), can recur in the allograft. Recurrent FSGS occurs in 30% of allografts, and is thought to be mediated by a circulating 50 kDa factor that causes increased glomerular permeability.[70] Although controlled trials have not been performed, there are multiple case reports and case series describing the use of plasma exchange for recurrent FSGS.[71] In the majority of cases, improvement of disease (elimination or decrease in proteinuria and stabilization of renal function) was achieved. In most cases, treatment consisted of 6–14 exchanges over 1–2 weeks, initiated shortly after the reappearance of proteinuria. Alternatively, immunoadsorption with *Staphylococcus* protein A or anti-IgG columns have also been reported to be efficacious.[72,73]

Extracorporeal photoactive chemotherapy in transplantation

Photopheresis has been used in the setting of solid and hematopoietic transplantation. The postulated rationale for this therapy in the setting of transplantation is that rapidly expanding T-cell clones are preferentially targeted by the induced immune response. Most extensively studied is the use of photopheresis to treat acute rejection and for prophylaxis of rejection in cardiac transplantation. Anecdotal success has been described with acute rejection of cardiac allografts, and one small control study found equal efficacy with corticosteroid therapy (8 of 9 and 7 of 7 reversals

of rejection, respectively).[74–76] In the largest controlled trial to date of prophylactic photopheresis in cardiac transplantation, 60 patients received standard immunosuppression with or without photopheresis. A greater proportion of patients in the photopheresis group had one rejection episode or none (27 of 33) than in the standard-therapy group (14 of 27), and a smaller proportion of patients in the photopheresis group had two or more rejection episodes (6 of 33) than in the standard-therapy group (13 of 27, $p = 0.02$).[77] However, there was no significant difference in the time to a first episode of rejection, the incidence of rejection associated with hemodynamic compromise, or survival at 6 and 12 months.

Small uncontrolled case series in lung transplants with bronchiolitis obliterans and chronic rejection have reported improvement or stabilization of declining pulmonary function with photopheresis.[78,79] In one case of post-lung-transplantation Epstein–Barr virus-associated lymphoma, photopheresis combined with a moderate reduction in immunosuppression was associated with complete remission.[80] Similarly, uncontrolled reports of photopheresis suggesting a benefit in both renal transplant rejection and with acute and chronic graft-versus-host disease following allogeneic hematopoietic stem cell transplantation have been reported.[81–84]

Controlled clinical trials are necessary to establish the actual efficacy and optimal timing of photopheresis in these settings.

UNINTENDED CONSEQUENCES AND ADVERSE REACTIONS ASSOCIATED WITH APHERESIS

Drug clearance

An unintended consequence of hemapheresis is potential reduction in circulating drugs. In general, the drugs that are most affected have a small volume of distribution and are extensively protein-bound (similarly to drugs that are treated with plasma exchange in acute toxicity). Limited drug kinetic data in the context of hemapheresis suggest that supplemental dosing of prednisone, digoxin, cyclosporine, ceftriaxone, ceftazidime, valproic acid, and phenobarbital after plasma exchange is not necessary.[85,86] However, dosing of certain drugs such as salicylates and tobramycin should be supplemented, and phenytoin (for which there are conflicting reports of clearance) requires careful patient monitoring. In general, removal of a drug is likely to be increased during the distribution phase following administration. Therefore, whenever possible, drug doses should be administered following a hemapheresis procedure and not immediately before the exchange.

Effect on clotting following plasma exchange

Therapeutic plasma exchange is generally associated with the removal of large quantities of plasma and its associated coagulant proteins.[11,16,17,87–92] When non-coagulant-containing replacement fluids such as albumin, saline, and colloidal starches are used, this results in a 40–70% fall in clotting factor activity, associated with a small prolongation in measured prothrombin and activated partial thromboplastin times (PT and aPTT) (although such values frequently remain within the normal range). Fibrinogen, having a volume of distribution that is almost exclusively intravascular (80%), is the clotting factor that is most depleted.[11] Clotting factors levels generally return to normal within 1–2 days following exchange. In the absence of an underlying hemostatic defect or liver disease, the use of clotting-factor-free replacement solutions is well tolerated for 1–1.5 plasma exchange volumes.

An additional unintentional consequence of plasma exchange is a 9.4–52.6% reduction in circulating platelets.[88,90,93,94] Despite mean decreases in platelet counts of 52.6% following 1.6 plasma volume exchanged, Sultan et al[87] found that the platelets (as well as all clotting factors measured, with the exception of antithrombin III) had almost reached or even exceeded their initial values after 48–96 hours (just before the next plasma exchange). We have also observed normal platelet counts 48 hours after one-plasma-volume exchanges (just prior to the next plasma exchange).

In a hemostatically compromised patient or if large-volume daily exchanges are performed, hemostatic parameters should be monitored and the replacement supplemented with plasma or platelets as clinically indicated.

Adverse reactions

Adverse reactions associated with therapeutic apheresis are uncommon. A 1995 survey conducted by the American Association of Blood Banks and involving 18 centers and 3429 procedures reported 242 adverse events in 163 procedures (4.75% of all procedures, 6.87% of first-time procedures, and 4.28% of repeat

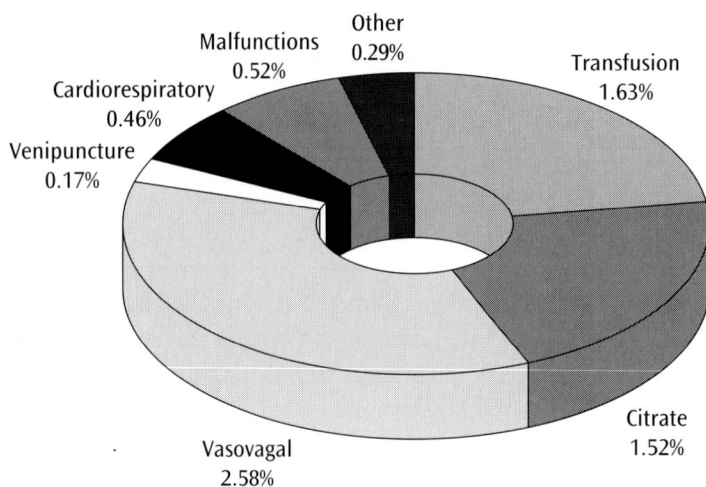

Malfunctions 0.52%
Other 0.29%
Cardiorespiratory 0.46%
Venipuncture 0.17%
Transfusion 1.63%
Citrate 1.52%
Vasovagal 2.58%

Figure 12.4
Relative frequency of adverse events associated with therapeutic apheresis procedures, based on data from 18 institutions in the USA encompassing 3421 procedures.[29]

procedures).[29] Mild reactions were not reported in this study. The types of reactions reported are summarized in Figure 12.4. Deaths occurring in patients being treated with hemapheresis are generally associated with the underlying disease, and mortality rates are largely a function of the patient population treated. For example, 10–20% of patients with TTP will die while receiving therapy.[46,52] Overall, the estimated mortality rates of patients receiving hemapheresis therapy range from 1 per 1000 to 3 per 10 000 procedures.[29,95]

The use of citrate anticoagulation can. lead to mild hypocalcemia characterized by tingling, oral paresthesias, or chest discomfort. Citrate reactions are usually mild and easily managed by slowing the infusion rate, increasing the acid–citrate–dextrose (ACD) ratio, or administering oral calcium. More severe reactions may be treated or prevented with intravenous calcium. Calcium chloride may be added to the replacement fluid (200 mg/l of 5% albumin or 3–6% HES) or given as a slow intravenous infusion (200 mg, diluted to at least 20 mg/ml and infused over 2 minutes) when replacing with FFP. Particular care must be taken with patients with liver failure and impaired ability to metabolize citrate.

Allergic-type reactions present in a spectrum ranging from mild urticaria to anaphylaxis, and are associated with replacement fluids, including plasma, HES, and albumin. Prophylactic administration of antihistamines may prevent allergic reactions; however, some patients will develop mild to severe reactions even with premedication. In such patients, premedication with an H_2 blocker such as hydroxyzine or cimetidine or the use of a continuous antihistamine drip may be effective in preventing breakthrough reactions.

Atypical allergic or anaphylactoid reactions have been described with ethylene oxide gas sterilization of tubing sets and with drug interactions between ACE inhibitors and albumin, respectively. Ethylene oxide reactions are usually characterized by periorbital edema with chemosis and tearing.[96] Double priming of the tubing is useful in the prevention of the recurrence of such a reaction. ACE-inhibitor reactions are associated with albumin infusion during plasma exchange.[14,15] It is thought that the symptoms are caused by rapid infusion of low levels of prekallikrein activator (PKA, which is a metabolite of clotting factor XII) found in the albumin product, which activates prekallikrein to bradykinin. The ACE inhibitor inhibits kininase II, leading to an accumulation of bradykinin. The patient may experience mild to severe facial flushing and hypotension. ACE-inhibitor therapy should be discontinued 24–48 hours prior to the start of plasma exchange. If the patient's condition is such that the procedure cannot be delayed for 24–48 hours, colloidal starch and saline may be used for replacement.

CONCLUSIONS

Hemapheresis has been largely successful in a variety of diseases. However, in general, its use has been largely supportive or adjunctive and rarely curative (a notable exception being TTP). Understanding of clinical indications for hemapheresis have been based on objective evidence of efficacy gleaned through published clinical and basic research. Nevertheless, many requests for hemapheresis continue to arise out of desperation or ignorance in diseases and conditions when therapeutic options have been exhausted and in diseases for which efficacy data are lacking. As hemapheresis is not without risk or cost, one must be judicious in its application, weighing the potential risks and benefits for the patient and insisting on a truly full informed consent. Additionally, clinical and basic research are essential to evaluate the efficacy of hemapheresis in those diseases for which such therapy seems rationale but for which efficacy data are lacking and to optimize therapy in those diseases for which efficacy has already been proven.

REFERENCES

1. Abel J, Rowntree LG, Turner BB. Plasma removal with return of corpuscles (plasmaphaeresis). *J Pharmacol Exp Ther* 1914; **5**: 62; *Transfus Sci* 1990; **11**: 166–77.
2. Adams WS, Bland WH, Bassett SH. A method of human plasmapheresis. *Proc Soc Exp Biol Med* 1952; **80**: 377–9.
3. Skoog WA, Adams WA. Plasmapheresis in a case of Waldenström's macroglobulinemia. *Clin Res* 1959; **7**: 96.
4. Schwab PJ, Fahey JL. Treatment of Waldenström's macroglobulinemia by plasmapheresis. *N Engl J Med* 1969; **263**: 574–9.
5. Solomon A, Fahey JL. Plasmapheresis therapy in macroglobulinaemia. *Ann Intern Med* 1963; **58**: 789–800.
6. Reynolds WA. Late report of the first case of plasmapheresis for Waldenström's macroglobulinemia. *JAMA* 1981; **245**: 606–7.
7. Hodgson WJB. Mercan S. Hemapheresis listening post. Optimal venous access. *Transfusion Sci* 1991; **12**: 274.
8. Leitman SF, Smith JW, Gregg RE. Homozygous hypercholesterolemia: selective removal of low density lipoproteins by secondary membrane filtration. *Transfusion* 1989; **29**: 341.
9. Belak M, Widder RA, Brunner R et al. Immunoadsorption with protein A sepharose or silica. *Lancet* 1994; **343**: 792–3.
10. Wolfe JT, Lessin SR, Singh AH, Rook AH. Review of imunomodulation by photopheresis: treatment of cutaneous T-cell lymphoma, autoimmune disease, and allograft rejection. *Artif Organs* 1994; **18**: 888–97.

11. McCullough J, Chopek M. Therapeutic plasma exchange. *Lab Med* 1981; **12**: 745–53.

12. Lasky LC, Finnerty EP, Glenis L, Polesky HF. Protein and colloid osmotic pressure changes with albumin and/or saline replacement during plasma exchange. *Transfusion* 1984; **24**: 256–9.

13. McLeod BC, Sassetti RJ, Stefoski D, Davis FA. Partial plasma protein replacement in therapeutic plasma exchange. *J Clin Apheresis* 1983; **1**: 115–18.

14. Owen, HG, Brecher ME. Atypical reactions associated with ACE inhibitors and apheresis. *Transfusion* 1994; **34**: 891–4.

15. Brecher ME, Owen HG. Washout kinetics of colloidal starch as a partial or full replacement for plasma exchange. *J Clin Apheresis* 1996; **11**: 123–6.

16. Owen HG, Brecher ME. Partial colloid replacement for therapeutic plasma exchange. *J Clin Apheresis* 1997; **12**: 87–92.

17. Brecher ME, Owen HG, Bandarenko N. Alternatives to albumin: starch replacement for plasma exchange. *J Clin Apheresis* 1997; **12**: 146–53.

18. Owen HG, Brecher ME, Howard JF, Bandarenko N. Minimizing hypovolemic reactions with 3% hetastarch replacment during therapeutic plasma exchange. *J Clin Apheresis* 1999; **14**: 91 (abst).

19. Gross AG, Weinstein R. Pentastarch as partial replacement fluid for therapeutic plasma exchange: effect on plasma proteins, adverse events during treatement, and serum ionized calcium. *J Clin Apheresis* 1999; **14**: 114–21.

20. Steinmuller DR. A dangerous error in the dilution of 25 percent albumin. *N Engl J Med* 1998; **338**: 1226–7.

21. Pierce LR, Gaines A, Varricchio F, Epstein J. Hemolysis and renal failure associated with the inappropriate use of sterile water to dilute human albumin 25%. *N Engl J Med* 1998; **338**: 1226–7.

22. Pierce LR, Gaines A, Finlayson JS et al. Hemolysis and acute renal failure due to the administration of albumin diluted in sterile water. *Transfusion* 1999; **39**: 110–11.

23. American Medical Association Council on Scientific Affairs. Current status of therapeutic plasmapheresis. *JAMA* 1985; **253**: 819–25.

24. Straus RG, Ciavarella D, Gilcher RO et al. Clinical applications of therapeutic hemapheresis: an overview of current management. *J Clin Apheresis* 1993; **8**: 189–94.

25. McLeod BC. Introduction to the Third Special Issue: Clinical Applications of Therapeutic Apheresis. *J Clin Apheresis* 2000; **15**: 1–5.

26. Leitman SF, Kucera E, McLeod BC et al. *Guidelines for Therapeutic Hemapheresis.* Bethesda, MD: American Association of Blood Banks, 1992.

27. Leitman SF, Ciavarella D, Kucera E et al. *Guidelines for Therapeutic Hemapheresis.* Bethesda, MD: American Association of Blood Banks, 1993.

28. Leitman SF, Ciavarella D, McLeod B et al. *Guidelines for Therapeutic Hemapheresis.* Bethesda, MD: American Association of Blood Banks, 1994.

29. McLeod BC, Sniecinski I, Ciavarella D et al. Frequency of immediate adverse effects associated with therapeutic apheresis. *Transfusion* 1999; **39**: 282–8.

30. McLeod BC (ed). Special Issue: Clinical Applications of Therapeutic Apheresis. *J Clin Apheresis* 2000; **15**: 1–159.

31. Kuroki S, Saida T, Nukina M et al. *Campylobacter jejuni* strains from patients with Guillain–Barré syndrome belong mostly to Penner serogroup 19 and contain β-N-acetylglucosamine residues. *Ann Neurol* 1993; **33**: 243–7.

32. Weinstein R. Therapeutic apheresis in neurologic disorders. *J Clin Apheresis* 2000; **15**: 74–128.

33. French Cooperative Group on Plasma Exchange in Guillain–Barré Syndrome. Efficiency of plasma exchange in Guillain–Barré syndrome: role of replacement fluids. *Ann Neurol* 1987; **22**: 753–61.

34. French Cooperative Group on Plasma Exchange in Guillain–Barré Syndrome. Plasma exchange in Guillain–Barré syndrome: one-year follow-up. *Ann Neurol* 1992; **32**: 94–7.

35. Guillain-Barré Syndrome Study Group. Plasmapheresis and acute Guillain–Barré syndrome. *Neurology* 1985; **35**: 1096–104.

36. Plasma Exchange/Sandoglobulin Guillain–Barré Syndrome Trial Group. Randomized trial of plasma exchange, intravenous immunoglobulin, and combined treatments in Guillain–Barré syndrome. *Lancet* 1997; **349**: 225–30.

37. Dyck PJ, Daube J, O'Brien P et al. Plasma exchange in chronic inflammatory demyelinating polyradiculoneuropathy. *N Engl J Med* 1986; **314**: 461–5.

38. Hahn AF, Bolton CF, Pillay N et al. Plasma-exchange therapy in chronic inflammatory demyelinating polyneuropathy. A double-blind, sham-controlled, cross-over study. *Brain* 1996; **119**: 1055–66.

39. Dyck PJ, Litchy WJ, Kratz KM et al. A plasma exchange versus immune globulin infusion trial in chronic inflammatory demyelinating polyradiculoneuropathy. *Ann Neurol* 1994; **36**: 838–45.

40. Choudhary PP, Hughes RAC. Long-term treatment of chronic inflammatory demyelinating polyradiculoneuropathy with plasma exchange or intravenous immunoglobulin. *Q J Med* 1995; **88**: 493–502.

41. Maselli RA. Pathophysiology of myasthenia gravis and Lambert Eaton syndrome. *Neurol Clin North Am* 1994; **12**: 285–303.

42. Weinstein R. Therapeutic apheresis in neurologic disorders. *J Clin Apheresis* 2000; **15**: 74–128.

43. Antozzi C, Gemma M, Regi B et al. A short plasma exchange protocol is effective in severe myasthenia gravis. *J Neurol* 1991; **238**: 103–7.

44. Gadjos P, Chevret S, Clair B et al. Clinical trial of plasma exchange and high-dose intravenous immunoglobulin. *Ann NY Acad Sci* 1993; **681**: 563–6.

45. Cohen JA, Brecher ME, Bandarenko N. Cellular source of serum lactate dehydrogenase elevation in patients with thrombotic thrombocytopenic purpura. *J Clin Apheresis* 1997; **13**: 16–19.

46. Brailey L, Brecher ME, Bandarenko N. Thrombotic thrombocytopenia purpura. *Therapeutic Apheresis* 1999; **3**: 20–4.

47. Furlan M, Robles R, Gabusera M et al. Von Willebrand factor-cleaving protease in thrombotic thrombocytopenic purpura and the hemolytic–uremic syndrome. *N Engl J Med* 1998; **339**: 1578–84.

48. Tsai H-M, Chun-Yet Lian E. Antibodies to von Willebrand factor-cleaving protease in acute thrombotic thrombocytopenic purpura. *N Engl J Med* 1998; **339**: 1585–94.

49. Rock G, Shumak KH, Sutton DM et al. Cryosupernatant as replacement fluid for plasma exchange in thrombotic thrombocytopenic purpura. *Br J Haematol* 1996; **94**: 383–6.

50. Harrison CN, Lawrie AS, Iqbal A et al. Plasma exchange with solvent/detergent-treated plasma of resistant thrombotic thrombocytopenic purpura. *Br J Haematol* 1996; **94**: 756–8.

51. Moake J, Chintagumpala M, Turner N et al. Solvent/detergent-treated plasma supresses shear-induced platelet aggregation and prevents episodes of thrombotic thrombocytopenic purpura. *Blood* 1994; **84**: 490–7.

52. Bandarenko N, Brecher ME. United States Thrombotic Thrombocytopenic Purpura Apheresis Study Group (US TTP ASG): multicenter survey and retrospective analysis of current efficacy of therapeutic plasma exchange. *J Clin Apheresis* 1998; **13**: 133–41.

53. McGrath MA, Penny R. Paraproteinemias: blood viscosity and clinical manifestations. *J Clin Invest* 1976; **58**: 1155–62.

54. Grima KM. Therapeutic apheresis in hematological and oncological diseases. *J Clin Apheresis* 2000; **15**: 28–52.

55. Motulsky AG. Frequency of sickling

disorders in US Blacks. *N Engl J Med* 1973; **188**: 31–3.

56. Castro O, Finke-Castro H, Coats D. Improved method for automated red cell exchange in sickle cell disease. *J Clin Apheresis* 1986; **3**: 93–9.

57. Cuttner J, Holland JF, Norton L et al. Therapeutic leukapheresis for hyperleukocytosis in acute myelocytic leukemia. *Med Pediatr Oncol* 1983; **11**: 76–8.

58. Hester JP, McCredie KB, Freireich EJ. Response to chronic leukapheresis procedures and survival of chronic myelogenous leukemia patients. *Transfusion* 1982; **22**: 305–7.

59. Goldfinger D, Capostagon V, Lowe C et al. Use of long-term leukapheresis in the treatment of chronic lymphocytic leukemia. *Transfusion* 1980; **29**: 450–4.

60. Owen HG, Brecher ME. Therapeutic apheresis of the pregnant patient. In: *Obstetrical Transfusion Practice* (Brecher ME, Sacher RA, eds). Bethesda, MD: American Association of Blood Banks, 1993: 95–115.

61. Traube D, Palmer A, Welsh K et al. Removal of anti-HLA antibodies prior to transplantation: an effective and successful strategy for highly sensitized renal allograft recipients. *Transplant Proc* 1989; **21**: 694–5.

62. Backman U, Fellstrom B, Frodin L et al. Successful transplantation in highly sensitized patients. *Transplant Proc* 1989; **21**: 694–5.

63. Alarabi A, Backman U, Wikstrom B et al. Plasmapheresis in HLA-immunosensitized patients prior to kidney transplantation in highly sensitized patients. *Transplant Proc* 1989; **21**: 762–3.

64. Takahashi K, Yagisawa T, Sonda K et al. ABO-incompatible kidney transplantation in a single center trial. *Transplant Proc* 1993; **25**: 271–3.

65. Aswad S, Mendez R, Mendez RG et al. Crossing the ABO blood barrier in renal transplantation. *Transplant Proc* 1993; **25**: 267–70.

66. Allen NH, Ayer P, Geoghegan T et al. Plasma exchange in acute renal allograft rejection: a controlled trial. *Transplantation* 1983; **32**: 425–8.

67. Kirubakaran MG, Disney APS, Norman J et al. A controlled trial of plasmapheresis in the treatment of renal allograft rejection. *Transplantation* 1981; **32**: 164–5.

68. Bonomini V, Vangelista A, Frasca GM et al. Effects of plasmapheresis in renal transplant rejection: a controlled study. *Trans Am Soc Artif Intern Organs* 1985; **31**: 698–700.

69. Blake P, Sutton D, Cardella C. Plasma exchange in acute renal transplant rejection. *Prog Clin Biol Res* 1990; **3**: 249–52.

70. Savin VJ, Sharma R, Sharma McCarthy ET et al. Circulating factor associated with increased glomerular permeability to albumin in recurrent focal segmental glomerulosclerosis. *N Engl J Med* 1996; **334**: 878–83.

71. Winters JL, Pineda AA, McLeod BC, Grima KM. Recurrent focal and segmental glomerulosclerosis. *J Clin Apheresis* 2000; **15**: 62–3.

72. Haas M, Godfrin Y, Oberbaurer R et al. Plasma immunoadsorption treatment in patients with primary focal segmental glomerulosclerosis. *Nephrol Dial Transplant* 1998; **13**: 2013–16.

73. Dantal J, Testa S, Bigot E, Soulillou JP. Disappearance of proteinuria after immunoadsorption in a patient with focal glomerulosclerosis. *Lancet* 1990; **336**: 190.

74. Costanzo-Nordin MR, Hubbell EA, O'Sullivan EJ et al. Photopheresis versus corticosteroids in the therapy of heart transplant rejection. Preliminary clinical report. *Circulation* 1992; **86**(5 Suppl): II242–50.

75. Wieland M, Thiede VL, Strauss RG et al. Treatment of severe cardiac allograft rejection with extracorporeal photochemotherapy. *J Clin Apheresis* 1994; **9**: 171–5.

76. Dall'Amico R, Livi U, Milano A et al. Extracorporeal photochemotherapy as adjuvant treatment of heart transplant recipients with recurrent rejection. *Transplantation* 1995; **60**: 45–9.

77. Barr ML, Meiser BM, Eisen HJ et al. Photopheresis for the prevention of rejection in cardiac transplantation. *N Engl J Med* 1998; **339**: 1744–51.

78. Villanueva J, Bhorade SM, Robinson JA, Husain AN, Garrity ER Jr. Extracorporeal photopheresis for the treatment of lung allograft rejection. *Ann Transplantation* 2000; **5**: 44–7.

79. O'Hagan AR, Stillwell PC, Arroliga A, Koo A. Photopheresis in the treatment of refractory bronchiolitis obliterans complicating lung transplantation. *Chest* 1999; **115**: 1459–62.

80. Schoch OD, Boelher A, Speich R, Nestle FO. Extracorporeal photochemotherapy for Epstein–Barr virus-associated lymphoma after lung transplantation. *Transplantation* 1998; **68**: 1056–8.

81. Dall'Aminco R, Murer L, Montini G et al. Successful treatment of recurrent rejection in renal transplant patients with photopheresis. *J Am Soc Nephrol* 1998; **9**: 121–7.

82. D'incan M, Kanold J, Halle P et al. Extracorporeal photopheresis as an alternative therapy for drug-resistant graft versus host disease: three cases [in French]. *Ann Dermatol Venereol* 2000; **127**: 166–70.

83. Greinix HT, Vole-Platzer B, Rabitsch W et al. Successful use of extracorporeal photochemotherapy in the treatment of severe acute and chronic graft-versus-host disease. *Blood* 1998; **92**: 3098–104.

84. Salerno CT, Park SJ, Kreykes NS et al. Adjuvant treatment of refractory lung transplant rejection with extracorporeal photopheresis. *J Thorac Cardiovasc Surg* 1999; **117**: 1063–9.

85. Pramodini BK-B, Woo MW. A review of the effects of plasmapheresis on drug clearance. *Pharmacotherapy* 1997; **17**: 684–95.

86. Stigelman WH, Henry DH, Talbert RL, Townsend RJ. Removal of prednisone and prednisolone by plasma exchange. *Clin Pharm* 1984; **3**: 402–7.

87. Sultan Y, Bussel A, Maisonneuve P et al. Potential danger of thrombosis after plasma exchange in the treatment of patients with immune disease. *Transfusion* 1979; **19**: 558–93.

88. Orlin JB, Berkman EM. Partial plasma exchange using albumin replacement: removal and recovery of normal plasma constituents. *Blood* 1980; **56**: 1055–9.

89. Wood L, Jacobs P. The efect of serial therapeutic plasmapheresis on platelet count, coagulation factors, plasma immunoglobulin and complement levels. *J Clin Apheresis* 1986; **3**: 124–8.

90. Flaum MA, Cueo RA, Appelbaum FR et al. The hemostatic imbalance of plasma-exchange transfusion. *Blood* 1979; **54**: 694–702.

91. Simon TL. Coagulation disorders with plasma exchange. *Plasma Ther Transfus Technol* 1982; **3**: 147–53.

92. Domen RE, Kennedy MS, Jones LL, Senhauser DA. Hemostatic imbalances produced by plasma exchange. *Transfusion* 1984; **24**: 336–9.

93. Wood L, Jacobs P. The effect of serial therapeutic plasmapheresis on platelet count, coagulation factors, plasma immunoglobulin and complement levels. *J Clin Apheresis* 1986; **3**: 124–8.

94. Owen HG, Koo A, McAteer M, Brecher ME. Evaluation of platelet loss during TPE on the COBE SPECTRA. *J Clin Apheresis* 1997; **12**: 28.

95. Huestis DW. Complications of therapeutic apheresis. In: *Therapeutic Hemapheresis* (Valbonesi M, Pineda AA, Bigs JC, eds). Milan: Wichtig Editore, 1986: 179–86.

96. Leitman SF, Boltansky H. Alter HJ et al. Allergic reactions in healthy plateletpheresis donors caused by sensitization to ethylene oxide gas. *N Engl J Med* 1986; **315**: 1192–6.

13 Transfusion service management

James P AuBuchon, Dafydd W Thomas

INTRODUCTION

The management of a transfusion service laboratory and the practice of transfusion medicine in a hospital setting offer intriguing and stimulating combinations of direct patient care opportunities and sophisticated challenges in medical management. While working within a system that extends from donor to patient and charged with managing resources for the good of tens or hundreds of patients, one is also expected to provide individualized care and ensure that each patient's hemotherapy advances their health to the greatest extent possible. Combining knowledge of technical particulars with medical acumen and business skills requires a wide array of training and experiences and offers a multitude of opportunities to be personally and clinically involved in patient management. This chapter will detail some of the key features of transfusion service management and the practice of transfusion medicine in the setting of a hospital to highlight necessary skills, useful approaches, and critical parameters for success.

THE ROLE OF A TRANSFUSION SERVICE

The underlying tenets of a transfusion service must be rooted in patient safety and blood supply adequacy. While these are no different than the charges undertaken by the blood supply agency, they take on different meanings in a transfusion service setting. Patient safety moves from an intensive focus on viral transmission to a broad perspective of *transfusion* safety; the issue is no longer blood *product* safety but rather transfusion *process* safety with recognition of all the steps in the entire transfusion process that must be completed accurately and in a timely manner to ensure a transfusion event without complications. The adequacy of the blood supply takes on different guises. As the hospital transfusion service usually depends on an external supplier, it is not in a position to be responsible for adequacy (other than through timely ordering or coordinating supplies with other hospitals in the area). Adequacy then depends on factors such as projecting near- and long-term component needs, encouraging conservative use of supplies as medically appropriate, and using short-dated inventories wisely to gain optimal advantage with available resources.

Issues such as these are evident to a transfusion service on a daily basis. Periodic examination of all their constituent parts, their interactions, and their ramifications is important to ensure that the service is meeting its clinical requirements. Such discussion and ultimate definitions of service requirements are the first step in ensuring successful performance in a measurable manner. (This is critical to quality management strategies, and will be elaborated upon later.)

A transfusion service, however, involves

much more than the transfusion service *laboratory*. Although often referred to by the common sobriquet 'blood bank', the broader definition of medical services subsumed in designating the operation a 'transfusion service' can set the stage for expanded clinical service and improved patient care. Transfusion medicine specialists have long fought against the concept of the distribution of blood components in the manner that a pharmacy dispenses medications. As with any prescribed drug, there may be side-effects as a result of the administration, and this makes it essential that the clinical gain is judged to be worth the risk. The extensive and detailed knowledge possessed by any specialist working in a support capacity – whether a pharmacist, a medical technologist, or a transfusion medicine specialist – may fill in crucial gaps in the clinical physician's knowledge base and help redirect therapy toward a more beneficial outcome or even avert a catastrophe. Therefore, the physician with specialized knowledge in transfusion and the medical technologist skilled in immunohematology may often hold the keys to improve hemotherapy for a patient.

A transfusion service should assess the role it expects to play in transfusion therapy. The provision of a supply of components adequate for clinical needs that are immunohematologically compatible would be included on this list as given. The further beyond these technical requirements the service is comfortable in extending its involvement in transfusion therapy, the greater assistance it offers patient care.[1,2] Some of these opportunities are highlighted in the following sections. For some physicians, these extra-laboratory services may represent challenges to go beyond the limited role that many transfusion service medical directors have assumed in the past. However, these opportunities represent the true reasons that physicians rather than technologists alone are in charge of transfusion services; they define ways in which physicians can share their skills with patients who will benefit from them. They represent opportunities for a trained physician to pass on knowledge to one lacking as much information in this specialized field, so that patient safety and transfusion therapy are optimized.[3]

TRANSFUSION SERVICE FUNCTIONS

Blood component supply

Maintaining an adequate supply of all components used in a facility is a basic requirement of any transfusion service. How this is accomplished may differ according to geography and according to national or regional norms.

Most commonly, a hospital transfusion service 'outsources' the provision of components to a blood center that specializes in this aspect of the transfusion chain. In some circumstances, the transfusion service may be a part of a regional blood center, and some hospitals collect some or all of the components they use. Regardless of the specific arrangement, the service must have clear understandings with the suppliers of the components about the type and quantity of components that are required, the qualifications of the donors and the testing performed on their units, and the availability and delivery schedules. Ideally, all suppliers of blood components should work to national or internationally agreed standards. Additional 'logistic' issues can also affect operations significantly, including the return policies for components, the availability of couriers or other deliverers of emergency needs, and plans for rotating components to reduce outdating. Furthermore, the blood supplier will want assurances of access to certain information, such as reports of post-transfusion infection, that are important in completing its role of ensuring the virologic safety of the blood supply.

These many details highlight the importance of a having a clear, mutually agreeable, written understanding of the requirements of both the supplier and the user of the components. Such a contract is important for specifying prices and volumes, and allowing both the blood supplier and the hospital to plan its details is important to avoid misunderstandings that may affect patient care. Documentation of these details is an important step in 'supplier qualification' which is an integral part of 'good manufacturing practices' and common sense for ensuring that the transfusion service will have available the material needed to complete its functions.

The specifications of the components to be supplied should be set with an eye on clinical requirements, financial resources, and supplier capabilities. The type of processing utilized routinely may traditionally have been selected by the blood supplier, depending on the capabilities of the service or the transfusing facility and its physicians, based on their practice of transfusion medicine. To avoid conflicts when the needs of these two entities diverge, the relationship should be clarified so that it is understood who is in control of decisions relating to use of additive solution storage systems, leukoreduction, etc. The transfusion service may require special modi-

fications for a proportion of units for special applications (e.g. intrauterine or neonatal transfusion), and the ability of the supplier to provide them in the necessary time frame should be determined. Expectations regarding how antigen-negative units will be identified should also be clarified.

Discussions regarding component selection need to be undertaken with the institution's medical staff. For example, what is the role to be played by units that have been treated by a pathogen-inactivation system? Not only does such treatment entail additional cost, but also it may carry with it additional, new risks (e.g. reagent toxicity or pooling) that will have to be weighed against the potential benefits. Will platelets be supplied in pools or by apheresis techniques? If the former approach is used, to what extent will the blood supplier or the transfusion service laboratory be responsible for converting the individual units into a transfusible pooled form? Careful consideration of all these issues and the potential for collaboration with the blood supplier will be necessary to ensure that clinical requirements can be met.

In many regions, transfusion services are not just at the periphery of simple spokes with the blood center at the central hub. Often, there is a web of interconnections between hospitals, allowing smaller ones access to a supply larger than is supportable on the basis of their usage volume but requiring them to rotate units after several weeks to larger facilities where their use can be assured. This rotation undoubtedly reduces outdating while maintaining access to adequate inventory in small facilities, but it requires hospitals to be aware of their impact on their neighbors.

Similarly, hospitals need to be very aware

of the structure of the system for returning blood components. At first, this may appear to be primarily an economic issue. If the blood center allows either crediting a certain proportion of the ordered units as returns or only when a certain numbers of days of shelf life remain, then there is a clear financial reason to adhere to the criteria and reduce outdating. However, regardless of which party *appears* to pay for outdated units, the *regional system* as a whole must bear the cost of these outdates, and any credit systems used by the blood center merely serve to distribute these costs amongst all hospitals.

Compatibility testing

Most hospital transfusion services would state their primary purpose in terms of pretransfusion testing: patient typing, antibody screening, and unit crossmatching. Indeed, it was around these purposes that hospital laboratories became involved in the delivery of transfusion care, and these remain their major functions. The manner in which these functions are provided varies among hospitals and across healthcare systems, but their purposes are similar. Also similar is their need to accomplish these tests rapidly with consistent accuracy.

The growing awareness amongst both clinicians and the general public has resulted in a high level of interest in transfusion matters. While the general public will always demand zero risk from the transfusion of blood components, this is impossible to achieve. As a result, there has been a need for transfusion specialists to develop a role that relates more directly to the clinical use of these components. The developing role of such clinicians aims to increase awareness about the whole process in an attempt to come closer to the public's demand for minimal risk. Since audits have shown that compatibility systems are a source of many of the mistakes that lead to mistransfusion, this area rightfully deserves careful scrutiny.[4,5]

Just as compatibility *testing* begins with a properly labeled sample, a reliable *system* for ensuring compatible blood must include oversight and assurance of the phlebotomy process. While most transfusion service laboratories do not use their own personnel to collect the samples, the transfusion service should be fully involved in establishing and evaluating the collection of samples and their labeling. While mislabeled samples account for only about 10% of the errors resulting in mistransfusion, this proportion amounts to well over 100 deaths in developed countries annually. Most of these errors could be eradicated with relatively simple 'systems' solutions.[6] These include the establishment of criteria for patient and sample identification with strict adherence to them, and appropriate staff training. The transfusion service would rightfully be involved in issues pertaining to patient identification systems, and it would also be the responsibility of the transfusion service to advocate the introduction of process controls to reduce the risk of mistransfusion. At least two of these exist commercially at present. One is a mechanical barrier system that interdicts transfusion to a patient other than the one giving the pretransfusion specimen; the other is a system that uses a small handheld computer to read a barcoded wristband, print a tube label, and match patient and unit identification at the bedside immediately prior to transfusion. These devices have been successfully implemented in a number of facilities,[7,8] but have not achieved the market penetration commensurate with the risk of mortality associated with the ongoing problem of mistransfusion. This risk is estimated at greater than 1 in 1 million units, which exceeds those of the major viral pathogens that continue to capture attention.[4] This important area requires more financial investment to ensure that safety is improved. The use of a scanning device may provide a quick and easy method of checking the component to be transfused, the patient due to receive the blood, and the healthcare worker responsible for the transfusion. Such devices could also scan at the end of administration. This would lead to a complete recording of that transfusion event, and would be invaluable in any audit examination should the need arise to look in a retrospective manner. The contemporary nature of the data recording would also make information almost immediately available, providing transfusion records for individual patients.[9]

The laboratory must decide on the most appropriate scheme for conducting ABO and Rh determinations and for crossmatching. Automation – long believed too expensive for transfusion services – has become more widely implemented in the last four years with the introduction of lower-volume (and lower-cost) equipment. Even laboratories transfusing less than 10 000 red cell units annually have found some of these pieces of equipment cost-saving. At the same time, they allow reduced dependence on staff, who may be difficult to recruit in many countries, since they can interface with laboratory information systems and the handheld devices mentioned above to reduce errors. For smaller laboratories, semiautomated devices are available to provide increased objectivity and throughput, reducing error potential. Multiple options exist in manual testing, since the variety of new methods introduced in the last decade can complement traditional tube testing. Each laboratory will need to decide on the most appropriate system based on the availability and skill of the workforce, the availability of capital resources, the performance in on-site comparative testing, and personal preferences. However, accepting the status quo 'because that's the way we've always done it' appears to be an assumption well worth challenging.

The next set of questions to be addressed pertains to the protocol for pretransfusion testing. The concept of 'type and screen' (T&S) prior to immediate spin crossmatching for patients without a history of clinically significant antibodies has been in use for over 20 years and has been shown to provide a reasonable combination of patient safety and laboratory efficiency. While it is recognized that perhaps one of every 30 000 transfusions given under this system is incompatible owing to the presence of an antibody against an antigen not represented on the screening cells and thereby missed, these undetected incompatible transfusions appear to be associated with morbidity extremely rarely.[10] Nevertheless, about half of the transfusion services in the USA reported in 1997 that they continued to employ an antiglobulin phase crossmatch for all patients.[11] It is argued that reduced efficiency and increased cost are usually incurred in smaller hospitals, where staff work in the transfusion service laboratory less often and are more prone to error. The regulated and monitored potency of reagents and the consistently high performance of laboratories on proficiency surveys, such as those produced through the College of American Pathologists, suggests that the concept of T&S followed by an immediate spin crossmatch for a patient who is not alloimmunized is widely applicable.

As more hospitals implement sophisticated laboratory information systems, expanded use of 'electronic crossmatching' can also be expected. As with systems that use an 'immediate spin' crossmatch, these protocols depend also on the antibody screen to detect alloimmunization. However, they allocate the responsibility of ABO-compatibility checks to means other than direct mixing of patient sera with donors' red cells. Most commonly, requirements for implementation of a computerized compatibility system include two independent determinations of the patient's ABO group and of the unit's. Knowing that ABO incompatibility may be missed by serologic testing in some circumstances[12,13] and that manual records have a greater likelihood of fallibility than validated electronic ones, an appropriately constructed electronic crossmatching system may offer improved patient safety when verifying ABO compatibility. Patients with a history of red cell alloimmunization, however, will continue to receive units selected to be phenotypically negative and crossmatched at the antiglobulin phase to ensure compatibility.

Beyond routine pretransfusion testing, the laboratory must decide how deeply to delve into immunohematologic examination of more complex patient problems. The extent to which a laboratory may wish to maintain an inventory of necessary reagents (e.g. antibody identification panels and phenotyping reagents) as well as specially trained technolo-

gists will depend on the frequency with which antibody problems are encountered in the patient population served. It will also depend on the availability of prompt, accurate, and financially reasonable reference laboratory services. While the local availability of a serologist with expert knowledge of the investigation of red cell antibody problems becomes more critical as more complex problems are tackled, less-completely trained laboratory personnel may be able to offer useful assistance, *providing there is* a 'local expert' able to interpret the results. The ability to share results electronically or by facsimile or the capability of seeing agglutination characteristics by digital image transmission would allow this expert to be at a remote location.

Similarly, the transfusion service will have to decide which other services it wishes to provide on-site and which it can or desires to have provided by its blood supplier. The economics of the healthcare system in which the facility operates and the clientele it serves will probably comprise the major issues in making this decision. Whether to have a gamma-irradiator available to prevent graft-versus-host disease in susceptible patients or whether to maintain a sterile connecting device to allow aliquoting for pediatric transfusions are examples of these issues. How frequently and in what situations are different components requested, such as pooled cryoprecipitate, and should special arrangements be created to ensure that the needed components are rapidly available?

The transfusion service need not restrict its testing to red cell transfusions. Platelet transfusions can be complicated by poor response that necessitates investigation to provide a transfusion approach that will secure hemostasis for the thrombocytopenic patient. Screening patients for platelet or HLA antibodies can readily be accomplished by several means with excellent sensitivities and specificities in hospital laboratories.[14] While most laboratories do not have the capabilities to conduct lymphocytotoxicity testing against panels of lymphocytes, to determine the exact specifics of HLA antibodies, some of the test kits for HLA-antibody screening include a sufficient number of reagent cells to allow a good appreciation of which HLA phenotype(s) will and will not be compatible. Similarly, most laboratories will be unable to identify definitively the specificity of most platelet-specific antibodies, but will be able to identify that one is present. This information, coupled with knowledge of the phenotypes of units involved in successful and unsuccessful transfusions, should allow a laboratory to deduce which (antigen-negative) units will provide clinical utility in future transfusions.

While few readers of this chapter would ever be in a situation of creating a transfusion service de novo and having to make all these decisions at once, all operations would benefit from their transfusion medicine specialists periodically surveying operations and opportunities critically to identify opportunities for improvement.

Centralization

Some of the most discussed issues in transfusion service management in the 1990s were centralization and outsourcing of services.[15,16] These involved two different approaches – both intended to reduce cost and improve service. One approach was to centralize the pretransfusion testing from multiple hospitals to a single one (usually the most active transfusion facility or the local blood center). Handling a larger number of samples in a single location (or a reduced number of laboratories for a metropolitan area) allowed the use of standardized procedures, highly trained dedicated technologists, automation, and laboratory information services – none of which might have been financially feasible for a small laboratory. There is a 'trade-off' with these systems in terms of accessibility to blood components, although potential problems were usually readily handled by dedicated couriers, remote-release capabilities (managed by a computer system), or decentralized inventories of group O Rh-negative red cells for emergency transfusions. Transfusion medicine specialists could similarly provide more consultation in the smaller facilities than would otherwise be feasible. In the USA, these concepts grew out of longstanding centralized crossmatching capabilities provided by blood centers such as those in Seattle and Tampa, and came to be implemented (less completely) in many other cities. Those facilities that no longer performed pretransfusion testing in-house would consider to have 'outsourced' this function, but another approach to outsourcing is the contractual provision of technical and medical staff to run a facility's transfusion service. This is a newer concept that remains under commercial development. It may provide many of the same advantages as centralization (except for concentration of volumes in a single central laboratory) while keeping the transfusion functions housed in the facility.

Consultation in hemotherapy

Extension of the 'laboratory' physician's domain to the bedside of the patient has been a key development of transfusion medicine over the last generation. This represents the potential for improving transfusion practice and patient care. Establishment of a system to accomplish this requires a few prerequisites, but holds the promise of inestimable clinical rewards.

To begin, the physician charged with management of the transfusion service must be knowledgeable in transfusion medicine. The extent of special knowledge or training in transfusion medicine need not be monumental before one can offer clinically valuable assistance. Given the woeful lack of hemotherapy education acquired by clinicians in most countries, a modicum of formal training in the subject coupled with careful and ongoing perusal of the transfusion literature will make this physician a valued source of information and advice among his or her colleagues.

The second prerequisite is disposition. This is not readily taught although it is certainly capable of being reinforced. The transfusion service physician who desires to be active clinically must be willing to use clinical experience and knowledge in clinical situations, responding in an appropriate manner at a useful time. This implies clinical acumen as well as skill in interpersonal interactions.

Finally, a system must be established to alert the transfusion specialist of the potential for providing assistance and a framework for this assistance must be delineated either explicitly or by local custom. Protocols for 'automatic consultation' have been developed whereby certain clinical situations – such as massive transfusions or the request for components that are most frequently misused – prompts the transfusion medicine specialist to interact with the clinician.[17] Depending on the circumstances, the clinician may (or may not) be predisposed to listen to an 'outsider's' opinion, and the advice offered will be received most readily if the transfusion specialist is acknowledged locally as giving sound advice with the patient's best interest at heart. The healthcare reimbursement system or hierarchy will also help determine the circumstances in which the transfusion specialist may become involved in a case, but the more opportunities that are explored, the greater the potential for improvement in patient hemotherapy.

Integration of companion services

The transfusion service may have the opportunity to improve patient care by expanding its involvement in other, related services. This will require the cooperation of those administering these other services, but their integration – functionally if not administratively – with the transfusion service holds the potential for improvement in patient care. This added involvement and integration can be facilitated by the hospital transfusion committee. The meetings can be a useful forum to highlight areas of common interest in patient care. Handled sensitively the meetings can be of great educational value.

Other laboratory services that relate frequently to transfusion medicine include hematology and coagulation. A process as simple as notification from the hematology laboratory to the transfusion service that a new diagnosis of acute leukemia has been made may allow the transfusion service to place appropriate component restrictions within their records. Coagulation testing may identify patients with certain diseases or with particular coagulopathic states that may require the assistance of the transfusion service (or its consulting physician). These intralaboratory connections may appear obvious, but their codification may transfer information that will improve patient care and take stress out of the provision of blood components.

The integration of related services may profitably extend the transfusion service beyond its walls. For example, the hospital may offer perioperative red cell salvage services for some surgeries. Even if the service is staffed by persons who are not administratively linked to the laboratory, the transfusion service may be able to offer valuable assistance in a number of aspects of this operation. For example, detailing labeling requirements and storage times and conditions for units would be simple for blood bankers but possibly confusing for nursing or operating room staff. The transfusion service staff would also be able to offer advice regarding appropriate quality control checks and perhaps offer to integrate the red cell collection service into the ongoing quality assurance activities centered in the transfusion service. This sharing of expertise can ensure that appropriate (and required) oversight of the operation is instituted.

INTEGRATION OF QUALITY IMPROVEMENT SYSTEMS: TAKING A HOSPITAL-WIDE VIEW OF THE TRANSFUSION PROCESS

The importance of integrated, all-encompassing quality improvement systems has come to be widely recognized as valuable in transfusion medicine. A full description of such a system is beyond the scope of this chapter, and full explanations of the structure and function of such systems can be found elsewhere. Of special note in the context of this discussion is the scope of the program.

The intention of a quality assurance – improvement in patient care – will be best accomplished if the quality improvement system takes a broad view of the functions of the transfusion service. Certainly, the internal operations of the transfusion service laboratory need to be included in the quality improvement system. This system must be able to ensure that the validated procedures of the laboratory are being followed by competent, trained, proficient staff using controlled, qualified reagents on acceptable samples to yield outcomes that meet requirements. Furthermore, the system should be structured to capture as many relevant deviations as possible and ensure that their thorough evaluation leads to improvements in the system to prevent their recurrence.[18,19] However, just as compatibility testing involves more than crossmatching, quality assurance should extend from the vein of the patient's arm back to that vein at the time of transfusion.[20] Oversight of the entire process of transfusion should be included in the transfusion service's quality improvement plan, encompassing phlebotomist and nursing training and qualification, patient identification systems, sample labeling, transfusion procedures, and clinical follow-up. Many, if not all, of these functions are likely to be performed by staff who do not report within the administrative structure of the transfusion service, and the medical director or supervisor of the transfusion service cannot expect to simply command attention on request. However, once the purpose and concept of quality improvement is understood by those performing the extra-laboratory portions of transfusion operations, it is likely that they will welcome the assistance of the transfusion service team. This assistance should begin with a joint analysis of what is expected of all parties and the key elements of the process that need to be accomplished in each major step. Once responsibilities have been agreed upon, the transfusion service staff may be able to assist in the writing of procedures and training of staff. For example, there can be confidence that patient identification will be verified at the time of sampling, and that pretransfusion samples will have been properly labeled. Careful explanation of the rationale behind common blood banking labeling standards may facilitate compliance with procedures to be performed at the time of transfusion and help ensure that appropriate clinical follow-up is provided to the transfusion recipient. (This may include obtaining post-infusion laboratory tests that will aid assessment of the effectiveness of the transfusion.) Finally, once the system has been implemented, the transfusion service staff may be able to help design and implement a periodic audit process so that the function of the system can be assessed.

The importance of extending the concept of quality assurance beyond the walls of the transfusion service cannot be overemphasized. Since over half of all fatal mistransfusions are related to errors committed at the patient's bedside – either at the time of pretransfusion sampling or at the time of transfusion – a quality assurance system that pertains only to the technical details of laboratory processes will miss the largest source of errors currently existing in most systems.[4,5] Given that mistransfusion represents the greatest mortality risk involved in red cell transfusion (at approximately 1–2 per million) and that sampling labeling errors (at 2900 samples)[21] and transgressions of transfusion protocols (at 1 in 400 transfusions)[22] are all far more common than other risks that receive much more attention, extending quality improvement concepts and systems throughout the transfusion process should provide dramatic improvements in patient care.

Of course, extending quality assurance functions beyond the technical aspects of transfusion medicine has long been practiced with respect to review of transfusion decisions. While this function is usually handled outside the framework of the other quality assurance functions of the transfusion service, it represents an important tool for improving patient care.

UTILIZING THE TRANSFUSION COMMITTEE

A transfusion committee can serve numerous important functions for its institution, its patients, and the transfusion service that services them. The presence of a transfusion committee is universal in US hospitals and is now regarded as essential in all UK hospitals (as suggested in an NHS Executive Health

Circular). However, its function is often limited to or highly focused on review of blood utilization. While this is an important function, this delimitation fails to engage the committee in other important functions that offer great opportunities for improvement in the transfusion process in the institution. The objective analysis of decisions to transfuse and the benefit or detriment to patient outcome has been poorly assessed in the past.[23] The transfusion committee should ensure that the whole transfusion process is made as safe as possible. The committee should provide a source of current transfusion opinion and be responsible for the implementation of national and international guidelines where appropriate.

The structure and composition of the committee should be given careful consideration. Representatives from all departments or services frequently using the transfusion service should be included, and they should be persons appropriately placed in their departments to be aware of clinical trends and to effect changes sought by the committee. There should also be representation of the transfusion service laboratory, hospital administration, risk management, and other key functions to ensure good communication and cooperation. Education of new members in the operation of the committee and the function of the transfusion service may be fruitful. The chair of the committee may or may not be the medical director of the transfusion service; arguments have been advanced in both directions, and their local resolution is probably highly dependent on personalities and the administrative structure of the hospital. In any case, the committee should have a defined reporting relationship to the medical staff

organization and medical director of the institution, through which charges, reports, and official communications may be channeled effectively.

Component usage review

Review of the practices of ordering and administering blood components is required by accrediting or regulatory agencies in some countries and is a common practice of peer review in others. This review should encompass all aspects of clinical transfusion, including component ordering criteria, distribution and administration of the units, and evaluating the effects of the transfusion. The first of these is usually the focus of review efforts, and the remainder are appropriate targets of consideration for the transfusion service's quality assurance system (and reviewed within the transfusion committee). Detailed reviews of the process, including suggested audit criteria and suggestions for improvement of the process, have been published; some key elements will be highlighted here.

At the outset, and repeatedly during the administration of the process, the committee and those working on its behalf should remind themselves that the process is intended to be helpful to patients and to be educational for physicians, not punitive. The committee will undoubtedly learn much about the transfusion practices of the physicians of the institution, and this information can be used to direct educational efforts through lectures and laboratory newsletters. Interactions with individual physicians who appear not to be practicing in a manner analogous to their colleagues can redirect their practice patterns, but such interactions must be handled with skill and diplomacy to avoid defensive posturing and incomplete acceptance of the committee's information. The accent on a 'blame-free' process allows open discussion and prevents the withdrawal of a physician's cooperation with this ongoing audit of transfusion practice.

Engagement of a transfusion committee in the process of reviewing clinical transfusion decisions should begin with establishment of audit criteria. These are usually derived from transfusion 'triggers', suggesting acceptable indications for transfusion based on specific clinical situations. These are best developed from review of the growing literature regarding evidence-based transfusion practices. Prior to implementation in the institution, modifications may need to be made to the guidelines allowing a gradual change in local practice. A too-hurried approach by the committee is less successful than one that allows the guided change of clinical practice towards an eventual goal over time. Ideally, the audit process should concentrate on the improvement in practice achieved by each physician's practice when judged against historical performance rather than against a national standard of best practice. This offers reward for sometimes only minimal but important change. This will require more effort than tracking the composite practice of a particular service or of all physicians in the institution, but may be more useful in highlighting those physicians whose practice deviates from that of the remainder.

Importantly, the audit criteria should be distinguished from clinical indications; if they are made to be the same, there will be no latitude between situations in which transfusion essentially must be given and those where the

audit process will be activated. This will result in a large proportion of audit case investigations resulting in a conclusion on review by the committee that the clinical situation justified the transfusion; most facilities have staff restrictions that will require a more targeted approach. For example, if the institution's physicians felt that patients with anemia to a hemoglobin of 8 g/dl or below warranted red cell transfusion and this number were adopted as the *audit* criterion, then many transfusions occurring when patients' hemoglobins were in the 8–9 g/dl range would occur and on investigation would be likely to result in a determination that special clinical circumstances were present that justified the transfusion. Placing the audit criterion at a higher level, say 10 g/dl in this example, would result in some inappropriate transfusions being excluded from the audit review process, but a larger proportion of transfusions that were included would probably be adjudged to be inappropriate. At the same time, consideration should be given to establishing criteria to detect undertransfusion, ensuring that concerns about transfusion risks do not prevent transfusion when it is indicated.

Once the audit criteria have been developed with input and agreement from all 'transfusing' departments, they should be reviewed and approved by the governing medical body of the institution. They should then be disseminated widely to begin the process of encouraging uniform and evidence-based decisions on transfusion use.

Transfusion decisions can be reviewed at several different points, and the transfusion committee will need to decide which ones to utilize. At the same time, the resources of the institution to review the cases entered into the auditing system need to be considered to determine not only the methods to be used but also the proportion of transfusions to be subjected to analysis against the audit criteria and, if necessary, subsequent investigation.

The most common form of transfusion audit is retrospective in nature. After the transfusion, a computer program or a trained staff person identifies those cases falling outside an audit trigger. These are researched – usually first by a staff person and then by a physician – and the ordering physician is invited to provide input if a reasonable indication is not identified from the patient's record. All of this information is considered by the transfusion committee, which adjudicates the clinical indication.

While the retrospective approach may be aided by knowledge of the outcome of the case, it is difficult to capture the urgency and uncertainty of the moment of decision. Furthermore, these reviews often take place long after the event, straining recall and limiting the educational impact of the case; most importantly, they can only improve care for future patients, not the one involved in the transfusion. Therefore, concern has been expressed about the overall value of retrospective audits, although they have been reported to achieve large changes in transfusion practice [23]

Prospective audits insert a reviewer in the process before delivery of the component. These have a greater potential for improving patient care immediately,[23-25] but hold the potential for confrontational exchanges. 'In the heat of battle' may not be the best time for a clinician to assimilate new information on hemotherapy indications. While generally accepted as the most powerful approach, this is also the least utilized, since it requires a knowledgeable physician (whose authority is accepted by colleagues) to be available to discuss cases and suggest alternative approaches. Accommodations are usually built into the system for rapid response in cases of emergency, such as beginning to thaw plasma when requested from the operating room; ensuring clinicians that the review process will not delay needed therapy will be important in gaining their acceptance of a new prospective audit system.

A combination of approaches may also be useful to implement.[23,26] If an institution finds that certain components – such as those that are ordered infrequently – are more likely to be utilized without appropriate indications, then a prospective audit system may be most beneficial for patient care. The amount of clinical information that can be captured for review before the transfusion must also be considered. As clinicians heed the call for individualization of hemotherapy, access to laboratory data alone will be less useful in judging the appropriateness of a transfusion decision. Finally, the volume of requests for a particular component (e.g. red cells) may overwhelm staff attempting to conduct prospective review of transfusion requests. Audits may also be targeted to particular clinical services, rotated periodically among services, or restricted to a proportion of all requests.

Review of a case that has been selected for audit is strongly encouraged to be conducted by an impartial but knowledgeable party. Sending all audited cases involving surgeons, for example, to the Department of Surgery for review and adjudication may allow for the review to be conducted by someone who would be most attuned to the problems faced by the clinician who ordered the transfusion. However, abdication of the investigation and review by the transfusion committee to the transfuser's department may mean that those reviewing the case are no more knowledgeable of the transfusion literature and therapeutic alternatives to be applied than the clinician who placed the order. Furthermore, the transfusion committee will be deprived of detailed knowledge of the thought processes and practice patterns of transfusing physicians if not directly engaged in the process. It is important that representatives of the transfusion committee attend these various audits to give an informed opinion in a friendly way. Only by attending regularly and offering helpful advice will the committee's involvement be realized to be non-punitive.

Once the transfusion committee has completed its review, the physician(s) involved in the patient's care should be made aware of the decision of the committee and the rationale behind that decision. Again, focus on the educational aspects of this intervention and the target of improved patient care should help maximize internalization of the committee's mindset. A report of the findings relayed to the departmental chair, the quality assurance committee, or the credentialing committee of the institution may alert them of physicians recalcitrant to these educational attempts in order to ensure that other forces are brought to bear to effect remediation. (Labeling these communications as privileged and as part of quality assurance efforts may, in some jurisdictions, protect them from legal discovery and ease fears about this process leading to legal liability.) The composite results of the committee's efforts should be tracked to verify that improvements in transfusion decisions are being achieved. (The extent of the review effort, in terms of the proportion of transfusions reviewed, will determine the strength of the conclusions about the wisdom of the physicians' decisions.)

Transfusion incidents

Another role of the committee is to ensure that there is effective monitoring of transfusion incidents. These include administration of incompatible components, misidentification, serious morbidity, or even mortality associated with the transfusion of blood components at the institution. These reports can then contribute in a confidential manner to regional or national registers recording the hazards associated with blood component use and lead to improved care beyond the institution.

Ongoing education and in-service training of staff (both new appointments and existing staff) should be encouraged by the transfusion committee. The various steps of the transfusion process should be constantly reviewed. The committee needs to review the parameters of the ongoing quality assurance system to ensure that the standard operating policies are being followed. This would include blood collection from the laboratory, adequate checking of the patient and blood component to be given, and the recording of its administration both on the patient's chart and a contemporary entry in the notes explaining the reason for transfusion.

Policy and process review

The transfusion committee's other functions may be summarized in terms of oversight of the operation of the transfusion service and input from its users to improve patient care. This amounts to allowing the 'customers' of the service an inside view of the operation of the service in order to help direct its policies. By seeing the outcomes of its processes, they can also gain confidence in the operation. Reports allowing feedback relating to errors and accident reports may allow clinicians to see how the transfusion service detects and responds to problems. This involvement may lead them to suggest improvement in the service or changes in clinical operations at their interface with the service, with an intent to improve operations overall. Some of these improvements may not have been evident to those not working primarily in the clinical sphere, and the simplest solution to the problem may not have been achieved without this clinical input.

The transfusion committee can also serve as a useful sounding board for new policies that the transfusion service would like to implement, and the committee can recommend to the medical staff certain key decisions regarding the institution's approach to transfusion therapy. For example, conversion to an electronic crossmatching procedure may be greeted with skepticism or outright refusal by the medical staff without the committee's prior review of all the theory behind it by and acceptance of the groundwork and validation of software performed by the laboratory. The transfusion committee can also serve as a review committee for the medical staff, looking carefully at new options in transfusion, such as virally inactivated components, and recommending to them a course of action for the institution.

Therefore, the transfusion committee can serve numerous important functions beyond reviews of transfusion. Their medical expertise and in-depth study of transfusion issues can help guide other physicians' practice and recommend therapeutic options for the institution.

REFERENCES

1. AuBuchon JP. The role of transfusion medicine physicians. A vanishing breed? *Arch Pathol Lab Med* 1999; **123**: 663–7.
2. Popovsky MA, Moore SB, Wick MR et al. A blood bank consultation service: principles and practice. *Mayo Clin Proc* 1985; **60**: 312–14.
3. Williams RL, McLellan D, Lees S, Dunlop D. Improving transfusion practices in a busy teaching hospital. *J R Coll Surg Edin* 1997; **42**: 314–16.
4. Linden JV, Paul B, Dressler KP. A report of 104 transfusion errors in New York State. *Transfusion* 1992; **32**: 601–6.
5. Sazama K. Reports of 355 transfusion-associated deaths: 1976 through 1985. *Transfusion* 1990; **30**: 583–90.
6. Wenz B, AuBuchon JP, Mercuriali F. Practical methods to improve transfusion safety by using novel blood unit and patient identification systems. *Am J Clin Pathol* 1997; **107**(suppl 4): S12–16.
7. Wenz B, Burns ER. Improvement in transfusion safety using a new blood unit and patient identification system as part of safe transfusion practice. *Transfusion* 1991; **31**: 401–3.
8. AuBuchon JP, Littenberg B. A cost-effectiveness analysis of the use of a barrier system to reduce the risk of mistransfusion. *Transfusion* 1996; **36**: 222–6.
9. Langeberg AF, Berg M, Novak SC, Sandler SG. Evaluation of the Immucor I-Trac system for positive patient, blood sample and blood unit identification. *Transfusion* 1999; **39**: 25S–26S.

10. Meyer EA, Shulman IA. The sensitivity and specificity of the immediate-spin crossmatch. *Transfusion* 1989; **29**: 99–102.

11. Maffei LM, Johnson ST, Shulman IA, Steiner EA. Survey on pretransfusion testing. *Transfusion* 1998; **38**: 343–9.

12. Shulman IA, Meyer EA, Lam HT, Nelson JM. Additional limitations of the immediate spin crossmatch to detect ABO incompatibility. *Am J Clin Pathol* 1987; **87**: 677.

13. Shulman IA, Calderon C. Effect of delayed centrifugation or reading on the detection of ABO incompatibility by the immediate-spin crossmatch. *Transfusion* 1991; **31**: 197–200.

14. Leach MF, AuBuchon JP. Comparison of ELISA and solid phase red cell adherence methods for detection of HLA and platelet antibodies – a blinded study. *Transfusion* 2000; **40**: 104S.

15. Triulzi DJ. Advantages of outsourcng the transfusion service. *Transfus Sci* 1997; **18**: 559–64.

16. Domen RE. The transfusion service is an integral and important component of the hospital and should not be outsourced. *Transfus Sci* 1997; **18**: 565–74.

17. Tomasulo PA, Lenes BA, Noto TA et al. Automatic special case consultations in transfusion medicine. *Transfusion* 1986; **26**: 186–93.

18. Kaplan HS, Battles JB, Van der Schaaf TW et al. Identification and classification of the causes of events in transfusion medicine. *Transfusion* 1998; **38**: 1071–81.

19. Battles JB, Kaplan HS, Van der Schaaf TW, Shea CE. The attributes of medical event-reporting systems: experience with a prototype medical event-reporting system for transfusion medicine. *Arch Pathol Lab Med* 1998; **122**: 231–8.

20. Shulman IA, Lohr K, Derdiarian AK, Picukaric JM. Monitoring transfusionist practices: a strategy for improving transfusion safety. *Transfusion* 1994; **34**: 11–15.

21. Lumadue JA, Boyd JS, Ness PM. Adherence to a strict specimen-labeling policy decreases the incidence of erroneous blood grouping of blood bank specimens. *Transfusion* 1997; **37**: 1169–72.

22. Baele PL, De Bruyere M, Deneys V et al. Bedside transfusion errors. A prospective study by the Belgium SAnGUIS group. *Vox Sang* 1994; **66**: 117–21.

23. Toy PT. Effectiveness of transfusion audits and practice guidelines. *Arch Pathol Lab Med* 1994; **118**: 435–7.

24. Simpson MB. Prospective–concurrent audits and medical consultation for platelet transfusions. *Transfusion* 1987; **27**: 192–5.

25. Marconi M, Almini D, Pizzi MN et al. Quality assurance of clinical transfusion practice by implementation of the privilege of blood prescription and computerized prospective audit of blood requests. *Transfus Med* 1996; **6**: 11–19.

26. Stehling L, Luban NL, Anderson KC et al. Guidelines for blood utilization review. *Transfusion* 1994; **34**: 438–48.

Index

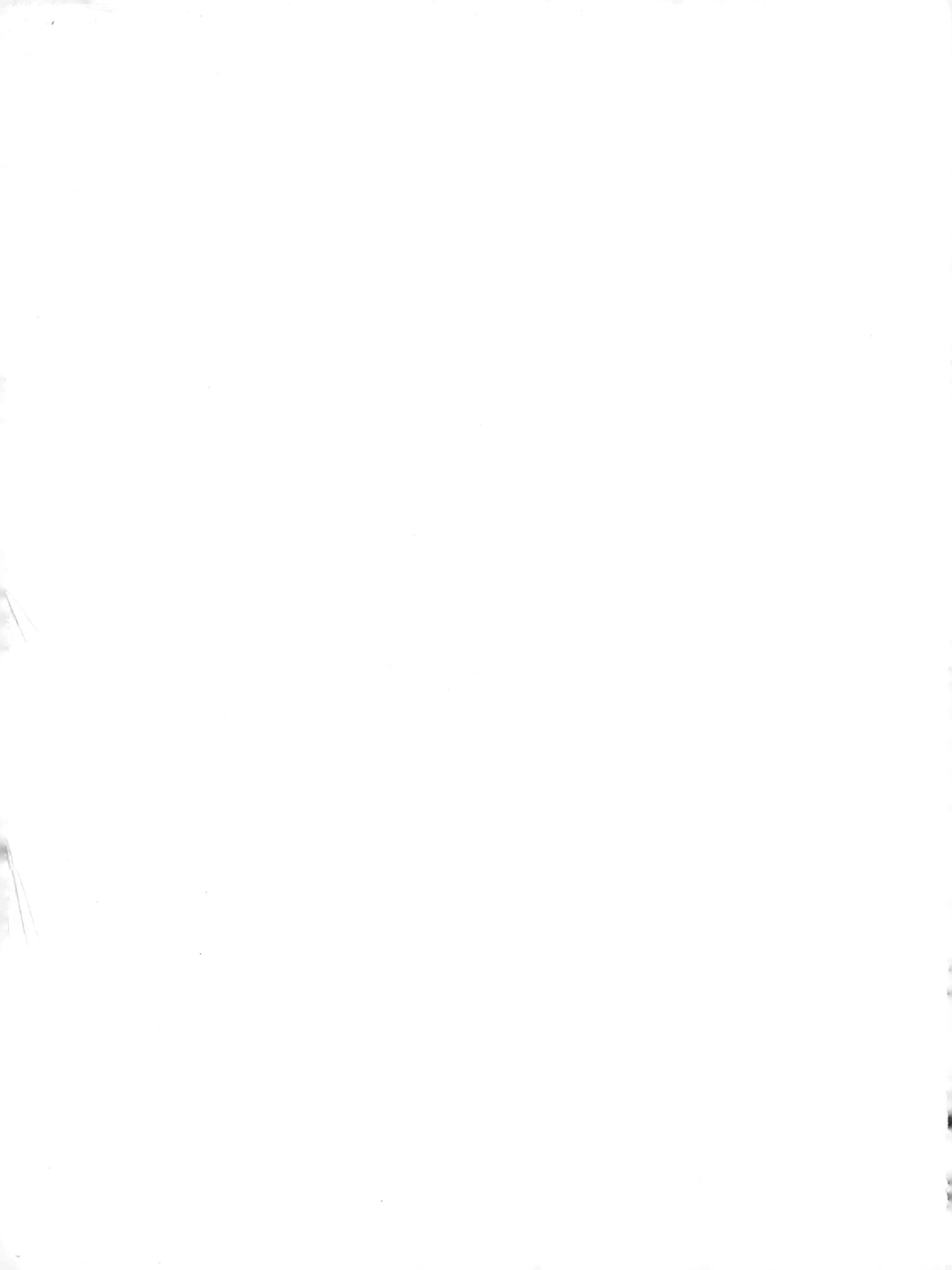